# 经自然腔道取标本手术
# 基础与培训——
# 胃肠外科

主　　编 | 王锡山　丁克峰　Petr V. Tsarkov（俄罗斯）

副 主 编 | Jim Khan　Cüneyt Kayaalp　Sergey Efetov
王贵玉　周海涛　胡军红　王丹波　张　卫
韩方海　刘　正　关　旭　蒙家兴

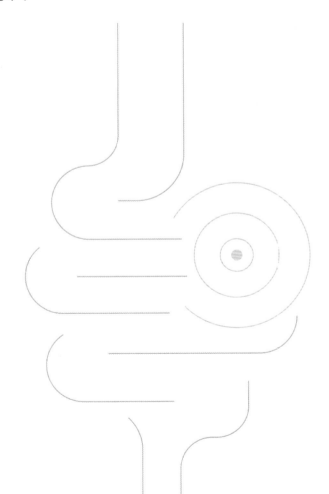

人民卫生出版社
·北 京·

**图书在版编目（CIP）数据**

经自然腔道取标本手术基础与培训．胃肠外科 ：汉英对照/王锡山，丁克峰，（俄罗斯）彼得·察尔科夫主编．－－北京 ：人民卫生出版社，2025．8．－－ ISBN 978-7-117-38387-5

Ⅰ．R730.56

中国国家版本馆 CIP 数据核字第 2025FZ8728 号

| 人卫智网 | www.ipmph.com | 医学教育、学术、考试、健康，购书智慧智能综合服务平台 |
| 人卫官网 | www.pmph.com | 人卫官方资讯发布平台 |

**策划编辑** 刘岩岩　吴桐菲　　　　**责任编辑** 吴桐菲　刘岩岩

**数字编辑** 赵奕涵　　　　　　　　**书籍设计** 惠亦凡

开开此层获取权益

0002 0004 7524 6191

使用说明

**经自然腔道取标本手术
基础与培训——胃肠外科**

Jing Ziran Qiangdao Qu Biaoben Shoushu
Jichu yu Peixun——Weichang Waike

主　　编：王锡山　丁克峰　Petr V.Tsarkov（俄罗斯）
出版发行：人民卫生出版社（中继线 010-59780011）
地　　址：北京市朝阳区潘家园南里 19 号
邮　　编：100021
E - mail：pmph @ pmph.com
购书热线：010-59787592　010-59787584　010-65264830
印　　刷：北京华联印刷有限公司
经　　销：新华书店
开　　本：889×1194　1/16　　　印张：19　　字数：629 千字
版　　次：2025 年 8 月第 1 版　　印次：2025 年 8 月第 1 次印刷
标准书号：ISBN 978-7-117-38387-5
定　　价：159.00 元

打击盗版举报电话：010-59787491　E-mail：WQ @ pmph.com
质量问题联系电话：010-59787234　E-mail：zhiliang @ pmph.com
数字融合服务电话：4001118166　　E-mail：zengzhi @ pmph.com

# 编 者 名 单
（以姓氏汉语拼音为序）

| | |
|---|---|
| Cüneyt Kayaalp | Private Gastrointestinal Surgery Clinic, Istanbul, Turkiye |
| Jim Khan | University of Portsmouth |
| Petr V.Tsarkov | Sechenov First Moscow State Medical University |
| Sergey Efetov | Sechenov First Moscow State Medical University |
| 包满都拉 | 中国医学科学院肿瘤医院 |
| 陈海鹏 | 中国医学科学院肿瘤医院 |
| 陈龙翊 | 中国医学科学院肿瘤医院 |
| 陈田力 | 中国医学科学院肿瘤医院 |
| 陈瑛罡 | 中国医学科学院肿瘤医院深圳医院 |
| 丁克峰 | 浙江大学医学院附属第二医院 |
| 冯 波 | 上海交通大学医学院附属瑞金医院 |
| 关 旭 | 中国医学科学院肿瘤医院 |
| 韩方海 | 广东省第二人民医院 |
| 何国栋 | 复旦大学附属中山医院 |
| 何庆泗 | 山东大学齐鲁医院 |
| 侯文运 | 中国医学科学院肿瘤医院 |
| 胡军红 | 郑州大学第一附属医院 |
| 胡茜玥 | 中国医学科学院肿瘤医院 |
| 黄 亮 | 中山大学附属第六医院 |
| 黄 睿 | 哈尔滨医科大学附属第二医院 |
| 江 波 | 山西省肿瘤医院 |
| 姜 争 | 中国医学科学院肿瘤医院 |
| 金英虎 | 哈尔滨医科大学附属第二医院 |
| 李大为 | 哈尔滨医科大学附属第二医院 |
| 李太原 | 南昌大学第一附属医院 |
| 李月刚 | 中国医学科学院肿瘤医院 |
| 刘 骞 | 中国医学科学院肿瘤医院 |
| 刘 正 | 北京美中爱瑞肿瘤医院 |
| 刘恒昌 | 中国医学科学院肿瘤医院 |
| 刘家良 | 中国医学科学院肿瘤医院 |
| 刘金超 | 淄博市市立医院 |
| 刘瑞延 | 陕西省人民医院 |
| 卢 召 | 中国医学科学院肿瘤医院 |
| 吕靖芳 | 中国医学科学院肿瘤医院 |
| 马 丹 | 陆军军医大学第二附属医院 |
| 马天翼 | 哈尔滨医科大学附属第二医院 |
| 蒙家兴 | 香港明德国际医院 |
| 莫显伟 | 广西医科大学附属肿瘤医院 |
| 彭 健 | 中南大学湘雅医院 |
| 乔天宇 | 哈尔滨医科大学附属第二医院 |
| 权继传 | 中国医学科学院肿瘤医院 |
| 孙 鹏 | 中国医学科学院肿瘤医院深圳医院 |
| 汤坚强 | 中国医学科学院肿瘤医院 |
| 汤庆超 | 哈尔滨医科大学附属第二医院 |
| 田艳涛 | 中国医学科学院肿瘤医院 |
| 王 松 | 淄博市市立医院 |
| 王丹波 | 中国医科大学肿瘤医院 |
| 王贵玉 | 哈尔滨医科大学附属第二医院 |
| 王锡山 | 中国医学科学院肿瘤医院 |
| 王效明 | 淄博市市立医院 |
| 王泽军 | 贵州医科大学附属肿瘤医院 |
| 韦 烨 | 复旦大学附属华东医院 |
| 熊德海 | 重庆大学附属三峡医院 |
| 熊治国 | 湖北省肿瘤医院 |
| 燕 速 | 青海大学附属医院 |
| 尹叶锋 | 中国医学科学院肿瘤医院 |
| 于 刚 | 淄博市市立医院 |
| 于冠宇 | 海军军医大学第一附属医院（长海医院） |
| 俞少俊 | 浙江大学医学院附属第二医院 |
| 郁 雷 | 哈尔滨医科大学附属第二医院 |
| 袁子茗 | 哈尔滨医科大学附属第二医院 |
| 张 骞 | 中国科学院大学附属肿瘤医院 |
| 张 卫 | 海军军医大学第一附属医院（长海医院） |
| 张金珠 | 中国医学科学院肿瘤医院 |
| 张明光 | 中国医学科学院肿瘤医院 |
| 张铁民 | 海南医学院第二附属医院 |
| 张筱倩 | 中国医学科学院肿瘤医院 |
| 赵志勋 | 中国医学科学院肿瘤医院 |
| 郑朝旭 | 中国医学科学院肿瘤医院 |
| 周海涛 | 中国医学科学院肿瘤医院 |
| 朱晓明 | 海军军医大学第一附属医院（长海医院） |
| 庄 孟 | 中国医学科学院肿瘤医院 |

**编写秘书** 刘家良 刘 正 胡茜玥

# 序 一

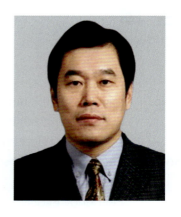

近年来,随着外科学的不断发展,肿瘤手术的目标已经不再局限于根治性切除,对微创效果和器官功能保留的追求,已成为手术的更高境界。在此背景下,锡山教授为推动外科微创治疗、提升外科技术水平作出了杰出贡献。作为我国结直肠肿瘤领域的领军人物,他的多项技术创新,特别是经自然腔道取标本手术(natural orifice specimen extraction surgery,NOSES),已成为引领行业发展的典范。

锡山教授在推动 NOSES 方面做了大量工作,牵头制定十余部国际及中国 NOSES 专家指南与共识,为世界范围内 NOSES 的开展建立了行业标准。为丰富 NOSES 理论体系,NOSES 的适应证范围不断拓展。从第 1 版的结直肠肿瘤,扩充至第 2 版的胃肠肿瘤,再延伸到第 3 版的腹盆腔肿瘤,到第 4 版,胸部肿瘤及食管癌等手术也被规范地纳入其中。他的著作先后被多位国际著名专家译为英、韩、俄、日、法等多种语言进行全球推广,这客观反映了 NOSES 的可行性和其巨大的社会价值,也反映出中国 NOSES 在国际上的威望与地位,更再次诠释了 NOSES 的广阔应用前景。

为更好地促进 NOSES 的规范化应用,建立完善的培训体系及编撰规范的培训教程至关重要。因此,锡山教授组织编写了中英文 NOSES 国际结构化培训与认证教程《经自然腔道取标本手术基础与培训——胃肠外科》。这部专著涵盖了 NOSES 核心理论及手术要点。其目的在于帮助国内外医生系统掌握 NOSES 的精髓,使这一微创技术不仅在理论层面上得以不断完善,更在全球范围内得以实践推广。值得一提的是,该专著内容系统、细致,涵盖了从术式选择到术中操作及术后管理的每一关键步骤,对全球外科医生均具有重要的参考价值。

这部专著的出版,不仅是中国 NOSES 发展历程中的一大里程碑,也是将 NOSES 推向全球的坚实一步。我深信,这部专著必将为全球外科领域带来深远的影响。

2024 年 12 月

# 序 二

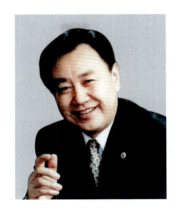

　　在整合医学理念的推动下,各学科之间的深度融合使现代医学朝着整体视角下优化诊疗手段的方向快速发展。锡山教授敏锐地捕捉到这一趋势,历经十余年的不断探索与实践,带领国内与国际同道成功构建了系统化的 NOSES 整合理论技术体系,为微创手术开辟了新的高度,使其更具创新性和临床应用价值。

　　作为一项外科技术,NOSES 不仅在微创治疗上取得突破,还实现了横向整合和纵向整合的全面发展。横向整合方面,NOSES 将胃肠外科、肝胆胰脾外科、胸外科、妇科和泌尿外科等多个学科紧密联系,推动了 NOSES 在多学科协作和融合中的深入发展;纵向整合方面,NOSES 系统化地整合了从基础理论到手术操作、患者管理等知识体系,全面覆盖了临床应用的每一环节。这一系统化体系不仅帮助医生在无腹部切口的情况下对患者实现高效治疗,更显著提高了患者的生活质量与治疗体验。NOSES 体现了从患者整体出发的诊疗思路,彰显出锡山教授对整合医学理念的深刻理解和践行,不仅限于医学技术本身,还触及心理学、社会学等领域的交融,开创了全新诊疗视角。

　　由锡山教授主编的《经自然腔道取标本手术基础与培训——胃肠外科》在内容上更加全面、实用、接地气,尤其注重手术的操作细节和临床规范,极具指导价值。同时,本部专著采用中英文双语呈现,为国内、国际同道学习、培训 NOSES 提供了方便,也搭建了交流的桥梁,有助于推动 NOSES 全球规范普及。这一创新性著作不仅是临床操作指南,更是传播 NOSES 理念的重要载体,为外科医生应用 NOSES 提供了切实支持。

　　由本部专著作为指引,NOSES 必将助力我国微创外科在内科与外科交汇处绽放光彩。我期待此书能为各位同道在 NOSES 领域的探索提供宝贵参考,助力 NOSES 不断攀登国际前沿,造福更多患者。

2024 年 12 月

# 前　言

　　岁月不居，时节如流。回首 NOSES 概念被提出十余年，经历了萌芽阶段、起步阶段、发展阶段和成熟阶段。全国同道共同致力于 NOSES 技术体系和理论体系的不断完善，大家都付出了智慧与辛劳，而我杖乡之年，在 NOSES 发展道路上经历了新奇、灵感、努力、付出、质疑、诋毁、赞誉、掌声、鲜花……感悟颇多。这不只是一个技术体系和理论体系的问题，更是人性、江湖、人生的思辩。与此同时，深感科技与学术之发展，教学与培训之重要，思考与传承之力量。肩负造福病人之使命，培养人才之责任，学科发展之担当，故愿将感悟收集于此，分享给学员。

## 1. 创新与反思
- 我们现有的知识、经验，以及惯性思维，往往是我们创新的最大敌人，也是我们否认别人的理由。
- 在规范中创新，在创新中务实，在务实中求真，在求真中前行。
- 你可限制我动手，但无法限制我动脑，因此思考才是一个外科医生必备素养之一。
- 人类机体的完美弥补了医学的不足和我们的自以为是。

## 2. 个人成长与职业发展
- 个人吃一堑，行业长一智。
- 一个外科医生敢于否定自己的那一天，才是真正成长起来。
- 当我们的努力过程变成成绩的那一刻，成绩就代表过去，我们要向新的目标起航。
- 实力是唯一的话语权，实干是唯一的兴邦路。
- 欲望激发潜能，目标诞生活力。
- 智者天下，善者未来。
- 用技术赢得天下，靠德行赢得未来。

## 3. 医德与职业文化
- 用欣赏的眼光看待别人的成绩，用挑剔的目光看待自己的不足。
- 当你没有成绩之前，没有自尊可言，因为你的自尊与患者的生命相比一文不值!
- 善良感动不了卑鄙，正直也消融不了无耻，但我们不能因此而不善良、不正直。
- 团队文化
- 两个一

　　一个座右铭：德不如佛者不可为医，技不如仙者不可为医。

　　一个目标：以自身健康和所医治的患者康复为目标。
- 两个二

　　两感：一个医生时刻要有成就感和内疚感。成就感是我们事业执着前行的动力；内疚感可以为我们的事业纠偏。

　　两追求：外科医生的每一个动作都要透射出智慧；外科医生要有立体的解剖思维。

· 两个三

  行医三原则:依法行医——原则性;人文行医——灵活性;科学行医——科学性。

  做医三境界:匠——用"手"看病;家——用"脑"看病;师——用"心"看病。

## 4. 医学与社会洞察

· 医学的发展依赖其他学科的发展,如光学、电学、工程学、药学、美学等,医学是科技进步、社会进步及人类文明的复合体。

· 图恩不施报,施报不图恩。

· 让人感恩一辈子很难;让人恨一辈子很容易。

· 旁观者之所以清是因为不涉及自己利益。

· 文明源于文化的积累与传承;传承源于民族的自信与使命;感恩源于内心的虔诚与敬畏,发展源于国家的创新与信仰。

· 医生六真理念:信仰要真、本领要真、合作要真、传授要真、发力要真、情感要真。

· 人要成功很难,需要无数个因素有利于他,而失败很简单,只需要一个因素。

　　以上为我不同时期的感悟及铭记的名言,其中一些正是我心路历程的记录。我愿将其分享,如能对读者有所裨益,我甚感欣慰! 此次编写《经自然腔道取标本手术基础与培训——胃肠外科》中英一体本旨在为国内外学员提供学习、运用和推广 NOSES 提供参考,希望所有学员成为有爱心、有情怀、有温度、有哲思,造福患者、福佑社会、推动外科前行的国际 NOSES 人。

　　NOSES 是中国的,更是世界的!

　　敬心尊道是为前言!


2024 年 12 月

# 目 录

**第四章**
**腹腔镜下胃 NOSES 的标准化流程**   |   **133**

**第五章**
**消化道 NOSES 常见并发症及处理**   |   **170**

# 视频目录

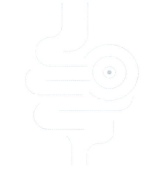

# 第一章

# NOSES 总论

随着微创理念的深入人心和外科技术的飞速发展，如今的微创外科已经毫无争议地成为当下外科舞台上的耀眼新星。经自然腔道内镜手术（natural orifice translumenalendoscopic surgery，NOTES）颠覆了人们的传统观念，让微创手术走向"无切口"的极致。近年来，经自然腔道取标本手术（natural orifice specimen extraction surgery，NOSES）作为微创外科的一名新秀，逐渐引起国内外学者的广泛关注和热议。众所周知，NOSES 巧妙地结合了 NOTES 的"无切口"理念和常规腹腔镜技术的操作技巧，既表现出了完美的微创效果，又兼具良好的安全性和可操作性。目前，NOSES 不仅应用于结直肠领域，在胃肠、肝胆、胰脾、泌尿、妇科，以及胸外科的治疗中也开始逐渐推广普及，这反映出 NOSES 的强大生命力和推广潜力。

## 第一节　NOSES 定义与分类

NOSES 是指使用常规腹腔镜器械、经肛门内镜微创手术（transanal endoscopic microsurgery，TEM）、软质内镜或机器人辅助手术平台等设备完成腹腔内手术操作（切除、重建），经自然腔道（直肠、阴道或口腔）取出病灶标本的腹壁无辅助切口手术。该手术与常规腹腔镜手术最大的区别就在于病灶标本经自然腔道取出，避免了腹壁取标本的辅助切口，术后腹壁仅存留几处微小瘢痕（图 1-1-1）。

根据取标本的不同途径，NOSES 主要分为三种，即经肛门取标本、经阴道取标本、经口腔取标本（图 1-1-2）。目前临床应用最广的是前两种方式，尤其是经肛门取标本。经肛门取标本主要适用于标本较小，容易取出的患者；经阴道取标本主要适用于标本较大，经肛门取出困难的女性患者。由于食管管腔狭长、管壁弹性差，术者在开展经口腔取标本手术时，一定要严格把握适应证。

根据取标本的不同手术方式，NOSES 又可分为三类，分别是标本外翻体外切除（外翻切除式）、标本拉出体外切除（拉出切除式）、标本体内切除拖出体外（切除拖出式）（图 1-1-3）。不同手术方式具有不同的

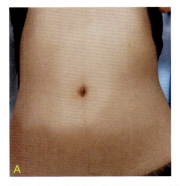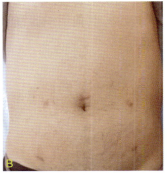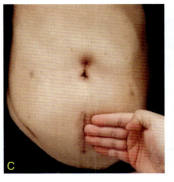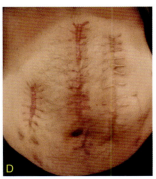

图 1-1-1　直肠癌术后腹壁切口瘢痕对比

A. 直肠癌 NOTES 后腹壁；B. 直肠癌 NOSES 后腹壁；C. 常规腹腔镜直肠癌手术后腹壁；D. 复发直肠癌开腹手术后腹壁。

Figure 1-1-1　Comparison of abdominal wall incision scars after rectal cancer surgery

A. Abdominal wall after NOTES for rectal cancer; B. Abdominal wall after NOSES for rectal cancer; C. Abdominal wall after conventional laparoscopic surgery of rectal cancer; D. Abdominal wall after open surgery for radical resection of recurrent rectal cancer.

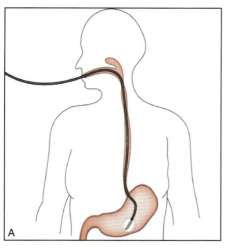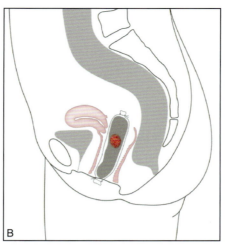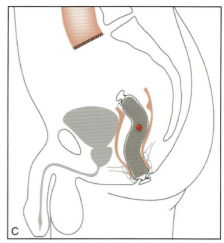

图 1-1-2　取标本的不同途径

A. 经口腔取标本；B. 经肛门取标本；C. 经阴道取标本。

Figure 1-1-2　Different routes for specimen extraction

A. Transoral specimen extraction；B. Transanal specimen extraction；C. Transvaginal specimen extraction.

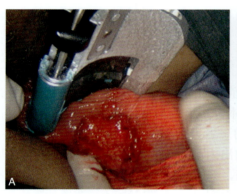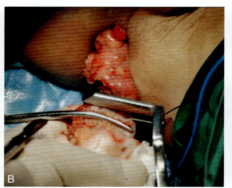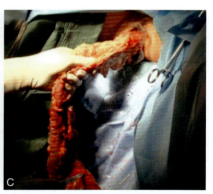

图 1-1-3　取标本的不同手术方式

A. 外翻切除式；B. 拉出切除式；C. 切除拖出式。

Figure 1-1-3　Different procedures of specimen extraction

A. Eversion-resection procedure；B. Extraction-resection procedure；C. Resection-extraction procedure.

操作特点和技巧，但影响术式选择的决定性因素是肿瘤位置。在结直肠 NOSES 中，外翻切除式主要适用于低位直肠肿瘤，拉出切除式主要适用于中位直肠肿瘤，而切除拖出式的适应范围最为广泛，包括高位直肠、乙状结肠、左半结肠、右半结肠及全结肠。除结直肠以外，其他组织器官的标本取出方式都是采用切除拖出式。

## 第二节　开展 NOSES 的理念与原则

　　肿瘤外科发展与 NOSES 诞生之间的关系可以看作是一个循序渐进的技术演变过程，肿瘤外科从传统开腹手术到腹腔镜、机器人辅助手术，经历了多次技术进步，这为 NOSES 的诞生奠定了基础。技术的进步、微创理念的深化、患者需求的转变共同推动肿瘤外科领域催生了 NOSES，而 NOSES 的诞生又进一步推动了肿瘤外科微创技术的发展。NOSES 继承了肿瘤外科的核心理念，即肿瘤学安全性与器官功能保留,同时通过创新的标本取出方式,将微创手术提升到一个新的高度,进而满足了患者对手术创伤小、恢复快的需求。NOSES 是肿瘤根治术式及结直肠外科术式的一部分,因此,该技术操作必须满足根治术与结直肠外科手术的三个理念和两个原则。三个理念指的是肿瘤功能外科理念(function preservation in oncology surgery concept,FPOSC)、手术损伤效益比理念(surgical risk-benefit balance concept,SRBBC)与无菌无瘤理念(concept of aseptic and tumor-free surgical practice,CATFSP);两个原则指的是要符合全直肠系膜切除术(total mesorectal excision,TME)原则和全结肠系膜切除术(complete mesocolic excision,CME)原则。

## 一、三个理念

1. FPOSC　NOSES 因其诸多的优势,已成为很多肿瘤患者的外科治疗选择。胃肠肿瘤 NOSES 手术切除范围选择必须遵循 FPOSC 理念,即最大限度地切除肿瘤保证根治和最大限度地保留正常组织和器官功能。该理念体现了外科医生的权衡能力。例如,同样行经肛门外翻式切除肿瘤手术,一例患者外翻肠管长度为 3~4cm,另一例患者外翻肠管长度为 10cm 以上(图 1-2-1)。虽然两者均进行了 NOSES,但前者对,后者错,错误在于后者不符合 FPOSC 理念。再比如右半结肠切除术中对中结肠动脉的保留,以及直肠 NOSES 中对盆底神经功能的保护都体现了 FPOSC。肿瘤外科手术时遵循的 FPOSC 不仅在于根治肿瘤与保留功能并重,还关注肿瘤患者的临床结局,尤其是术后生活质量。切忌为了手术而手术。

2. SRBBC　到目前为止,对于大多数实体瘤来说,手术依然是实现肿瘤治愈的关键手段,因此,术式的合理选择就显得尤为重要。SRBBC 是指手术切除肿瘤造成的机体创伤、损伤、打击与组织、器官、身体承受力、总体获益的比较判定,即哪些患者该做手术,该做什么样的手术,让患者在最小的损伤耐受下获得最大的受益。如果标本既可经肛门也可经阴道取出,要选择经肛门取标本,这样可以避免阴道不必要的损伤,也更符合 SRBBC。SRBBC 体现了外科医生的抉择能力,通过准确评估能够确保适宜的手术应用于合适的患者,在保障患者安全且同时也维护了自身的操作安全。切忌出现成功的手术、失败的治疗。

3. CATFSP　为确保 NOSES 成功实施,无菌术与无瘤操作是其操作的基本要求。第一,术者要具有基本的 CATFSP,严格遵循探查由远及近、不接触隔离技术、整块切除原则、血管优先处理原则,并尽量锐性分离。第二,术前必须进行充分肠道和阴道准备。第三,必须掌握一定的手术操作技巧,重视手术团队的整体配合,尤其是消化道重建和标本取出环节,这是完成高质量 NOSES 的核心步骤。第四,合理使用抗肿瘤药及抗菌药。对有高危复发风险的结直肠癌患者,特别是有肿瘤侵及浆膜、淋巴结转移、腹腔冲洗液细胞学检查游离癌细胞为阳性或可疑阳性、术中瘤体被过度挤压或瘤体破裂等情况的患者,可进行腹腔用药。术中将化疗药物注入腹腔直接作用于腹腔内种植和脱落的癌细胞,维持腹腔内较高的有效药物浓度,是预防和治疗结直肠癌腹腔种植转移的重要手段之一。目前,临床常用的结直肠癌腹腔用药包括雷替曲塞、洛铂、肿瘤坏死因子、氟尿嘧啶植入剂等。

## 二、两个原则

1. TME 原则是用于直肠癌治疗的标准手术技术原则,通过在直肠系膜外的膜解剖平面内精确切除直肠及其系膜组织,以确保完整的肿瘤切除和淋巴结清扫。TME 注重切除范围的完整性和自主神经的保护,

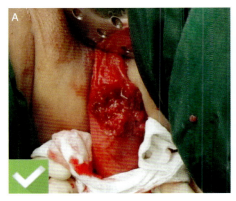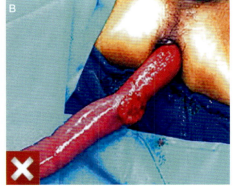

图 1-2-1　两例外翻式切除肿瘤的手术图片

Figure 1-2-1　Intraoperative images of two cases undergoing transanal external resection of tumors

既可确保肿瘤的根治性,又可减少术后功能障碍,如性功能或排尿功能的损失,有效降低了局部复发率并改善患者的生活质量。

2. CME 原则是一种基于解剖学用于结肠癌治疗的标准手术技术原则,通过在膜解剖平面内完整切除结肠及其系膜组织,以确保包括肿瘤周围的淋巴结在内的所有相关组织被彻底切除。CME 强调高位结扎血管和彻底的淋巴结清扫,以降低局部复发的风险,同时保证无瘤操作,防止肿瘤细胞播散,从而提高结肠癌患者的无病生存率和整体预后。

## 第三节　NOSES 适应证选择

由于 NOSES 基于腹腔镜平台完成,因此,NOSES 适应证要满足腹腔镜手术的基本要求。通常来说,开展腹腔镜等微创手术需要满足以下条件:①手术医生具有腹腔镜操作经验;②不能用于局部晚期肿瘤;③不适用于肿瘤引起的急性肠梗阻和肠穿孔;④需要进行全腹腔探查;⑤需考虑术前对病灶进行定位。NOSES 的开展一定要满足腹腔镜手术适应证的基本要求。

此外,NOSES 涉及经自然腔道取标本这一环节,这也对 NOSES 适应证提出了特殊要求。新版《结直肠肿瘤经自然腔道取标本手术专家共识》中已明确指出,结直肠肿瘤 NOSES 的特有适应证主要包括:肿瘤浸润深度以 $T_2 \sim T_3$ 为宜,经肛门取标本的标本环周直径 <5cm 为宜,经阴道取标本的标本环周直径 5~7cm 为宜。相对禁忌证包括肿瘤局部病期较晚、标本较大、身体质量指数( body mass index,BMI )> $30kg/m^2$。由于目前尚无法证实阴道后穹隆切口是否会影响女性生育功能,因此,不建议对未婚或有生育要求的女性行经阴道取标本。NOSES 特有适应证主要是针对经自然腔道取标本这一操作环节所提及的,主要涉及三方面考虑因素,即标本大小、肿瘤浸润深度和 BMI。

对于结直肠癌伴有局部器官侵犯需行联合脏器切除的患者,以及结直肠癌伴有远处转移或其他部位病变需同时进行手术切除的患者,也可以选择复杂手术 NOSES。在联合脏器和多脏器切除中,NOSES 的手术适应证要更为严格,尤其对医生的操作技术提出了更为严格的要求。

## 第四节　经自然腔道取标本操作规范

经自然腔道取标本是 NOSES 最具特色的核心手术步骤,也是最受关注和热议的手术环节。经自然腔道取标本操作体现很强的个体差异,既与患者自然腔道解剖生理状况有关,也与医生对取标本的认知水平和操作经验有关。

### 一、经肛门取标本

经肛门这个自然通道取标本的手术方式有很多,广大医师也熟练掌握。概括起来,有以下三种方式。

1. 经肛门外翻式切除取标本　经肛门外翻式切除取标本适用于低位直肠肿瘤病灶较小、侵犯环周直径 <1/2 的患者。该方法是利用健侧肠壁的弹性,将包含肿瘤的远端直肠外翻于肛门外,然后使用碘附水进行大量冲洗,尤其是肠壁反折处。这样可在直视下清晰分辨肿瘤下切缘,确保在切缘安全的情况下离断肿瘤。

2. 经直肠残端取标本　经直肠残端取标本是目前结直肠 NOSES 应用最广、创伤最小的首选取标本途径。为兼顾取标本操作的安全性与可行性,对该操作规范要求如下:①术中取标本前必须进行充分扩肛。②用大量碘附水冲洗直肠断端。③取标本前需置入保护套避免标本与自然腔道接触。④取标本过程中需轻柔缓慢操作,避免暴力拉拽破坏标本完整性;如取标本阻力较大,可嘱麻醉医生适当给予肌肉松弛药,降低肛门括约肌张力。经直肠残端取标本是否会损伤肛门括约肌及影响排便功能,是 NOSES 关注的焦点问题。结合目前研究结果可知,只要符合适应证,就不会明显增加肛门损伤的风险。

3. 经直肠切口取标本　经直肠切口取标本主要适用于右半结肠或左半结肠或横结肠切除的患者。该取标本方式增加了一处直肠切口，增加了术后直肠漏风险，因此，术前必须与患者及家属进行充分沟通并取得同意才可开展该手术。经直肠切口取标本存在两处操作难点：第一，如何使标本顺利经肛门取出，操作要点与经直肠残端取标本一致。第二，如何选择直肠切口位置，以及具体操作规范。有条件的医疗单位可采用术中肠镜确认。

建议直肠切口位置选择在腹膜反折以上直肠中段前壁，切口大小 3~5cm，切口方向平行于肠管走行，注意切开肠管时勿损伤对侧肠壁。肠管切口缝合建议采用自切口远端向近端的连续缝合，缝合后需进行注水注气试验检测直肠切口是否缝合完整。有条件的医疗单位可采用术中肠镜来确认。

## 二、经阴道取标本

阴道切开与缝合是经阴道取标本的操作难点，推荐将阴道后穹隆作为阴道切口的优先选择。直肠子宫陷凹具有独特的解剖优势，在腹腔镜下容易寻找和显露，能有效减少副损伤的风险。同时，阴道后穹隆愈合能力良好，周围无重要的血管和神经，黏膜愈合后无瘢痕，对患者性生活的影响较小。阴道切开包括腹腔镜下切开和经阴道切开，术者可根据操作习惯进行选择。阴道切口长度建议 3~5cm，方向为横行切开，切开深度为阴道壁全层，完成标本取出后，需经腹腔冲洗阴道。阴道切口缝合包括经阴道腹腔外缝合和腹腔镜下缝合，缝合方式多采用倒刺线从阴道切口一端向另一端进行连续全层缝合，缝合后需行阴道指诊或肛门指诊，检查切口是否缝合确切及直肠是否有损伤。

## 三、经口腔取标本

除经肛门、经阴道取标本外，也有学者开始尝试开展经口腔取标本的 NOSES，包括袖状胃切除术、胃间质瘤切除术、肝活检术、胆囊切除术、脾切除术等。胃与食管、口腔相通，因此，对于病灶较小的胃肿瘤，可采取经口腔取标本。经口腔取标本无须再另辟蹊径，不涉及自然腔道的切开、缝合及标本的转运，主要操作要点为标本经食管、口腔取出。经口腔取标本过程中，建议将标本置入保护套中进行封闭，并在内镜全程指引下完成标本取出。但由于食管的管腔狭窄、管壁弹性差，术者在开展经口取标本手术时，一定要严格把握适应证。

## 四、经自然腔道取标本经验与技巧

1. 系膜优先法应用于经肛门外翻式切除取标本　在常规腹腔镜下直肠外翻切除式直肠癌手术中，若肿瘤较小且系膜较薄时，采用直接翻出法可轻松将远端直肠翻出。但对肿瘤较大或系膜肥厚的患者，此法容易导致外翻失败及肿瘤破碎。系膜优先法克服了肿瘤较大、系膜肥厚，以及聚集成团卡在肛门的困难。先剪开直肠前壁（约 3cm），将裁剪的系膜自直肠腔拉出肛门外，以减小翻出的压力，这样在采用外拉内推的方式将带肿瘤的肠管翻出时，操作就会容易得多。系膜优先法有很多技巧，如对标本采用外拉内推的方法就可以将肥胖及肿瘤较大者外翻成功。但要判定准确，切忌造成不必要的损伤。

2. 经肛门取标本操作技巧
（1）扩肛前给予肌肉松弛药是有必要的；
（2）保护套采用经 12mm 戳卡孔经腹置入方法；
（3）助手经肛门取标本时，优先夹持系膜根部；
（4）术者在取标本时避免牵拉保护套，此时保护套可起隔离和扩张支架的作用；
（5）当肿瘤环周最大处进入肛管时可收拢保护套，并连同保护套一起向外牵拉；
（6）腹腔镜下术者和助手经腹配合，收紧保护套内口，此时经腹操作的助手可用吸引器配合，防止标本向腹腔内渗液。

3. 经阴道取标本操作技巧
（1）切口选择：根据经验，可选用膀胱拉钩，经阴道外口置入阴道内，用其尖端顶住阴道后穹隆处。在膀胱拉钩的协助定位下，术者于腹腔镜下横行切开阴道后穹隆，切口长度为 3~5cm。由于阴道具有很强的延展性，在切口处上下牵拉扩展，将切口扩大至 5cm 即可满足取标本要求。
（2）切口缝合：可选择直视下经阴道缝合，也可选择腹腔镜下缝合。根据经验，体外缝合难度较低，尤其是对不能熟练掌握腹腔镜下缝合技巧的外科医生，体外缝合是首选方法。①体外缝合：由于阴道后穹隆位置深在，因此进行体外缝合时，充分显露阴道后穹隆切口十分必要。在临床实践中，常用阴道扩张器或直角拉钩等器械充分显露阴道，阴道后穹隆左右两端是重要部位，用两把 Allis 钳分别夹持阴道切口的上下缘，并适当向体外牵拉，而后间断或连续缝合数针，显露不满意时，考虑阴道切口全层开放缝合。缝毕阴道填塞纱布以免残腔积血影响愈合，压迫 24~48 小时后取出纱布。②腹腔镜下缝合：该缝合技术难度较大，对术者的操作能力提出很高要求。腹腔镜下缝合阴道切口需使用专用阴道倒刺线（15cm 即可，线太长会影响操作），多采用从阴道切口一端向另一端进行连续全层缝合。缝合后行阴道指诊或肛门指诊。缝合过程中需要将阴道切口上下缘向腹腔内牵拉，牵拉力量不宜过大，以防止阴道出血。

## 第五节　消化道重建操作规范

NOSES 需在全腹腔镜下进行消化道重建，这也是 NOSES 的重点和难点环节。建议 NOSES 消化道重建遵循开腹和常规腹腔镜手术的消化道重建原则，包括以下 4 个方面：①确保肿瘤根治性切除的前提下，根据切除消化道的范围，选择安全可行的消化道重建方式；②术中要确保吻合口张力小、血运好，并保证吻合口通畅无狭窄；③保证肿瘤功能外科理念，减少不必要组织损伤，并兼顾消化道生理功能；④对于低位直肠癌、超低位吻合保肛手术，如存在吻合口漏高危风险或患者进行了新辅助放化疗，建议酌情进行保护性回肠造口术。

### 一、消化道重建方式选择（结直肠）

结直肠的消化道重建主要分为三种方式，端端吻合、功能性端端吻合和功能性侧侧吻合。吻合手术方式包括结肠 - 直肠吻合、结肠 - 结肠吻合、回肠 - 结肠吻合、结肠 - 肛管吻合。结肠 - 直肠吻合可用于直肠 NOSES 消化道重建，推荐端端吻合。功能性侧侧吻合方式适用于横结肠、左半结肠、右半结肠切除手术。回肠 - 结肠吻合方式适用于右半结肠切除手术。功能性端端吻合方式多用于右半结肠切除手术（图 1-5-1）。

### 二、消化道重建注意事项

在消化道重建过程中，应注重手术器械的选择、吻合质量的检查，以及高危因素的防范。通过科学合理的步骤和对细节的严格把控，可有效提高手术成功率并降低并发症风险。

1. 手术器械的选择　对于 NOSES 消化道重建来说，选择手术器械对于腹腔镜下的手术操作至关重要。合理使用具有预置芯片技术的电动直线切割闭合器、具有 3D 吻合技术的电动环形吻合器和弧形头端吻合器等设备，有助于更为稳定和精确地完成吻合。这些器械操作便捷且性能稳定，能显著提高吻合效果，并降低术中及术后不良事件发生的可能性。

2. 吻合质量的检查　吻合前须检查肠壁血运、吻合口张力、系膜方向是否扭转；吻合后须检查吻合口是否有渗漏、出血，以及通畅程度等情况。在吻合质量评估中，可通过检查上下切缘吻合口的完整性、观察吻合钉是否有显露、指检评估吻合口是否存在缝钉反穿等情况评价吻合的确切程度。同时可以采用注水注气试验，检测吻合口是否存在渗漏。此外，术中肠镜检查也能提供有效的视野，便于判断吻合口的通畅程度、吻合钉环抱组织宽度和是否存在其他隐患。

3. 高危因素的防范　对于有高危因素的患者，需要采取额外措施来降低发生吻合口并发症的风险。例如，对于吻合不完全或有渗漏风险的情况，可以在腹腔镜下加固吻合口，常采用倒刺线连续缝合或使用可吸收线进行间断加固。在保肛手术中，还可以经肛门加固吻合口。对于"危险三角区"，通常使用"8"字缝合，进一步提高吻合口的稳定性。完成消化道重建后，需在吻合口旁放置引流管，并保持引流通畅，以降低吻合口并发症的发生率。

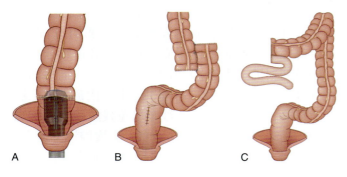

图 1-5-1　吻合方式

A. 端端吻合；B. 侧侧吻合；C. 功能性端端吻合。

Figure 1-5-1　Ways of anastomosis

A. End-to-end anastomosis; B. Side-to-side anastomosis; C. Functional end-to-end anastomosis.

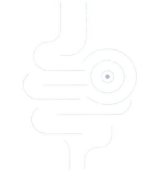

# 第二章

# NOSES围手术期准备

围手术期准备是胃肠外科手术前的常规程序。随着快速康复外科理念的推广，围手术期准备的内容也在不断调整改进。由于NOSES手术操作的特殊性，良好的围手术期准备尤为重要，涉及肠道准备、女性患者的阴道准备、手术团队及器械准备等诸多方面。只有做好各个方面的准备，才能达到最满意的手术效果。

## 第一节 肠道准备

与常规腹腔镜手术相比，NOSES在标本取出途径与消化道重建方式方面有很大区别，术中很多操作涉及无菌术的把控，因此，NOSES对肠道准备提出了很严格的要求。如术前准备不充分，肠内容物较多，很容易导致术中肠内容物进入腹腔，继而因腹腔污染发生感染，甚至出现吻合口漏等严重并发症。

肠道准备是指包括控制饮食、导泻、灌肠及联合口服抗生素的肠道准备方法。这一概念最早在20世纪50年代提出，主要认为肠道准备可以减少或清除粪块、降低感染和吻合口并发症发生率。传统的肠道准备理念认为，理想的肠道准备应具备以下特点：①使结肠完全空虚；②操作安全、便捷、迅速；③可有效降低肠道内细菌数量；④可减少抗生素用量；⑤不影响水电解质平衡；⑥刺激性小，患者耐受程度好；⑦性价比高，患者顺应性好；⑧对肠道影响小，术后肠道功能恢复快。

肠道准备药物中，电解质溶液、甘露醇、复方聚乙二醇、硫酸镁、磷酸钠盐口服液、酚酞片等均属于作用程度较剧烈的药物，外科医生应留意水和电解质紊乱的情况，并根据需要进行补充。而蓖麻油、液态石蜡和小剂量番泻叶冲剂具有起效慢、作用缓和的特点，可配合流食联合应用于不完全性肠梗阻患者。

对于NOSES，肠道准备这一环节是不可缺少的，这是术中无菌操作的有力保障。参考《美国结直肠外科医师协会2019版肠道准备在择期结直肠手术中的应用临床实践指南》，对于择期结直肠切除术，通常建议采用机械肠道准备联合术前口服抗生素，以降低手术部位感染、吻合口漏及再入院的发生率。

拟行NOSES的患者行术前肠道准备，可参考如下方案：①饮食调整。术前3天开始半流质饮食，术前2天全流质饮食，术前1天禁食，根据患者营养状态给予至少1天静脉营养支持。②机械肠道准备联合术前口服抗生素。对于无梗阻症状患者，目前常用方法为术前1天口服复方聚乙二醇，并分次口服肠道不吸收或少吸收的覆盖革兰氏阴性菌和厌氧菌的抗感染药物，如新霉素、红霉素、甲硝唑等。

## 第二节 阴道准备

在经阴道NOSES中，由于阴道是取标本的主要途径，因此需要严格的消毒和准备。

拟行经阴道取标本的患者，可采用如下方案进行阴道准备和相关操作：①术前3天使用3‰碘附或1‰苯扎溴铵冲洗阴道，每天1次；②手术当天，冲洗阴道后，以3‰碘附消毒宫颈，用纱布球擦干阴道黏膜及宫颈，然后留置导尿管；③术区消毒时，外阴、阴道及肛门周围等部位需要在原有基础上再消毒 2 次；④术中需要严格按照无菌和无瘤原则进行操作；⑤术后可于阴道内留置一块碘附纱布，并于术后 48 小时取出。

## 第三节　手术团队及器械准备

要组建自己的团队，其核心是团队成员在手术操作过程中要协同合作、各司其职。在团队组建初期，会出现配合不顺畅的情况，尤其是主刀医生，容易不自觉地越位，频繁承担助手的工作。这一点需要特别注意，要给予助手机会，毕竟成长需要时间和实践的打磨。

众所周知，开腹手术可以单打独斗，主刀医生同进修医生或实习生一起就可完成手术，但腹腔镜手术不同于开腹手术，尤其是 NOSES，其操作需要很多技巧，这对术者与助手配合的默契程度提出了很高要求，尤其在无菌操作和无瘤操作方面。因此，需要建立一支固定的手术团队，团队成员只有长期的磨合和实践才能达到心领神会、人镜合一的境界。

巧妇难为无米之炊，要想高质量完成 NOSES，除了密切的团队配合外，还需进行手术平台、器械平台和能量平台的充分准备。NOSES 与常规腹腔镜手术的操作步骤差异主要表现在消化道重建方式和标本的取出方式。要完成这两个手术步骤，需做好器械准备。

不同的胃肠 NOSES 术式，消化道重建过程中使用的手术器械各不相同。在右半结肠 NOSES 中，其消化道重建多借助腹腔镜下直线切割闭合器（如 Endo-GIA）完成。横结肠 NOSES 手术中常采用"V 型三角吻合"方式，本质上属于侧侧吻合的一种变型，同样需使用腹腔镜下直线切割闭合器。对于左半结肠、乙状结肠和直肠 NOSES，根据肿瘤位置及医生操作习惯的不同，消化道重建方式也有很大区别，主要包括端端吻合和侧端吻合两种方式，这两种方式都必须使用管型吻合器，吻合器的型号需要根据肠管口径进行选择，如 3D 电动管型吻合器可保证吻合质量进而降低吻合口漏风险。在此，笔者强调一点，如肠管长度允许，尽量采用端端吻合，此举可减少侧端吻合中一侧肠管的盲端，降低吻合口漏的风险。另外，根据不同的吻合器设计，抵钉座从肠管的取出方式也有所不同。如抵钉座连接杆为空心，可以采用固定挤压法取出抵钉座；如抵钉座连接杆带有反穿刺针，建议采用绑线法取出抵钉座。

在取标本步骤中，与经腹操作一样，NOSES 也需要一个取标本的辅助装置，以最大限度确保无菌操作与无瘤操作的实施。根据检索文献及临床实践可知，用于辅助取标本的工具包括切口保护套、超声刀保护套、无菌标本袋、自制塑料套管、经肛微创手术套管及经肛内镜等（图 2-3-1）。虽然取标本装置的种类很多，但主要可以概括为硬质和软质两种，两种装置也各有优势。软质装置具有很好的可塑性和弹性，不受标本大小的限制，只要自然腔道条件允许，均可以取

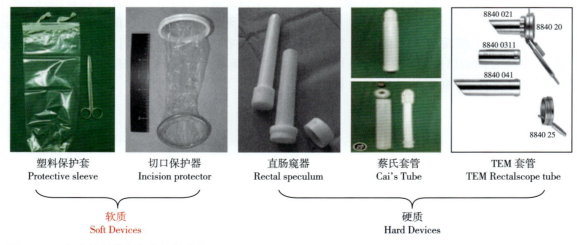

塑料保护套　　切口保护器　　直肠窥器　　蔡氏套管　　TEM 套管
Protective sleeve　Incision protector　Rectal speculum　Cai's Tube　TEM Rectalscope tube

软质　　　　　　　硬质
Soft Devices　　　　Hard Devices

图 2-3-1　经自然腔道取标本保护装置

Figure 2-3-1　Protective device for specimen extraction through the natural orifice

出。硬质装置具有很强的韧性，可以起到很强的支撑作用。如标本环周直径小于设备口径，可以很容易将标本取出，但如果标本环周直径大于设备口径，标本将很难取出。因此，在选择取标本装置时，一定要了解各种装置的特性，并且要根据标本大小及自然腔道的具体情况综合判断，只有这样，取标本时才能有的放矢、收放自如。

"工欲善其事，必先利其器。"NOSES 相关专用器械的研发一定是今后发展的重要方向，也是 NOSES 走向规范化的一个重要条件。

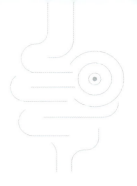

# 第三章

# 腹腔镜下结直肠 NOSES 的标准化流程

**第一节** 腹部无辅助切口经肛门外翻式切除取标本的腹腔镜下低位直肠癌根治术

（CRC-NOSES I 式 A 法和 B 法，外翻法）

## 【简介】

CRC-NOSES I 式主要适用于肿瘤较小的低位直肠癌患者。相比常规腹腔镜直肠癌根治术，CRC-NOSES I 式在手术范围、淋巴结清扫等方面无明显差异，其主要区别在于消化道重建和标本取出这两个环节。CRC-NOSES I 式的操作要点为经肛门将直肠外翻至体外，在体外直视下切除直肠肿瘤，再进行全腹腔镜下乙状结肠与直肠的端端吻合。此外，CRC-NOSES I 式还可以于直视下准确判断肿瘤下切缘到齿状线的距离，避免肿瘤下切缘阳性，并能够大大提高超低位保肛手术的可能性。目前，低位直肠癌 CRC-NOSES I 式主要包括两种消化道重建方法，即 CRC-NOSES I 式 A 法（图 3-1-1）和 B 法（图 3-1-2）。两种方法在操作方式上略有区别，A 法涉及无瘤操作的应用问题，B 法不涉及无瘤操作的应用问题，因此，B 法比 A 法适应证略宽一些，但二者均能达到相同的手术效果。CRC-NOSES I 式在保证肿瘤根治性切除的基础上，具有手术创伤小、恢复快、美容效果好等明显优势，是一个值得被外科医生掌握和推广的技术。

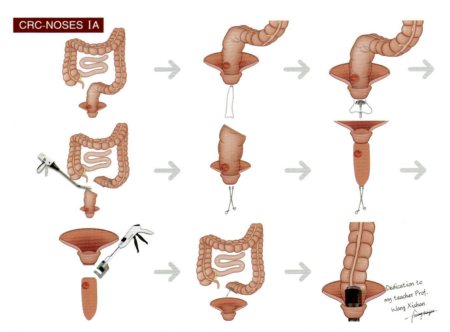

图 3-1-1 CRC-NOSES I 式 A 法标本取出及消化道重建的主要手术步骤
Figure 3-1-1 The main surgical steps of specimen extraction and digestive tract reconstruction in CRC-NOSES I A

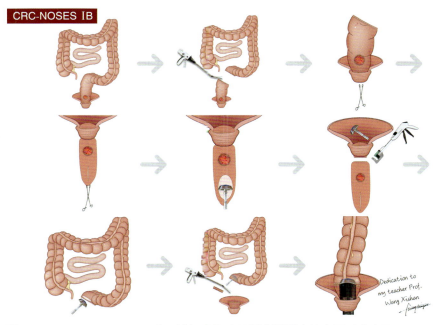

图 3-1-2　CRC-NOSES Ⅰ式 B 法标本取出及消化道重建的主要手术步骤

Figure 3-1-2　The main surgical steps of specimen extraction and digestive tract reconstruction in CRC-NOSES ⅠB

## 一、适应证与禁忌证

### 【适应证】

1. 低位直肠癌或良性肿瘤。
2. 浸润溃疡型肿瘤,且侵犯肠管 <1/2 周。
3. 隆起型肿瘤,肿瘤环周直径 <3cm。
4. 肿瘤下缘距齿状线 2~5cm 为宜。

### 【禁忌证】

1. 肿瘤侵犯肠管 >1/2 周。
2. 肿瘤环周直径 >3cm。
3. 黏液腺癌或印戒细胞癌,且术中无法明确下切缘状况。
4. 过于肥胖者(BMI>35kg/m$^2$)。

## 二、手术操作步骤、技巧与要点

### 【戳卡位置】

1. 腹腔镜镜头戳卡孔(10mm 戳卡)　脐上 1~2cm。
2. 术者主戳卡孔(12mm 戳卡)　放置于麦氏点偏下。
3. 术者辅助戳卡孔(5mm 戳卡)　脐右侧 10cm 左右。
4. 助手辅助戳卡孔(5mm 戳卡)　反麦氏点。
5. 助手主戳卡孔(5mm 戳卡)　脐水平左上方,靠内侧腹直肌外缘为宜(图 3-1-3)。

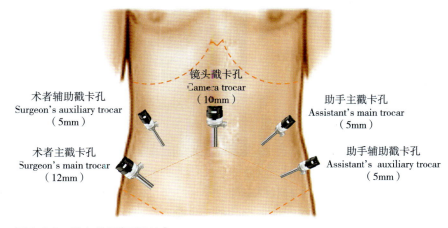

图 3-1-3　戳卡位置(五孔法)

Figure 3-1-3　Trocar placement(Five-port method)

## 【探查】

1. 常规探查　探查肝脏、胆囊、胃、脾脏、大网膜、结肠、小肠、直肠和盆腔。

2. 肿瘤探查　腹腔镜下常无法探及低位直肠肿瘤，术者可以用右手行直肠指检，与左手操作钳会合，来判定肿瘤位置及大小，是否适合行该手术。

3. 解剖结构的判定　包括对乙状结肠、直肠系膜肥厚程度，血管弓长度、预切除范围的判定。

## 【解剖与分离】

1. 第一刀切入点　在骶骨岬下方 3~5cm 通常有一菲薄处，用超声刀从此处切开系膜，进入 Toldt's 间隙。

2. 肠系膜下血管游离与离断　拓展 Toldt's 间隙，向头侧至肠系膜下动脉根部，向外侧至左侧生殖血管，清扫肠系膜下动脉根部淋巴结，结扎并切断血管。

3. 直肠后方的游离　沿 Toldt's 间隙向远端游离，进入直肠后间隙，切开直肠骶骨筋膜后进入肛提肌上间隙，继续向尾侧游离，直至肛提肌裂孔。

4. 直肠右侧的游离　沿直肠系膜与右侧盆壁的解剖界限分离至腹膜反折，并横行切开腹膜反折右侧。

5. 乙状结肠及直肠左侧的游离　打开乙状结肠与左侧腹壁的粘连，与内侧 Toldt's 间隙贯通，并向头侧游离，必要时游离结肠脾曲（结肠左曲）。向尾侧沿解剖边界游离至腹膜反折处与右侧会合。

6. 直肠前壁的游离　切开腹膜反折线向远端游离，进入直肠前间隙，尽量保证邓氏筋膜完整性，向尾侧游离直至肛提肌水平。游离至该位置已到达 TME

终点，此水平的直肠通常无系膜，无须裸化。

7. 乙状结肠系膜裁剪　可采取反向裁剪法，于系膜水平预切除线，由远端逆行向近端裁剪乙状结肠系膜。

## 【标本切除与消化道重建】

### CRC-NOSES　Ⅰ式 A 法（视频 3-1）

视频 3-1　CRC-NOSES Ⅰ式 A 法
Video 3-1　CRC-NOSES Ⅰ A

1. 标本切除　严格遵循无菌原则和无瘤原则，经肛门置入保护套，至肿瘤上方 5cm。用卵圆钳夹持抵钉座，经保护套内肿瘤的对侧滑入，至预切除线上方（图 3-1-4、图 3-1-5）。用直线切割闭合器在裸化的肠管预切除线处切割闭合乙状结肠（图 3-1-6），并将抵钉座留在乙状结肠肠腔内。用碘附纱布消毒断端。经肛门置入卵圆钳伸至直肠断端，夹持肠系膜断端及肠壁，将直肠外翻拉出肛门外（图 3-1-7、图 3-1-8）。标本翻出体外后，肿瘤位置清晰可见。用碘附盐水冲洗，确认无误后用直线切割闭合器在肿瘤下缘 1~2cm 处切断直肠（图 3-1-9）。移除标本，直肠断端可自行还纳回腹腔。

2. 消化道重建　充分进行扩肛，经肛门注入碘附盐水，在腹腔镜下观察直肠断端有无渗漏；在乙状结肠断端将抵钉座连接杆取出（图 3-1-10）。经肛门置入环形吻合器，完成乙状结肠 - 直肠端端吻合（图 3-1-11、图 3-1-12）。

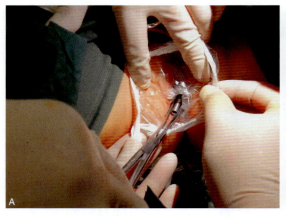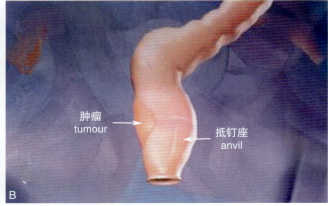

图 3-1-4　抵钉座通过直肠

A. 经肛门置入抵钉座；B. 将抵钉座从肿瘤的对侧置入肠腔

Figure 3-1-4　The anvil is delivered through the rectum

A. Inserting the anvil through the anus; B. Placing the anvil into the bowel lumen at the opposite side of the tumor

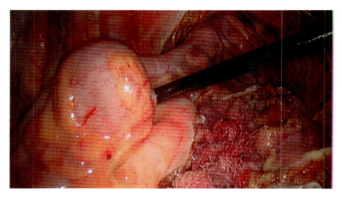

图 3-1-5　将抵钉座送入乙状结肠

Figure 3-1-5　Placing the anvil into the sigmoid colcn

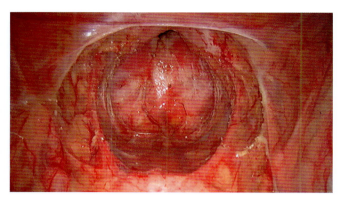

图 3-1-8　标本翻出后盆腔展示

Figure 3-1-8　Pelvic display after specimen eversion

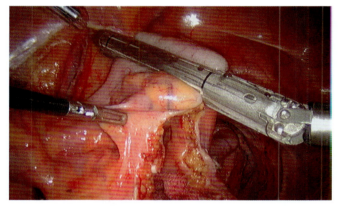

图 3-1-6　切割闭合乙状结肠

Figure 3-1-6　Resecting and closing the sigmoid colon

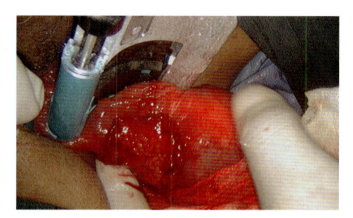

图 3-1-9　体外切除标本

Figure 3-1-9　Extracorporeal removal of the specimen

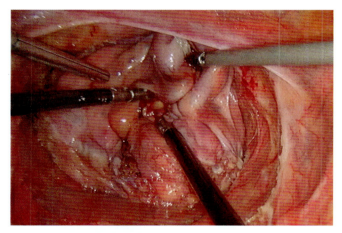

图 3-1-7　经肛门将直肠外翻拉出体外

Figure 3-1-7　Everting the specimen through the anus outside of the body

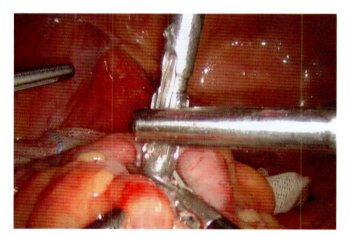

图 3-1-10　取出抵钉座连接杆

Figure 3-1-10　Removal of the anvil shaft

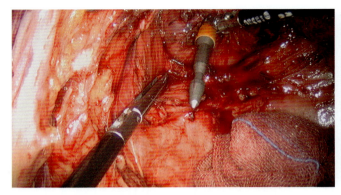

图 3-1-11　经肛门置入环形吻合器并旋出吻合器穿刺针

Figure 3-1-11　Transanal insertion of the circular stapler and removal of   the puncture needle from the stapler

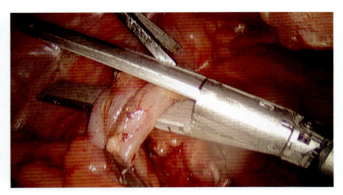

图 3-1-13　切割闭合乙状结肠

Figure 3-1-13　Transecting and closing the sigmoid colon

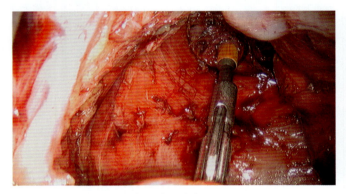

图 3-1-12　乙状结肠 - 直肠端端吻合

Figure 3-1-12　End-to-end anastomosis of the sigmoid colon and rectum

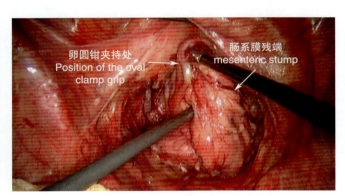

卵圆钳夹持处
Position of the oval clamp grip

肠系膜残端
mesenteric stump

图 3-1-14　经肛门将标本翻出体外

Figure 3-1-14　Everting the specimen through the anus

## CRC-NOSES　Ⅰ式 B 法（视频 3-2）

视频 3-2　CRC-NOSES Ⅰ式 B 法
Video 3-2　CRC-NOSES Ⅰ B

1. 标本切除　用直线切割闭合器在裸化的肠管预切除线切割闭合乙状结肠（图 3-1-13），用碘附纱布消毒断端。助手将卵圆钳经肛门伸至直肠断端，夹持肠系膜断端及肠壁。将直肠匀速外翻拉出肛门外（图 3-1-14）。外翻后切开肠壁（图 3-1-15），经外翻后的肠壁通道将抵钉座送入盆腔（图 3-1-16）。用碘附盐水冲洗标本，无误后在肿瘤下缘 1~2cm 处切断直肠（图 3-1-17、图 3-1-18）。移除标本。

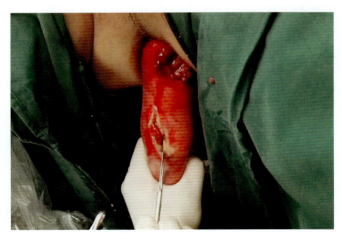

图 3-1-15　切开直肠壁

Figure 3-1-15　Incising the rectal bowel wall

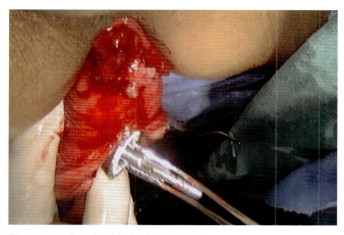

图 3-1-16　经肛门将抵钉座送入盆腔

Figure 3-1-16　Introducing the anvil into the pelvic cavity through the anus

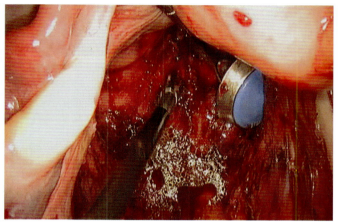

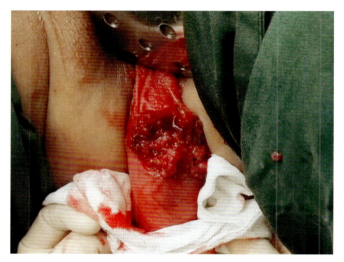

图 3-1-17　充分显露肿瘤下缘

Figure 3-1-17　Fully exposing the inferior margin of the tumor

2. 消化道重建　在乙状结肠断端处肠壁切开一小口，并用碘附纱布进行消毒（图 3-1-19），将抵钉座置入乙状结肠肠腔内（图 3-1-20），用直线切割闭合器关闭乙状结肠切口（图 3-1-21）。在乙状结肠断端将抵钉座连接杆取出（图 3-1-22）。经肛门置入环形吻合器，旋出吻合器穿刺针，行乙状结肠 - 直肠端端吻合（图 3-1-23）。并通过注水注气试验检查吻合口通畅确切，生理盐水冲洗，确切止血，分别经左、右下腹戳卡孔放置引流管（图 3-1-24、图 3-1-25）。对于超低位保肛患者，也可经肛门对吻合口进行加固缝合（图 3-1-26）。

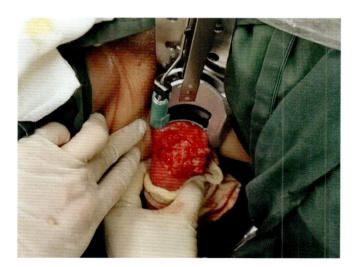

图 3-1-18　体外切除标本

Figure 3-1-18　Extracorporeal removal of the specimen

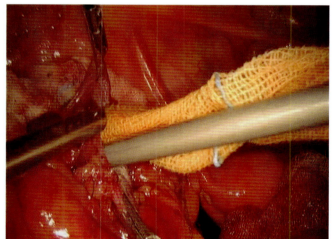

图 3-1-19　切开乙状结肠肠壁并进行消毒

Figure 3-1-19　Incising and disinfecting the sigmoid colon wall

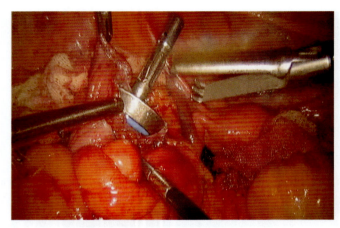

图 3-1-20　将抵钉座置入乙状结肠肠腔内

Figure 3-1-20　Placement of the anvil into the lumen of the sigmoid colon

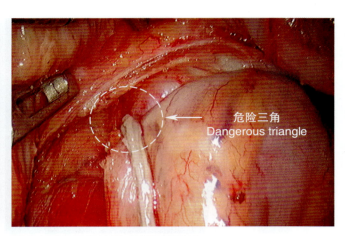

危险三角
Dangerous triangle

图 3-1-23　乙状结肠 - 直肠端端吻合

Figure 3-1-23　End-to-end anastomosis of the sigmoid colon and rectum

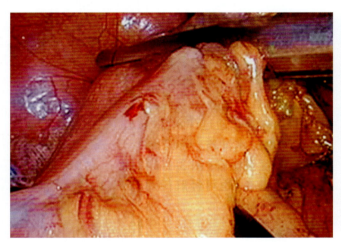

图 3-1-21　闭合乙状结肠肠壁

Figure 3-1-21　Closure of the sigmoid colon wall

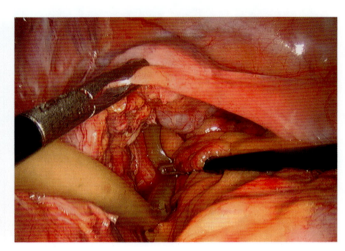

图 3-1-24　置入左侧引流管

Figure 3-1-24　Placement of a drainage tube on the left side

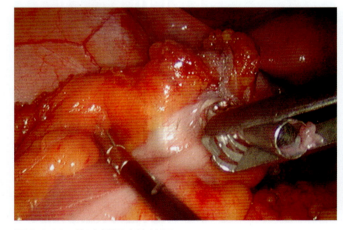

图 3-1-22　取出抵钉座连接杆

Figure 3-1-22　Removal of the anvil shaft

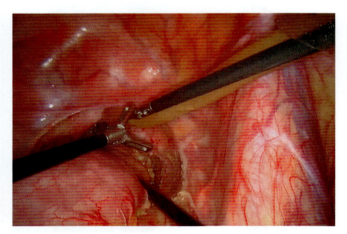

图 3-1-25　置入右侧引流管

Figure 3-1-25　Placement of a drainage tube on the right side

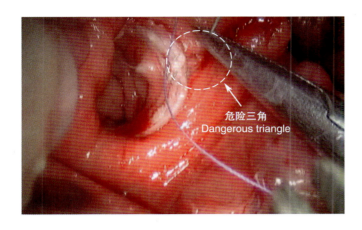

图 3-1-26　经肛门对吻合口进行加固缝合

Figure 3-1-26　Reinforcing and suturing the anastomosis through the anus

# 第二节　腹部无辅助切口经肛门取标本的腹腔镜下低位直肠癌根治术

## （CRC-NOSES Ⅰ式 C 法，Parks 法）

### 【简介】

低位直肠癌的特殊解剖位置增加了保肛手术的难度。虽然双吻合器吻合技术增加了保肛的机会，但由于吻合器尺寸的限制，对骨盆狭窄及肥胖患者，很难实现盆底肌平面切断闭合直肠。Parks 于 1982 年提出了经腹直肠癌切除术，经肛门结肠 - 肛管吻合的术式，后经许多学者应用证实了该术式在不影响长期疗效的前提下，不仅为更多直肠癌患者提供保肛机会，还可弥补双吻合器在低位直肠癌保肛手术中的不足。CRC-NOSES Ⅰ式 C 法，即腹部无辅助切口经肛门切断拉出标本、乙状结肠 - 肛管单层吻合的腹腔镜下低位直肠癌根治术（图 3-2-1，视频 3-3），既是对传统 Parks 法的升华，也是对低位直肠 NOSES 理论体系的完善。该术式特点鲜明：①在保证直肠癌根治的前提下，充分发挥了 NOSES 微创的优势，术后损伤小、疼痛轻、

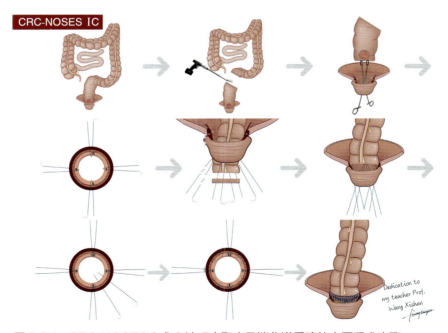

图 3-2-1　CRC-NOSES Ⅰ式 C 法标本取出及消化道重建的主要手术步骤

Figure 3-2-1　The main surgical steps of specimen extraction and digestive tract reconstruction in CRC-NOSES ⅠC

视频 3-3　CRC-NOSES I 式 C 法

Video 3-3　CRC-NOSES I C

恢复快；②经肛门切断取出标本、乙状结肠 - 肛管单层吻合，使用可吸收线缝合两端，因可吸收线组织相容性好，可减少吻合钉与组织相容性不良的弊端，进而降低吻合口炎症反应，减少吻合口狭窄的可能；③该术式最大限度保护肛门内外括约肌，保留肛门功能，充分保证了术后控便功能。

## 一、适应证与禁忌证

### 【适应证】

1. 低位直肠癌或良性肿瘤。
2. 肿瘤侵犯肠管 >1/2 周，标本无法经肛门外翻取出者。
3. 隆起型肿瘤，肿瘤环周径 <3cm。

4. 肿瘤下缘距齿状线 2~3cm 为宜。

### 【禁忌证】

1. 肿瘤局部浸润较重者。
2. 肿瘤环周径 >3cm，经肛门拖出困难者。
3. 黏液腺癌或印戒细胞癌，且术中无法明确下切缘状况。
4. 过于肥胖者（BMI>35kg/m²）。

## 二、手术操作步骤、技巧与要点

### 【戳卡位置】

1. 腹腔镜镜头戳卡孔（10mm 戳卡）　脐上 1~2cm。
2. 术者主戳卡孔（12mm 戳卡）　麦氏点偏下。
3. 术者辅助戳卡孔（5mm 戳卡）　脐右侧 10cm 左右。
4. 助手辅助戳卡孔（5mm 戳卡）　反麦氏点。
5. 助手主戳卡孔（5mm 戳卡）　脐水平左上方，靠内侧腹直肌外缘为宜（图 3-2-2）。

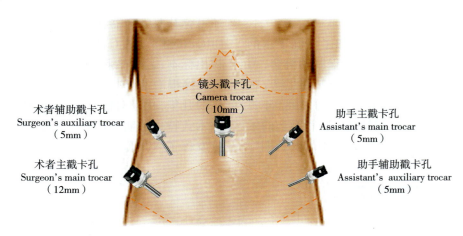

图 3-2-2　戳卡位置（五孔法）

Figure 3-2-2　Trocar placement（five-port method）

### 【探查】

1. 常规探查　探查肝脏、胆囊、胃、脾脏、大网膜、结肠、小肠、直肠和盆腔。
2. 肿瘤探查　术者可通过直肠指检判断肿瘤的位置、大小，并判断进行该手术的可能性。
3. 解剖结构的判定　乙状结肠及其系膜长度和肥厚程度，是否适合经肛门拉出体外。

### 【解剖与分离】

1. 第一刀切入点　在骶骨岬下方 3~5cm 通常有一菲薄处，用超声刀从此处切开系膜，进入 Toldt's 间隙。
2. 肠系膜下血管游离与离断　拓展 Toldt's 间隙，

向头侧至肠系膜下动脉根部，向外侧至左侧生殖血管，清扫肠系膜下动脉根部淋巴结，结扎并离断血管。

3. 直肠后方的游离　沿 Toldt's 间隙向尾侧游离，进入直肠后间隙，切开直肠骶骨筋膜后进入肛提肌上间隙，继续向尾侧游离，直至肛提肌裂孔。

4. 直肠右侧的游离　沿直肠系膜与右侧盆壁的解剖界限分离至腹膜反折，并横行切开腹膜反折右侧。

5. 乙状结肠及直肠左侧的游离　打开乙状结肠与左侧腹壁的粘连，与内侧 Toldt's 间隙贯通，并向头侧游离，必要时游离结肠脾曲。向尾侧沿解剖边界游离至腹膜反折处与右侧会合。

6. 直肠前壁的游离　切开腹膜反折线向尾侧游

离，进入直肠前间隙，尽量保证邓氏筋膜完整性，向尾侧游离直至肛提肌水平。游离至该位置已到达 TME 终点，此水平的直肠通常无系膜，无须裸化。

7. 乙状结肠系膜裁剪　可采取反向裁剪法，于系膜水平预切除线，由远端逆行向近端裁剪乙状结肠系膜。

**【标本切除与消化道重建】**

1. 标本切除　腹腔镜下将直肠充分游离后，于肿瘤上方预切除线处用直线切割闭合器将乙状结肠切断（图 3-2-3）。腹部操作结束后开始进行会阴部操作。应用肛门牵开器或膀胱拉钩完全展开肛门显露直肠，用碘附纱布对直肠肠腔进行充分消毒（图 3-2-4）。在齿状线上 0.5cm 切开直肠，电刀离断直肠全层（避免损伤肛门内括约肌）（图 3-2-5）。在切断直肠壁过程中，可以直视下判断下切缘位置，并保证下切缘的安全性（图 3-2-6）。经肛门拉出近端肠管及肠系膜（图 3-2-7），切除标本送检术后病理。

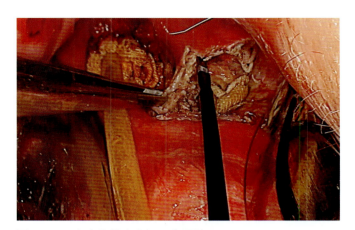

图 3-2-5　在齿状线上方切开直肠壁

Figure 3-2-5　Incising the rectal wall above the dentate line

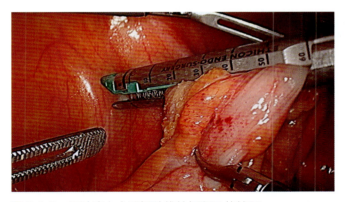

图 3-2-3　于肿瘤上方预切除线处切断乙状结肠

Figure 3-2-3　Transection of the sigmoid colon at the pre-cut line above the tumor

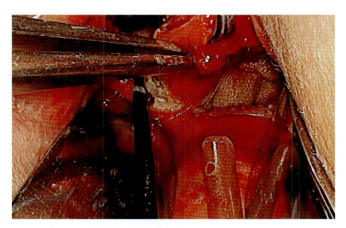

图 3-2-6　直视下判断下切缘位置

Figure 3-2-6　Direct visualization to determine the location of the lower resection margin

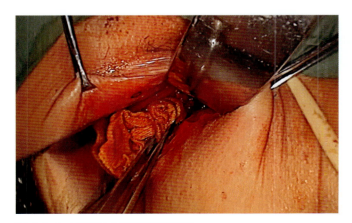

图 3-2-4　碘附纱布消毒直肠肠腔

Figure 3-2-4　Disinfecting the rectal lumen with the iodoform gauze

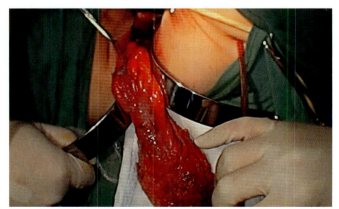

图 3-2-7　经肛门将近端肠管及肠系膜拉出体外

Figure 3-2-7　Pulling the proximal bowel and mesentery out through the anus

2. 消化道重建　以碘附盐水冲洗盆腔，探查无出血后开始进行消化道重建，行乙状结肠 - 肛管手工单层吻合。分别于肛管的 3 点、6 点、9 点、12 点方向全层缝入预留线（图 3-2-8），将预留线向四个方向展开备用（图 3-2-9）。经肛门置入卵圆钳，在腹腔镜下将乙状结肠拉出肛门外，仔细检查系膜方向无扭转后，在肛门外将乙状结肠断端打开，吻合备用。通过肛管处 4 根预留线分别将乙状结肠全层缝合，将乙状结肠缓慢退回肛管后，将预留线打结固定。于两针之间再全层缝合 2~3 针进行加固（图 3-2-10）。4 个象限全部缝合结束后，检查吻合缝线疏密程度、吻合口是否通畅、有无出血，完成乙状结肠 - 肛管端端吻合（图 3-2-11）。

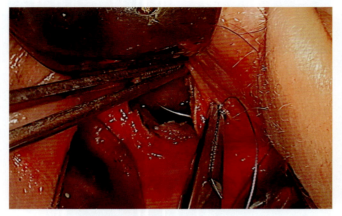

图 3-2-8　将预留线全层缝合至肛管断端
Figure 3-2-8　Full-thickness suturing of reserved sutures to the remnant of the anal canal

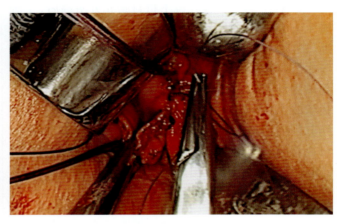

图 3-2-10　逐针加固缝合吻合口
Figure 3-2-10　Reinforcing the anastomosis stitch by stitch

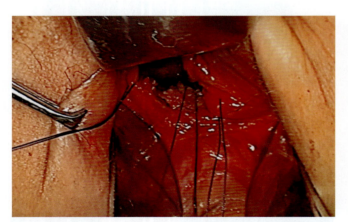

图 3-2-9　于 3 点、6 点、9 点、12 点方向在肛管缝合四针
Figure 3-2-9　Placement of four sutures at the 3, 6, 9, and 12 o'clock positions on the anal canal

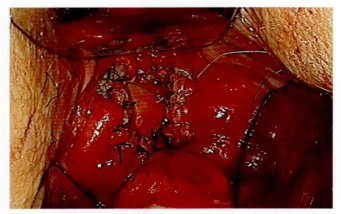

图 3-2-11　检查吻合口完整性
Figure 3-2-11　Checking the integrity of the anastomosis

## 第三节 腹部无辅助切口经肛门括约肌间切除标本的腹腔镜下超低位直肠癌根治术

### （CRC-NOSES I 式 D 法）

### 【简介】

CRC-NOSES I 式 D 法主要适用于下段和超低位直肠小肿瘤患者，其与常规的腹腔镜直肠癌根治术一样，应严格遵循 TME 原则。应在正确的平面进行解剖和切割，对盆腔底部的切割应更为充分，以便在括约肌间隙进行经会阴手术，这是准确完成该程序的关键。CRC-NOSES I 式 D 法的操作要点：腹腔镜下充分解剖后，于肛管内进行乙状结肠括约肌间切除，通过自然腔道提取标本，并将乙状结肠近端吻合至肛管。CRC-NOSES I 式 D 法不仅能确保彻底切除位于下段和超低位直肠的小肿瘤，还能最大限度地保护肛门功能，并避免在腹壁进行辅助切口。因此，该术式完全满足功能性手术和微创手术的要求（图 3-3-1，视频 3-4）。

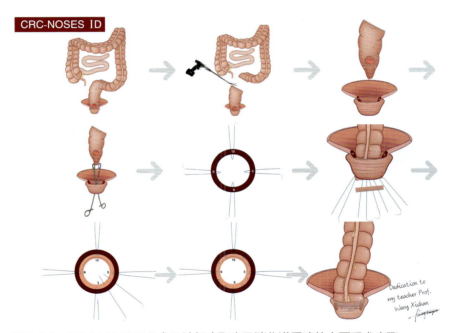

图 3-3-1 CRC-NOSES I 式 D 法标本取出及消化道重建的主要手术步骤
Figure 3-3-1 The main surgical procedures of specimen extraction and digestive tract reconstruction in CRC-NOSES I D

视频 3-4 CRC-NOSES I 式 D 法
Video 3-4 CRC-NOSES I D

## 一、适应证与禁忌证

### 【适应证】（图 3-3-2 ~ 图 3-3-4）

1. 超低位直肠癌。

2. 浸润型或溃疡型肿瘤，活动性良好。

3. 隆起型肿瘤，肿瘤厚度 <2cm。

4. 局部侵犯深度为 $T_1$ 或 $T_2$。

5. 病理类型为高中分化腺癌。

### 【禁忌证】

1. 肿瘤下缘位于齿状线至齿状线上 3cm 以内。

2. 肿瘤厚度 >3cm。

3. 直肠癌侵犯深度达 $T_3$。

4. 低分化或黏液腺癌，术中无法行快速冷冻病理确定下切缘状况者。

5. 过于肥胖者。

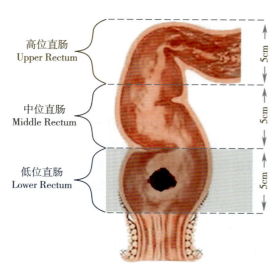

图 3-3-2　适用 I 式的肿瘤位置示意图

Figure 3-3-2　Illustrating the tumor location applicable to Type I

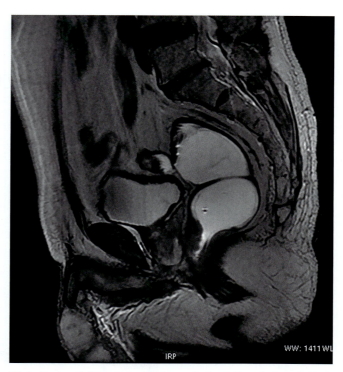

图 3-3-4　直肠 MRI：男性，$T_2$ 加权成像，肿瘤距齿状线 1.5cm，最大径 2.5cm

Figure 3-3-4　Rectal MRI：Male，$T_2$WI，located 1.5cm from the dentate line，with a maximum diameter of 2.5cm

## 二、手术操作步骤、技巧与要点

### 【戳卡位置】

1. 腹腔镜镜头戳卡孔（10mm 戳卡）　脐部正上方。

2. 术者主戳卡孔（12mm 戳卡）　麦氏点以下，使得超低位直肠操作更容易一些，尤其裸化超低位直肠壁时，可通过垂直角度切断肠系膜。

3. 术者辅助戳卡孔（5mm 戳卡）　脐右侧 10cm 左右，在直肠深部操作时，可减少与腹腔镜镜头的干扰。

4. 助手辅助戳卡孔（5mm 戳卡）　反麦氏点，主要通过此戳卡孔进行提拉，同时便于放置引流管。

5. 助手主戳卡孔（5mm 戳卡）　脐水平左上方，靠内侧腹直肌外缘为宜（图 3-3-5）。

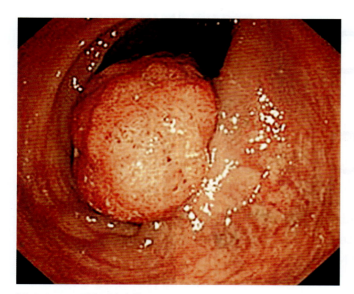

图 3-3-3　肠镜：肿瘤位于距肛门 2~4cm，隆起型，最大径为 2cm

Figure 3-3-3　Colonoscopy：The tumor is located 2-4cm from the anal verge，presenting as protuberant-type tumor，with a maximum diameter of 2cm

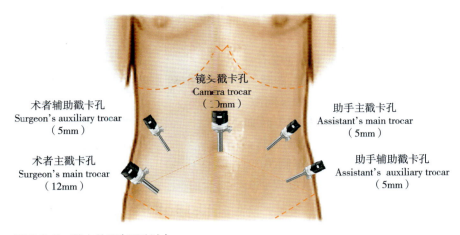

镜头戳卡孔
Camera trocar
（10mm）

术者辅助戳卡孔
Surgeon's auxiliary trocar
（5mm）

助手主戳卡孔
Assistant's main trocar
（5mm）

术者主戳卡孔
Surgeon's main trocar
（12mm）

助手辅助戳卡孔
Assistant's auxiliary trocar
（5mm）

图 3-3-5 戳卡位置（五孔法）

Figure 3-3-5 Trocar placement（five-port method）

## 【手术团队站位】

腹部操作：术者站位于患者右侧，助手站位于患者左侧，扶镜手站位于术者同侧；会阴部操作：术者站位于患者两腿之间，助手分别站位于患者左侧和右侧（图 3-3-6）。

## 【特殊手术器械】

超声刀、针式电刀、肛门牵开器。

## 【探查】

1. 常规探查 观察各脏器及腹膜表面有无种植转移等病变。

2. 肿瘤探查 根据肿瘤的位置、大小、侵犯深度，确定手术的可行性。

3. 解剖结构的判定 根据肿瘤位置决定是否保留肠系膜下血管及直肠上动脉。根据乙状结肠长度、系膜血管弓的长度、系膜肥厚程度，评估标本能否经肛门取出。

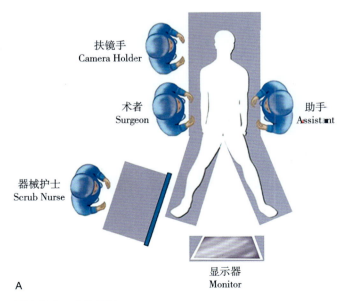

A

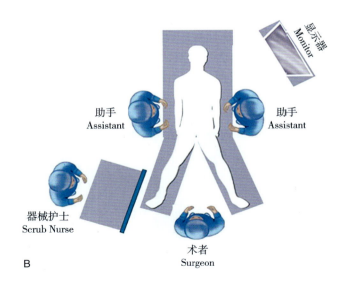

B

图 3-3-6 术者站位

A. 腹部操作；B. 会阴部操作。

Figure 3-3-6 Surgical team position

A. Abdominal operation B. Perineal procedure.

## 【解剖与分离】

1. 第一刀切入点　在骶骨岬下方 3~5cm 通常有一菲薄处,用超声刀从此处切开系膜,进入 Toldt's 间隙。

2. 肠系膜下血管游离与离断　拓展 Toldt's 间隙,向头侧至肠系膜下动脉根部,向外侧至左侧生殖血管,清扫肠系膜下动脉根部淋巴结,结扎并离断血管。

3. 直肠后方的游离　沿 Toldt's 间隙向尾侧游离,进入直肠后间隙,切开直肠骶骨筋膜后进入肛提肌上间隙,继续向尾侧游离,直至肛提肌裂孔。

4. 直肠右侧的游离　沿直肠系膜与右侧盆壁的解剖界限分离至腹膜反折,并横行切开腹膜反折右侧。

5. 乙状结肠及直肠左侧的游离　打开乙状结肠与左侧腹壁的粘连,与内侧 Toldt's 间隙贯通,并向头侧游离,必要时游离结肠脾曲。向尾侧沿解剖边界游离至腹膜反折处与右侧汇合。

6. 直肠前壁的游离　切开腹膜反折线向尾侧游离,进入直肠前间隙,尽量保证邓氏筋膜完整性,向尾侧游离直至肛提肌水平。游离至该位置已到达 TME 终点,此水平的直肠通常无系膜,无须裸化。

7. 乙状结肠系膜裁剪　可采取反向裁剪法,于水平系膜预切除线,由远端逆行向近端裁剪乙状结肠系膜。

## 【标本切除与消化道重建】

1. 标本切除　将肛门充分展开,在肿瘤远端 1~2cm 处确定下切缘,环形切开直肠壁(图 3-3-7)。沿骶后间隙从后壁到侧壁,最终到前壁向上进行解剖至盆腔(图 3-3-8、图 3-3-9)。然后将直肠和系膜经肛门提取出来,以确认切缘的完整性(图 3-3-10)。将卵圆钳插入肛门,拉动近端乙状结肠使其脱离体外,注意避免系膜扭转。操作应轻柔,以避免过度牵拉损伤括约肌。

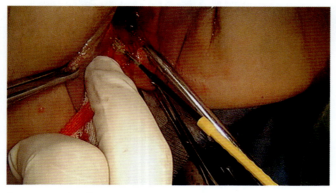

图 3-3-7　逐层切开肠壁

Figure 3-3-7　Sequentially incise the intestinal wall

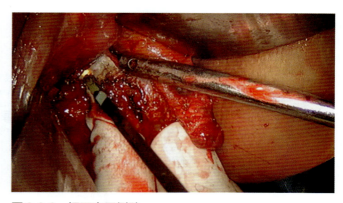

图 3-3-8　切开直肠侧壁

Figure 3-3-8　Incise the lateral wall of the rectum

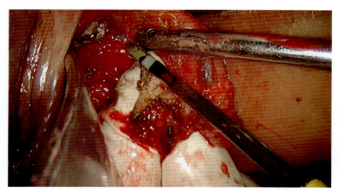

图 3-3-9　切开直肠前壁

Figure 3-3-9　Incise the anterior wall of the rectum

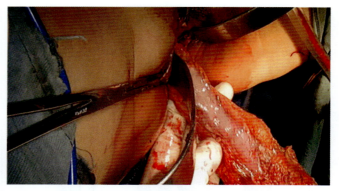

图 3-3-10　经肛门将标本拉出体外

Figure 3-3-10　Extract the specimen out through the anus

2. 消化道重建　打开拉出体外的近端乙状结肠断端(图 3-3-11),将乙状结肠断端与肛管间断缝合,完成吻合(图 3-3-12)。检查吻合确切无出血,局部消毒(图 3-3-13)。在盆腔内留置两根引流管,关闭戳卡孔。

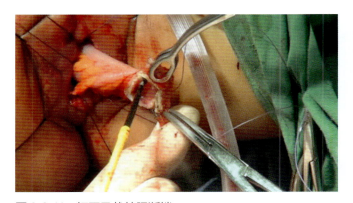

图 3-3-11　打开乙状结肠断端

Figure 3-3-11　Open the sigmoid colon stump

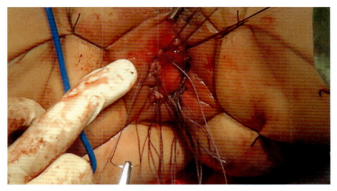

图 3-3-12　缝合乙状结肠断端与肛管

Figure 3-3-12　Suture the sigmoid colon stump to the anal canal

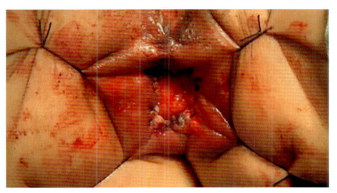

图 3-3-13　检查吻合口

Figure 3-3-13　Inspect the anastomosis site

## 第四节　腹壁无辅助切口经肛门取标本的腹腔镜下低位直肠癌根治术

### （CRC-NOSES I 式 E 法，Bacon 法）

【简介】

CRC-NOSES I 式 E 法是腹腔镜手术与改良的 Bacon 法的结合，主要适用于有大范围浸润的低位直肠癌患者。常规腹腔镜手术和 CRC-NOSES I 式 E 法之间的主要区别在于消化道重建和标本取出（图 3-4-1，视频 3-5）。CRC-NOSES I 式 E 法的手术特点如下：①根据 TME 原则，将直肠切割成括约肌的内外空间；②从肿瘤下方 1~2cm 和括约肌间沟上方开始环形缝合肛门；③环形切开直肠壁，然后向上解剖至腹腔层面；④从肛门取出直肠，保留正常直肠在 3~5cm 处，然后在肿瘤上缘 5~7cm 处切断直肠；⑤术后 2~3 周进行肛门成形术。这项技术要求术者和助手具备精湛的操作技巧，彼此之间配合默契。此外，必须严格遵守无菌原则和无瘤原则。CRC-NOSES I 式 E 法不仅能确保 R0 切除，还能在低位直肠癌中实现肛门功能保留，是符合功能外科要求的理想术式。

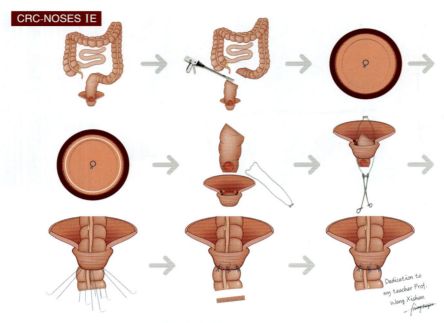

图3-4-1　CRC-NOSES I式 E 法标本取出及消化道重建的主要手术步骤

Figure 3-4-1　The main surgical procedures of specimen extraction and digestive tract reconstruction in CRC-NOSES I E

视频 3-5　CRC-NOSES I 式 E 法

Video 3-5　CRC-NOSES I E

## 一、适应证与禁忌证

### 【适应证】（图3-4-2~图3-4-4）

1. 低位直肠癌或内镜下不能切除的良性肿瘤。
2. 半周至环周生长的肿瘤,扁平型肿瘤最合适。
3. 肿瘤未侵及肛门括约肌。

4. 经肛门局部切除后需要补充根治切除,但常规腹腔镜器械无法吻合的低位直肠癌患者。

### 【禁忌证】

1. 肿瘤体积过大,无法经肛门取出。
2. 乙状结肠及系膜长度太短无法经肛门取出者。
3. 直肠系膜过于肥厚无法经肛门取出者。
4. 过于肥胖者（BMI>30kg/m$^2$）。
5. 直肠阴道瘘局部炎症较重者。

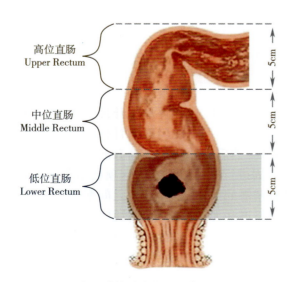

图3-4-2　适用I式 E 法的肿瘤位置示意图

Figure 3-4-2　Tumor location diagram for type I E

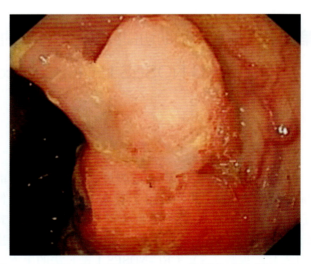

图3-4-3　肠镜:肿瘤距肛门2~4cm,隆起型,最大径为3.0cm

Figure 3-4-3　Colonoscopy: the tumor is located 2~4cm from the anal verge, protuberant-type tumor with a maximum diameter of 3cm

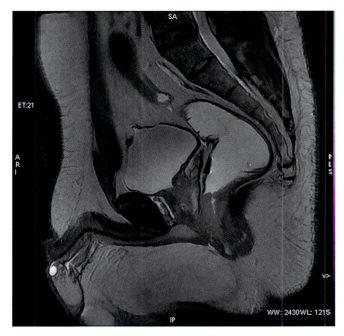

图 3-4-4　直肠 MRI：男性，$T_2$ 加权成像，距齿状线 0.5cm，最大径 3.0cm

Figure 3-4-4　Rectal MRI: Male, $T_2$WI, located 0.5cm from the dentate line, with a maximum diameter of 3cm

## 二、手术操作步骤、技巧与要点

### 【麻醉方式】

全身麻醉或全身麻醉联合硬膜外麻醉。

### 【患者体位】

患者取改良截石位，头低并向右侧倾斜，右侧大腿需稍平一些，有利于术者操作（图 3-4-5）。

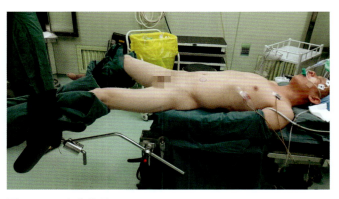

图 3-4-5　患者体位
Figure 3-4-5　Patient position

### 【戳卡位置】

1. 腹腔镜镜头戳卡孔（10mm 戳卡）　脐窗中或脐上 2cm 以内范围。
2. 术者主戳卡孔（12mm 戳卡）　麦氏点。
3. 术者辅助戳卡孔（5mm 戳卡）　右侧旁正中线脐上 5cm。
4. 助手辅助戳卡孔（5mm 戳卡）　反麦氏点。
5. 助手主戳卡孔（5mm 戳卡）　脐水平左腹直肌外缘（图 3-4-6）。

### 【手术团队站位】

腹部操作：术者站位于患者右侧，助手站位于患者左侧，扶镜手站位于术者同侧；会阴部操作：术者站位于患者两腿中间，助手分别站位于患者两侧（图 3-4-7）。

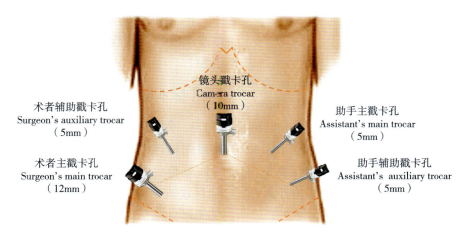

图 3-4-6　戳卡位置（五孔法）
Figure 3-4-6　Trocar site（five-port method）

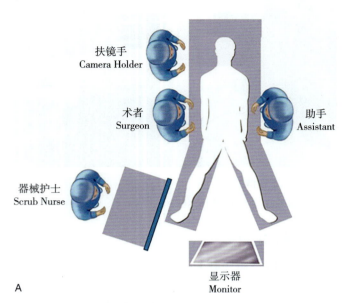

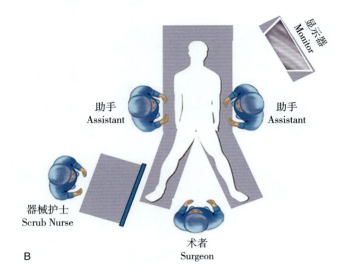

图 3-4-7　手术团队站位

A. 腹部操作；B. 会阴部操作。

Figure 3-4-7　Surgical team position

A. Abdominal procedure；B. Perineal procedure.

【探查】

1. 常规探查　观察各脏器及腹膜表面有无种植转移等病变。

2. 肿瘤探查　根据肿瘤的位置、大小、侵犯深度，确定手术的可行性。

3. 解剖结构的判定　根据肿瘤位置决定是否保留肠系膜下血管及直肠上动脉。根据乙状结肠长度、系膜血管弓的长度、系膜肥厚程度，评估标本能否经肛门取出。

【解剖与分离】

1. 第一刀切入点　在骶骨岬下方 3~5cm 通常有一菲薄处，用超声刀从此处切开系膜，进入 Toldt's 间隙。

2. 肠系膜下血管游离与离断　拓展 Toldt's 间隙，向头侧至肠系膜下动脉根部，向外侧至左侧生殖血管，清扫肠系膜下动脉根部淋巴结，结扎并离断血管。

3. 直肠后方的游离　沿 Toldt's 间隙向尾侧游离，进入直肠后间隙，切开直肠骶骨筋膜后进入肛提肌上间隙，继续向尾侧游离，直至肛提肌裂孔。

4. 直肠右侧的游离　沿直肠系膜与右侧盆壁的解剖界线分离至腹膜反折，并横行切开腹膜反折右侧。

5. 乙状结肠及直肠左侧的游离　切断乙状结肠与左侧腹壁的粘连，与内侧 Toldt's 间隙贯通，并向头侧游离，必要时游离结肠脾曲。向尾侧沿解剖边界游离至腹膜反折处与右侧会合。

6. 直肠前壁的游离　切开腹膜反折线向尾侧游离，进入直肠前间隙，尽量保证邓氏筋膜完整性，向尾侧游离直至肛提肌水平。游离至该位置已到达 TME 终点，此水平的直肠通常无系膜，无须裸化。

7. 乙状结肠系膜裁剪　可采取反向裁剪法，于水平系膜预切除线，由远端逆行向近端裁剪乙状结肠系膜。

【标本切除与消化道重建】

1. 会阴部操作　完全扩肛以显露齿状线（图 3-4-8）。用碘附棉球消毒肛管（图 3-4-9），并在距肿瘤下缘约 1cm 处荷包缝合肛门（图 3-4-10）。荷包缝合不仅可以有效减少肿瘤种植和肠内容物污染的风险，还可以确保远端切缘的安全距离。术者应在齿状线附近打开肠壁，保留肛门内括约肌，然后向上解剖以与腹腔中游离的结肠会合（图 3-4-11）。为了取出标本，将游离的结肠通过肛门提出体外，然后在距肿瘤上方 7~10cm 处切断肠管（图 3-4-12）。在此过程中，术者应遵循无菌和无瘤原则,轻柔操作,以避免对肠管和系膜的任何损伤。将多余的肠管固定到肛门需要缝合 5~8 针,注意避免缝合系膜血管,以免影响血供。最后,冲洗盆腔并在盆腔内放置引流管(图 3-4-13、图 3-4-14)。取出标本,用缝线将乙状结肠固定在肛门上(图 3-4-15)。

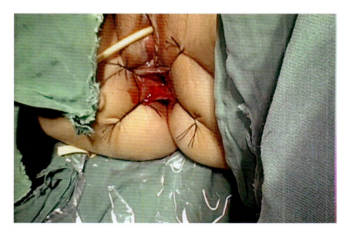

图 3-4-8　将肛门充分外展

Figure 3-4-8　Fully evert the anus

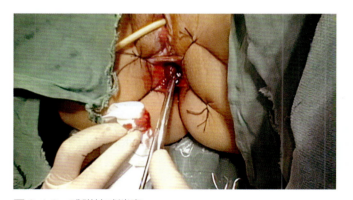

图 3-4-9　碘附棉球消毒

Figure 3-4-9　Disinfect with iodoform cotton ball

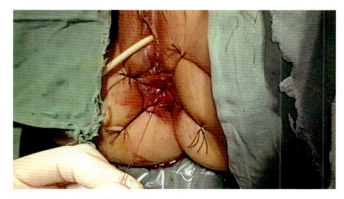

图 3-4-10　荷包缝合肛门

Figure 3-4-10　Suture by purse string

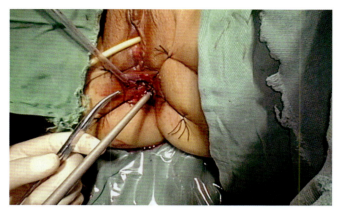

图 3-4-11　剥除白线上黏膜

Figure 3-4-11　Dissect the mucosa along the white line

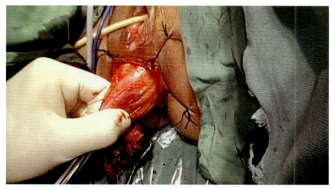

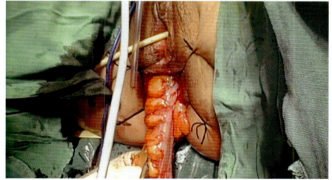

图 3-4-12　将结肠向肛门外拖出

Figure 3-4-12　Evert the colon outward toward the anus

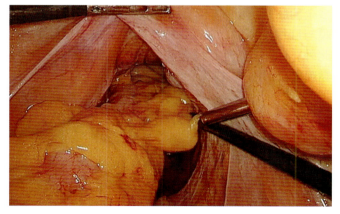

图 3-4-13　盆腔冲洗

Figure 3-4-13　Pelvic cavity irrigation

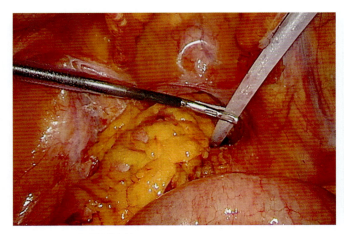

图 3-4-14　留置引流管

Figure 3-4-14　Placement of drainage tube

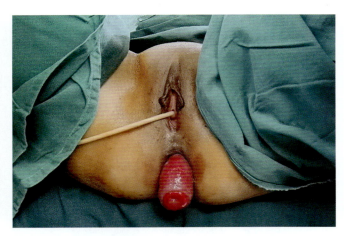

图 3-4-16　充分显露会阴部

Figure 3-4-16　Adequately expose the perineum

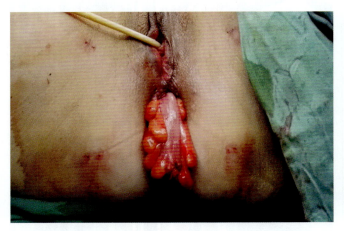

图 3-4-15　移除标本，缝线固定乙状结肠

Figure 3-4-15　Remove the specimen, secure the sigmoid colon with stitches

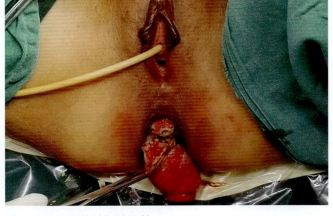

图 3-4-17　于体外切除肠管

Figure 3-4-17　Excise the bowel externally

　　2. 二期肛门成形术　术后 2~3 周可以进行二期肛门成形术。充分显露会阴部（图 3-4-16），并在肛缘处保留 0.5cm 的肠管，在保证良好血供的情况下切断多余的肠管（图 3-4-17）。需要注意的是，当缝合肠黏膜与肛缘皮肤时，应充分结扎和埋藏系膜侧的血管。此外，不应过度外翻肠黏膜，以避免发生黏膜坏死或黏膜脱垂（图 3-4-18）。

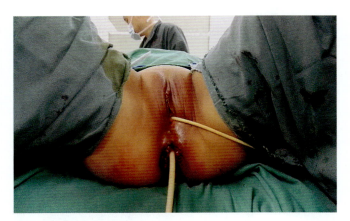

图 3-4-18　成形术后肛门

Figure 3-4-18　Post-anoplasty anus

## 第五节　腹部无辅助切口经肛门取标本的腹腔镜下低位直肠癌根治术

### （CRC-NOSES I 式 F 法,Petr 法）

### 【简介】

在低位直肠癌的外科治疗中,有几种通过肛门取出标本的方法,它们被统称为 CRC-NOSES I 式。在每种变体中,腹腔内切除近端结肠后,通过拉拽经肛门将直肠拉出或翻转以取出标本。切断肿瘤远端直肠;直肠残端用直线切割闭合器关闭,为吻合做好准备。CRC-NOSES I 式 F 法(图 3-5-1,视频 3-6)与上述技术有所不同,其特点是经腹外途径在肿瘤远近端离

断肠管。主要优势在于对远侧切缘的直视控制。由于没有腹腔内肠管切除,降低了腹腔污染的风险。CRC-NOSES I 式 F 法的主要步骤包括淋巴结清扫、血管切断、TME、乙状结肠游离,以及必要情况下结肠脾曲的游离。此外,它还包括经肛门翻转直肠、切断肿瘤近侧和远侧结肠,将环形闭合器的铁环安装在近侧结肠上,将其送回腹腔,关闭直肠断端并创建结直肠吻合口。CRC-NOSES I 式 F 法适用于中低位直肠的小肿瘤患者。

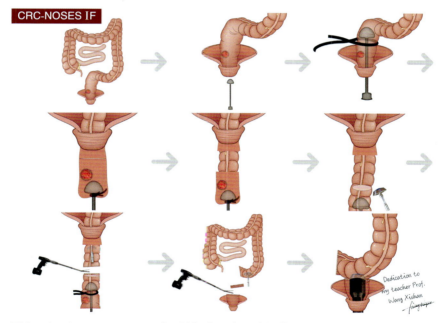

图 3-5-1　CRC-NOSES I 式 F 法标本取出及消化道重建的主要手术步骤
Figure 3-5-1　The main surgical procedures of specimen extraction and digestive tract reconstruction in CRC-NOSES I F

视频 3-6　CRC-NOSES I 式 F 法
Video 3-6　CRC-NOSES I F

## 一、适应证与禁忌证

### 【适应证】（图 3-5-2）

1. 肿瘤位于低位直肠。
2. 局限性肿瘤,肿瘤不侵出浆膜为宜。

3. 肿瘤环周直径 <3cm。
4. 肿瘤下缘距齿状线 3~5cm。

### 【禁忌证】

1. 局部晚期肿瘤。
2. 肿瘤直径 >3cm。
3. 黏液腺癌或印戒细胞癌。
4. 过于肥胖者（BMI>35kg/m$^2$）。

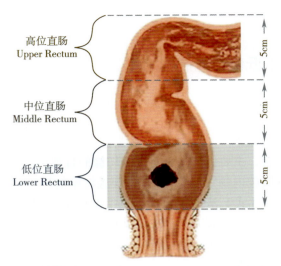

图 3-5-2　适用 CRC-NOSES I 式 F 法的肿瘤所在位置（示意图）

Figure 3-5-2　The location of tumors suitable for the CRC-NOSES IF（schematic diagram）

高位直肠 Upper Rectum

中位直肠 Middle Rectum

低位直肠 Lower Rectum

5cm

5cm

5cm

## 二、麻醉、体位、戳卡位置与手术团队站位

### 【麻醉方式】

全身麻醉或全身麻醉联合硬膜外麻醉。

### 【患者体位】

患者取功能截石位，右侧大腿需稍平一些（图 3-5-3）。

### 【戳卡位置】（图 3-5-4）

1. 腹腔镜镜头戳卡孔（10mm 戳卡）　脐窗中。

2. 术者主戳卡孔（12mm 戳卡）　脐与右髂前上棘连线中外 1/3 处，便于盆腔深部的手术及直线切割闭合器。

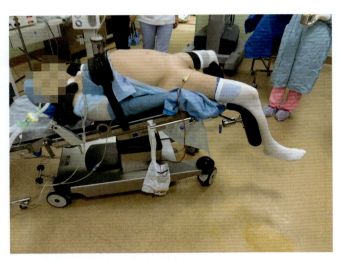

图 3-5-3　患者体位

Figure 3-5-3　Patient position

3. 术者辅助戳卡孔（5mm 戳卡）　脐下方 2cm、右侧 10cm 处，位置可根据患者情况进行调整，但两个相邻的戳卡间需保证足够的距离。

4. 助手主戳卡孔（5mm 戳卡）　脐水平左上方腹直肌外缘。

5. 助手辅助戳卡孔（5mm 戳卡）　脐与左髂前上棘连线中外 1/3 处。

### 【手术团队站位】

术者站位于患者右侧，助手站位于患者左侧，扶镜手站立于术者同侧（图 3-5-5）。

### 【特殊手术器械】

超声刀、外翻器械、29mm 环形吻合器、直线切割闭合器（可选）、腹腔镜抓钳。

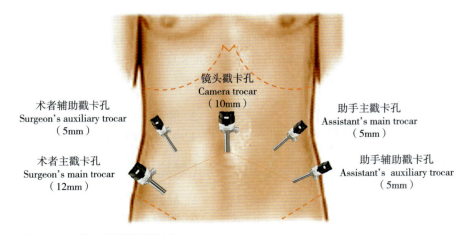

镜头戳卡孔
Camera trocar
（10mm）

术者辅助戳卡孔
Surgeon's auxiliary trocar
（5mm）

术者主戳卡孔
Surgeon's main trocar
（12mm）

助手主戳卡孔
Assistant's main trocar
（5mm）

助手辅助戳卡孔
Assistant's auxiliary trocar
（5mm）

图 3-5-4　戳卡位置（五孔法）

Figure 3-5-4　Trocar placement（five-port method）

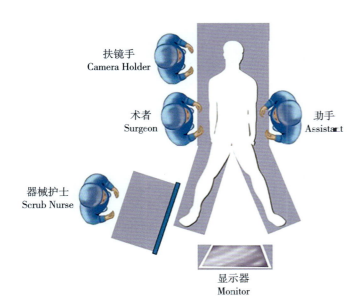

图 3-5-5　手术团队站位

Figure 3-5-5　Surgical team position

## 三、手术操作步骤、技巧与要点

### 【探查】

1. 常规探查　观察各脏器及腹膜表面有无种植转移等病变。

2. 肿瘤探查　根据肿瘤的位置、大小、侵犯深度，确定手术的可行性。

3. 解剖结构的判定　根据肿瘤位置决定是否保留肠系膜下血管及直肠上动脉。根据乙状结肠长度、系膜血管弓的长度、系膜肥厚程度，评估标本能否经肛门取出。

### 【解剖与分离】

1. 第一刀切入点　在骶骨岬下方 3~5cm 通常有一菲薄处，用超声刀从此处切开系膜，进入 Toldt's 间隙。

2. 肠系膜下血管游离与离断　拓展 Toldt's 间隙，向头侧至肠系膜下动脉根部，向外侧至左侧生殖血管，清扫肠系膜下动脉根部淋巴结，结扎并离断血管。

3. 直肠后方的游离　沿 Toldt's 间隙向尾侧游离，进入直肠后间隙，切开直肠骶骨筋膜后进入肛提肌上间隙，继续向尾侧游离，直至肛提肌裂孔。

4. 直肠右侧的游离　沿直肠系膜与右侧盆壁的解剖界限分离至腹膜反折，并横行切开腹膜反折右侧。

5. 乙状结肠及直肠左侧的游离　切断乙状结肠与左侧腹壁的粘连，与内侧 Toldt's 间隙贯通，并向头侧游离，必要时游离结肠脾曲。向尾侧沿解剖边界游离至腹膜反折处与右侧汇合。

6. 直肠前壁的游离　切开腹膜反折线向尾侧游离，进入直肠前间隙，尽量保证邓氏筋膜完整性，向尾侧游离直至肛提肌水平。游离至该位置已到达 TME 终点，此水平的直肠通常无系膜，无须裸化。

7. 乙状结肠系膜裁剪　可采取反向裁剪法，于水平预切除线，由远端逆行向近端裁剪乙状结肠系膜。

### 【标本切除与消化道重建】

1. 经肛门外翻直肠　在进行腹腔外切除标本的操作时，确保结肠长度足以进行经肛门取出标本非常重要。经肛门插入直肠外翻器直到其头部位于肿瘤的上方。使用一根线将直肠在其头部以下固定在棒周围（图 3-5-6）。

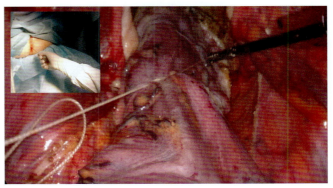

图 3-5-6　将直肠近端肠管结扎固定于直肠外翻器

Figure 3-5-6　Ligating and securing the proximal rectal stump with a rectal exteriorizer

小心地将金属棒拉出，将外翻的直肠拖到肛门外，形成一个双圆柱结构，其中直肠是外圆柱，乙状结肠是内圆柱。在这个外翻过程中，通过腹腔镜检查腹腔内结肠的长度，以防止其过度拉伸。外翻直肠直至肿瘤完全显露（图 3-5-7）。

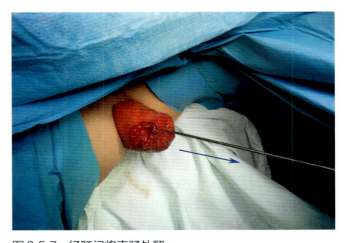

图 3-5-7　经肛门将直肠外翻

Figure 3-5-7　Evering the rectum through the anus

2. 标本切除　对直肠壁进行消毒。测量远端预切除线非常重要，它应该位于翻转的肿瘤向肛门的方向上方至少 2cm。在直视下，用电刀标记环形预切除线（图 3-5-8）。沿标记线小心离断直肠壁（图 3-5-9），注意不要损伤位于下方的乙状结肠肠壁。

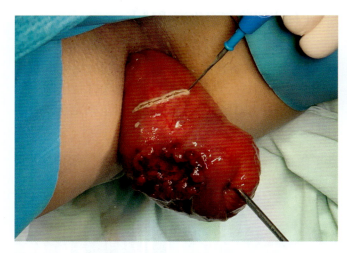

图 3-5-8　直视下标记环形预切除线
Figure 3-5-8　Marking the circular pre-cut line under direct vision

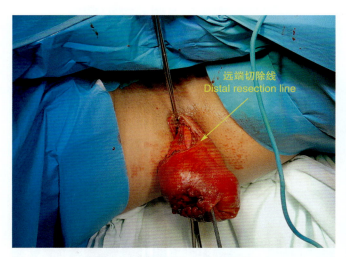

图 3-5-9　在肿瘤下方将外翻后的直肠壁离断
Figure 3-5-9　Transecting the everted rectal wall beneath the tumor

直视下切除外圆柱后，用 Alice 钳抓住残端远端边缘。另外，若行 TME，预切除线应尽可能靠近肠缘，以免残端残留直肠系膜细胞组织碎片。随后，规划肠管近端预切除线。将直肠展开使得标本恢复正常外观。用直线切割闭合器离断结肠。可采用端端吻合或侧端吻合来吻合肠管（图 3-5-10）。

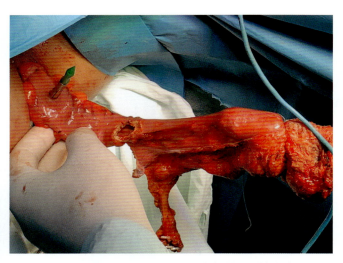

图 3-5-10　将抵钉座置入乙状结肠，准备进行侧端吻合
Figure 3-5-10　Placing the anvil into the sigmoid colon in preparation for end-to-side anastomosis

端端吻合时，在荷包线和直夹之间切断结肠，插入铁环，然后用荷包缝合将结肠环形缝合在抵钉座周围。侧端吻合时，通过小的远端切口将抵钉座轴插入肠腔，然后从侧面拉出抵钉座轴。

在先前所做的切口近端，用直线切割闭合器或连续缝合关闭肠腔（图 3-5-11）。消毒带有铁环的结肠残端并将其放回腹腔。对直肠残端进行荷包缝合并以环形直线切割闭合器固定。将一根细的聚合物管经肛门插入直肠，一端在肛门外，另一端伸出荷包线到腹腔外。在其周围荷包缝合关闭。

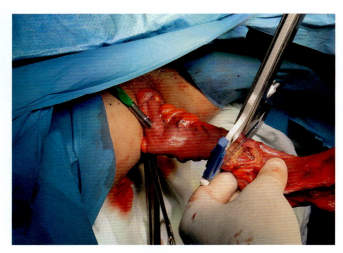

图 3-5-11　于预切线处切断闭合乙状结肠
Figure 3-5-11　Cutting and closing the sigmoid colon at the pre-cut line

3. 消化道重建　应用环形吻合器进行吻合。为确保环形吻合器穿刺针正确穿过直肠残端，可将其预先固定在先前插入的聚合物管上。以该管作为引导，

便于将环形吻合器穿刺针定位到荷包缝合的中心。通过其中一个吻合器穿刺针可将聚合物管拉出并取出（图 3-5-12、图 3-5-13）。

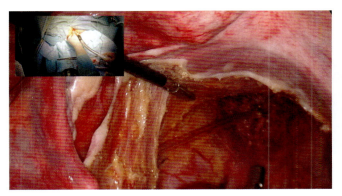

图 3-5-12　用聚合物管作为引导，将环形吻合器穿刺针插入腹部
Figure 3-5-12　Inserting the trocar of the circular stapler into the abdomen using a polymer tube

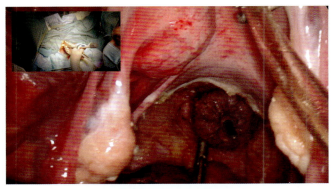

图 3-5-13　环形吻合器穿刺针与抵钉座连接
Figure 3-5-13　Connecting the trocar of the circular stapler to the anvil

在腹腔镜下完成结肠 - 直肠吻合（图 3-5-14），注意避免脂肪组织或其他结构被卷入吻合部位。

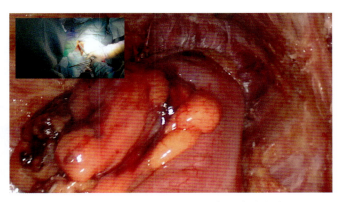

图 3-5-14　用环形吻合器行乙状结肠 - 直肠端端吻合
Figure 3-5-14　Performing end-to-end anastomosis of the sigmoid colon and rectum using a circular stapler

取出环形吻合器后，验证近端和远端切缘的完整性。通过注水注气试验检查吻合口的完整性（图 3-5-15）。通过右下腹戳卡将引流管置入盆腔内。

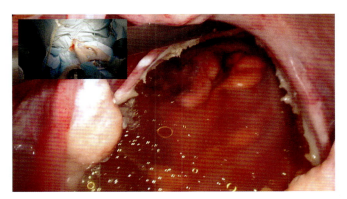

图 3-5-15　注水注气试验检查吻合口的完整性
Figure 3-5-15　Checking the integrity of the anastomosis by performing an air and water injection test

## 第六节　腹部无辅助切口经肛门取标本的腹腔镜下低位直肠癌适形根治术

### （CRC-NOSES I 式 G 法）

【简介】

腹腔镜下适形保肛手术联合经肛门取标本手术可以解决狭窄手术区域直肠切除的问题，并减少局部复发和并发症的发生率，以及显著改善肛门功能。内外括约肌间隙充满了神经纤维、弹性纤维和

Pacinian 小体，过度解剖可能损伤这些精细结构，进而影响术后肛门功能。有学者对接受适形保肛手术的 102 名患者的分析显示，肿瘤距肛缘距离的中位数为 3cm（3~4cm），距远端切缘距离的中位数为 0.5cm（0.3~0.8cm），局部复发率和远处转移率分别为 2% 和 10.8%，3 年生存率为 100%，无病生存率为 83.9%。回

肠造口还纳术后 12 个月 Wexner 评分和低位前切除综合征评分分别为 5.9 ± 4.3 和 29.2 ± 6.9。作为一种保肛手术，其优势在于能够在肿瘤学安全性和器官功能保留之间取得良好的平衡（图 3-6-1，视频 3-7）。

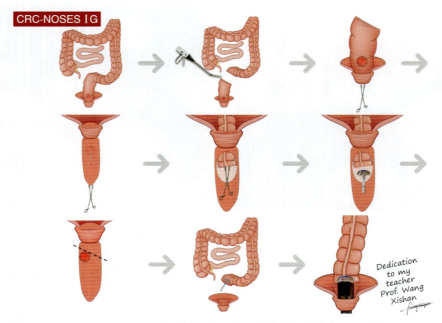

图 3-6-1　CRC-NOSES I 式 G 法标本取出及消化道重建的主要手术步骤

Figure 3-6-1　The main surgical procedures of specimen extraction and digestive tract reconstruction in CRC-NOSES IG

视频 3-7　CRC-NOSES I 式 G 法
Video 3-7　CRC-NOSES IG

## 一、适应证与禁忌证

### 【适应证】（图 3-6-2、图 3-6-3）

1. 术前电子结肠镜活检病理报告为高分化或中分化腺癌或间质瘤。
2. MRI 或 B 超检查提示，无外括约肌、耻骨直肠肌及肛提肌浸润，或者经新辅助放化疗后符合上述条件。
3. 直肠指检肿块可以推动，肿瘤直径 <3cm。
4. 肿瘤下缘距齿状线距离 ≤ 2cm。

### 【禁忌证】

1. 术前肛门失禁或肛门控便功能明显减退。
2. 腹腔严重粘连。
3. 心肺肝肾功能差，不能耐受腹腔镜手术。
4. 乙状结肠及系膜长度不足，无法经肛门取出标本。
5. 过于肥胖者（BMI>35kg/m²）。

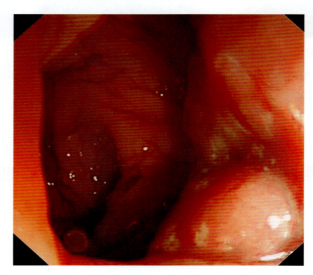

图 3-6-2　肠镜：距齿状线 1cm，溃疡型，最大径为 3cm

Figure 3-6-2　Colonoscopy: 1cm from the dentate line, ulcerative type, maximum diameter of 3cm

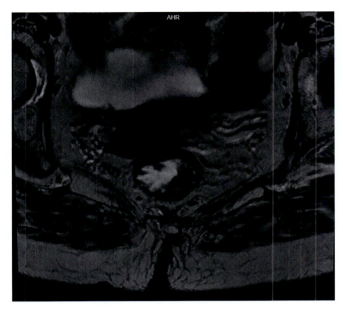

图 3-6-3　直肠 MRI: $T_2$, 距齿状线 1cm, 最大径 3cm

Figure 3-6-3　Rectal MRI: stage $T_2$, 1.0cm from the dentate line, maximum diameter of 3cm

## 二、手术操作步骤、技巧与要点

### 【麻醉方式】

全身麻醉或全身麻醉联合硬膜外麻醉。

### 【患者体位】

取膀胱截石位（图 3-6-4）。

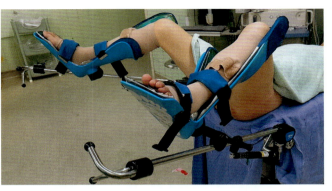

图 3-6-4　患者体位

Figure 3-6-4　Patient position

### 【戳卡位置】

1. 腹腔镜镜头戳卡孔（12mm 戳卡）　脐窗中。

2. 术者主戳卡孔（12mm 戳卡）　麦氏点。

3. 术者辅助戳卡孔（5mm 戳卡）　平脐右侧 10cm 处。

4. 助手主戳卡孔（5mm 戳卡）　脐水平左上方腹直肌外缘。

5. 助手辅助戳卡孔（5mm 戳卡）　反麦氏点，该操作较少，主要起提拉作用，靠外侧便于兼顾放置引流管（图 3-6-5）。

### 【手术团队站位】

术者站位于患者右侧，助手站位于患者左侧，扶镜手站立于术者同侧（图 3-6-6）。

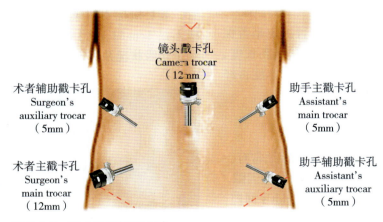

镜头戳卡孔
Camera trocar
（12mm）

术者辅助戳卡孔
Surgeon's
auxiliary trocar
（5mm）

助手主戳卡孔
Assistant's
main trocar
（5mm）

术者主戳卡孔
Surgeon's
main trocar
（12mm）

助手辅助戳卡孔
Assistant's
auxiliary trocar
（5mm）

图 3-6-5　戳卡位置（五孔法）

Figure 3-6-5　Trocar placement（five-port method）

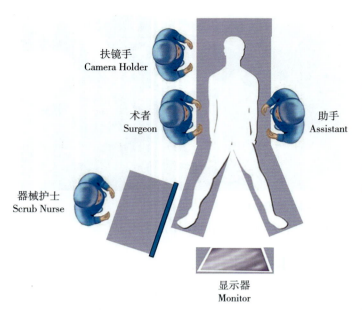

图 3-6-6　手术团队站位

Figure 3-6-6　Surgical team position

【特殊手术器械】

超声刀、60mm 直线切割闭合器、25mm 环形吻合器、直肠残端缝合线。

## 三、手术操作步骤、技巧与要点

【探查】

1. 常规探查　观察各脏器及腹膜表面有无种植转移等病变。

2. 肿瘤探查　根据肿瘤的位置、大小、侵犯深度，确定手术的可行性。

3. 解剖结构的判定　根据肿瘤位置决定是否保留肠系膜下血管及直肠上动脉。根据乙状结肠长度、系膜血管弓的长度、系膜肥厚程度，评估标本能否经肛门取出。

【解剖与分离】

1. 第一刀切入点　在骶骨岬下方 3~5cm 通常有一菲薄处，用超声刀从此处切开系膜，进入 Toldt's 间隙。

2. 肠系膜下血管游离与离断　拓展 Toldt's 间隙，向头侧至肠系膜下动脉根部，向外侧至左侧生殖血管，清扫肠系膜下动脉根部淋巴结，通常保留左结肠动脉后结扎、离断远端动脉及肠系膜下静脉。

3. 直肠后方的游离　沿 Toldt's 间隙向尾侧游离，进入直肠后间隙，切开直肠骶骨筋膜后进入肛提肌上间隙，继续向尾侧游离，直至肛提肌裂孔。

4. 直肠右侧的游离　沿直肠系膜与右侧盆壁的解

剖界线分离至腹膜反折，并横行切开腹膜反折右侧。

5. 乙状结肠及直肠左侧的游离　打开乙状结肠与左侧腹壁的粘连，与内侧 Toldt's 间隙贯通，并向头侧游离，必要时游离结肠脾曲。向尾侧沿解剖边界游离至腹膜反折处与右侧会合。

6. 直肠前壁的游离　切开腹膜反折线向尾侧游离，进入直肠前间隙，尽量保证邓氏筋膜完整性，向尾侧游离直至肛提肌水平。游离至该位置已到达 TME 终点，此水平的直肠通常无系膜，无须裸化。

7. 乙状结肠系膜裁剪　可采取反向裁剪法，于预切除线水平，由远端逆行向近端裁剪乙状结肠系膜。

【标本切除与消化道重建】

1. 标本切除　用直线切割闭合器在拟吻合处切断肠管。经肛门将远端直肠拖出：用碘附冲洗直肠肛管，扩肛至 3~4 指，使肛门括约肌充分松弛。用卵圆钳夹住直肠残端顶部，将肠管连同系膜一起插入直肠腔内，逐渐深入，并经肛门拖出。如果患者较肥胖或系膜肥厚，可先剔除多余的近端直肠系膜。经肛门钳夹经腹部推出的直肠，并向肛门外牵拉，将直肠完全翻转，拖出至肛门外，温水充分冲洗远端直肠，避免肿瘤与周围组织接触，操作时双手避免触摸肿瘤。

远端直肠适形切除吻合（图 3-6-7~ 图 3-6-9）：观察肿瘤后根据肿瘤位置设计预切除线，预切除线距肿瘤下缘及侧切缘至少 1cm，由肿瘤侧向对侧斜行向上，尽可能保留肿瘤对侧正常肠壁及齿状线。预切除线设计完毕后，在直视下从肿瘤侧沿预切除线环形切开直肠或肛管黏膜，逐层深入直至全层切开，直至离断肠管。如怀疑标本切缘安全性或因肿瘤位置低，远端切缘不足 1cm 时，应于吻合前行术中冷冻病理检查，以确定切缘状况并决定后续手术进程。

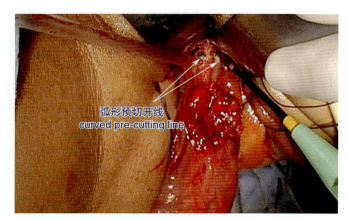

弧形预切开线
curved pre-cutting line

图 3-6-7　拖出后标记弧形预切除线

Figure 3-6-7　Marking the curved pre-cut line after pulling out

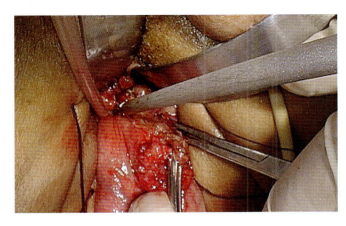

图 3-6-8　按预切除线切开肠管
Figure 3-6-8　Cutting the bowel along the pre-cut line

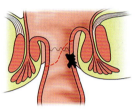
经肛拖出肿瘤
Tumor dragged out via the anus

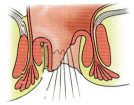
直视下斜行切除
Oblique resection under direct vision

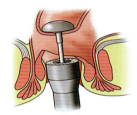
保留更多括约肌和齿状线
Preservation of more sphincter and dentate line

图 3-6-9　经肛门拖出式适形切除（示意图）
Figure 3-6-9　Rectal pull-through conformal resection through the anus（schematic）

2. 消化道重建　移出肿瘤后反复用温水冲洗封闭的直肠残端，再将乙状结肠残端拖出肛门外，放入吻合器抵钉座，冲洗消毒后，用卵圆钳将乙状结肠送回腹腔。然后用 3-0 可吸收线间断缝合直肠残端，肿瘤对侧可见多保留的肠管残端（图 3-6-10）。

重新建立气腹，经肛门置入吻合器器身，一般选用直径为 25mm 的环形吻合器，行直肠 - 乙状结肠端端吻合（图 3-6-11）。吻合时将肛门皮肤向外牵拉，并使吻合器尽量抵向盆腔，避免切除过多的肛门内括约肌、直肠、肛管皮肤。吻合结束后检查近、远端吻合口是否完整，并经肛门检查吻合口是否完整，对于吻合口不确切处，以 3-0 可吸收线间断缝合加固。

所有患者均行预防性末端回肠袢式造口术。

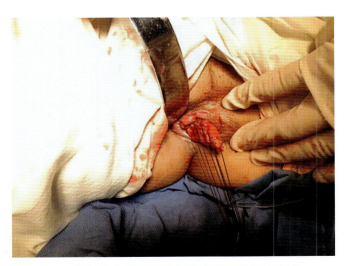

图 3-6-10　间断缝合直肠残端，可见多保留的肠管残端
Figure 3-6-10　Intermittent suturing of the rectal stump, showing the retained rectal stump

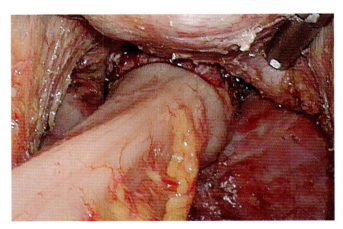

图 3-6-11　完成吻合
Figure 3-6-11　Completion of the anastomosis

## 第七节 腹部无辅助切口经直肠拉出标本的腹腔镜下中位直肠癌根治术

### （CRC-NOSES Ⅱ式 A 法）

【简介】

CRC-NOSES Ⅱ式 A 法主要适用于肿瘤较小的中位直肠癌患者。与常规腹腔镜直肠癌根治术一样，CRC-NOSES Ⅱ式 A 法需严格遵循 TME 原则，在正确的手术层面进行解剖和游离，这也是该手术能够快速安全进行的先决条件。CRC-NOSES Ⅱ式 A 法的操作特点：经肛门将直肠拉至体外，在体外切除直肠肿瘤标本后，再进行全腹腔镜下乙状结肠 - 直肠端端吻合（图 3-7-1，视频 3-8）。因此，对术者和助手二者之间配合默契程度提出很高要求。同时，应严格执行无菌操作和无瘤操作。CRC-NOSES Ⅱ式 A 法既能保证肿瘤根治效果，又能减少器官组织损伤，是符合功能外科要求的理想术式。

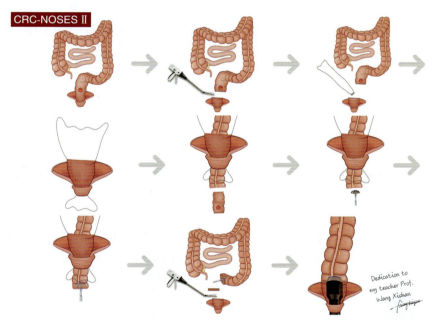

图 3-7-1　CRC-NOSES Ⅱ式 A 法标本取出及消化道重建的主要手术步骤
Figure 3-7-1　The main surgical procedures of specimen extraction and digestive tract reconstruction in CRC-NOSES ⅡA

视频 3-8　CRC-NOSES Ⅱ式 A 法
Video 3-8　CRC-NOSES ⅡA

## 一、适应证与禁忌证

【适应证】

1. 中位直肠癌或良性肿瘤。
2. 肿瘤环周直径 <3cm 为宜。

3. 肿瘤不侵出浆膜为宜。

【禁忌证】

1. 肿瘤体积过大，无法经肛门拉出。
2. 乙状结肠及系膜长度无法满足经肛门拉出。
3. 直肠系膜过于肥厚无法经肛门拉出。
4. 过于肥胖者（BMI>35kg/m²）。

## 二、手术操作步骤、技巧与要点

### 【戳卡位置】

1. 腹腔镜镜头戳卡孔（10mm 戳卡）　脐窗中。

2. 术者主戳卡孔（12mm 戳卡）　麦氏点。

3. 术者辅助戳卡孔（5mm 戳卡）　脐右旁正中线上 5cm。

4. 助手辅助戳卡孔（5mm 戳卡）　反麦氏点。

5. 助手主戳卡孔（5mm 戳卡）　脐水平左腹直肌外缘（图 3-7-2）。

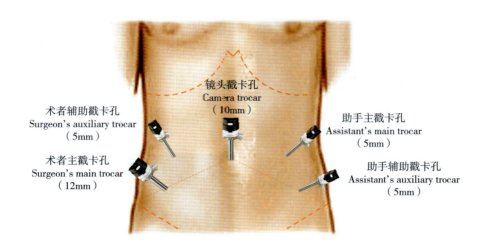

图 3-7-2　戳卡位置（五孔法）

Figure 3-7-2　Trocar placement（five-port method）

### 【探查】

1. 常规探查　观察各脏器及腹膜表面有无种植转移等病变。

2. 肿瘤探查　根据肿瘤的位置、大小、侵犯深度，确定手术的可行性。

3. 解剖结构的判定　判定乙状结肠及其系膜血管长度，判定中段直肠系膜肥厚程度，评估标本能否经直肠拉出。

### 【解剖与分离】

1. 第一刀切入点　在骶骨岬下方 3~5cm 通常有一菲薄处，用超声刀从此处开始操作，易于进入 Toldt's 间隙。

2. 肠系膜下血管根部游离与离断　逐层分离裸化肠系膜下血管，充分裸化后进行结扎并切断，系膜根部淋巴结清扫应采用整块切除，注意保护下腹下丛。

3. 直肠系膜的游离　打开乙状结肠系膜无血管区，向下向外游离至左侧髂总动脉分叉处，沿骶前间隙向下方分离至肿瘤下方 5cm 左右，注意保护左侧输尿管和左侧生殖血管。

4. 直肠右侧的游离　横行游离右侧腹膜反折，一般在肿瘤下方 5cm 即可。

5. 乙状结肠及直肠左侧的游离　切断乙状结肠外侧粘连，沿 Toldt's 筋膜向内侧游离，打开系膜向上继续分离；向下游离直肠左侧至腹膜反折处与右侧会合。

6. 裸化肿瘤下方肠管　在肿瘤下方 5cm 内进行肠壁裸化，约 3cm 范围。因此处直肠壁需进行两次切割，直肠系膜裸化范围应尽量充分。

7. 乙状结肠系膜裁剪　确定吻合预切除线，将系膜提起以确定其走行，沿肠系膜下血管走行进行裁剪，向预切除线分离至肠壁，裸化 2cm 范围，预判其游离长度是否满足经肛门拉出标本。

### 【标本切除与消化道重建】

1. 标本切除　充分扩肛冲洗后，可经肛门置入一碘附纱团于肿瘤下方（图 3-7-3）。在肠腔内纱布团指引下，术者用超声刀在肿瘤下方约 2cm 处横行切开肠管（图 3-7-4）。助手右手持吸引器，置于肿瘤下方约 2cm 处，当横行切开肠管时，及时吸尽肠内容物。助手经肛门置入卵圆钳，取出碘附纱布，随后经戳卡孔将无菌塑料套放入腹腔（图 3-7-5），并将保护套一端经肛门拉出体外，将直肠断端置入套内（图 3-7-6），最后经肛门用卵圆钳夹住近端直肠断端，缓慢经肛门拉出。将分离的标本拉出肛门，在肛门外乙状结肠预切除线处上荷包钳，切断直肠移去标本（图 3-7-7）。

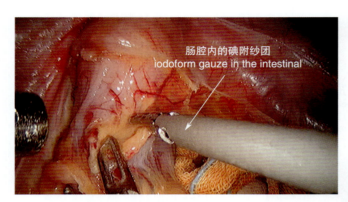

图 3-7-3　经肛门置入碘附纱团

Figure 3-7-3　Transanal placement of the iodoform gauze

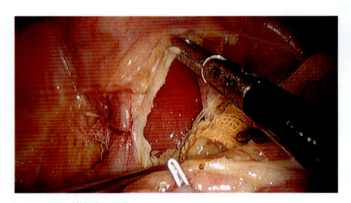

图 3-7-4　横行切开直肠

Figure 3-7-4　Transection of the rectum

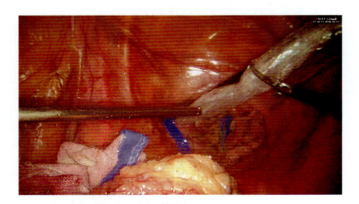

图 3-7-5　经戳卡孔置入无菌塑料套

Figure 3-7-5　Insertion of protective sleeve through the trocar

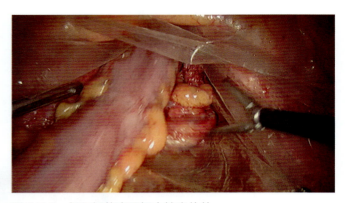

图 3-7-6　经肛门将直肠标本拉出体外

Figure 3-7-6　Transanal extraction of the rectal specimen

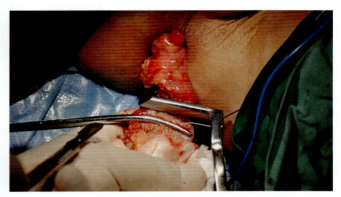

图 3-7-7　于肿瘤近端预切除线处切断直肠

Figure 3-7-7　Transection of the bowel at the pre-cut line above the tumor

2. 消化道重建　将抵钉座置入乙状结肠断端，收紧荷包，冲洗消毒后，用卵圆钳将其送回腹腔（图 3-7-8）。向腹腔内注入 1 000ml 碘附盐水冲洗腹腔并扩肛。用直线切割闭合器闭合直肠残端（图 3-7-9）。经肛门置入环形吻合器完成端端吻合（图 3-7-10、图 3-7-11）。注水注气试验检查吻合口完整性（图 3-7-12）。于盆腔放置两根引流管（图 3-7-13）。

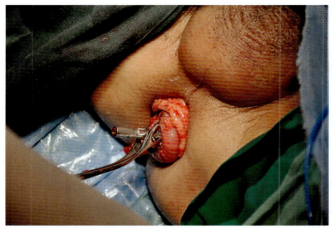

图 3-7-8　乙状结肠断端置入抵钉座

Figure 3-7-8　Inserting the anvil into the proximal sigmoid colon

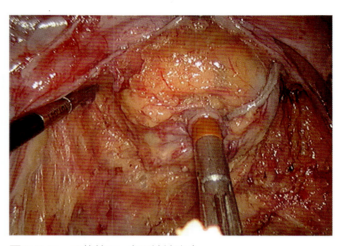

图 3-7-11　乙状结肠 - 直肠端端吻合

Figure 3-7-11　End-to-end anastomosis between the sigmoid colon and rectum

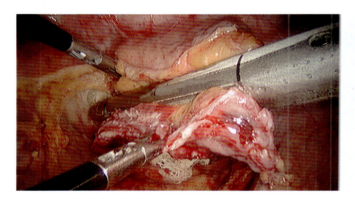

图 3-7-9　闭合直肠断端

Figure 3-7-9　Closing of the rectal stump

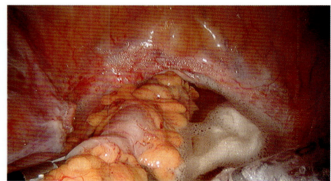

图 3-7-12　注水注气试验

Figure 3-7-12　air and water injection test

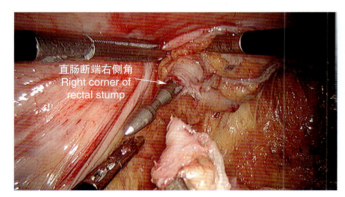

直肠断端右侧角
Right corner of rectal stump

图 3-7-10　于直肠断端一角旋出吻合器穿刺针

Figure 3-7-10　The anvil trocar needle is rotated out from one corner of the rectal stump

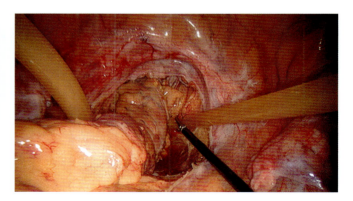

图 3-7-13　盆腔置入引流管

Figure 3-7-13　Two drainage tubes are placed in the pelvic cavity

## 第八节　腹部无辅助切口改良式经直肠拖出标本的腹腔镜下中位直肠癌根治术

### （CRC-NOSES Ⅱ式 B 法）

【简介】

CRC-NOSES Ⅱ式 B 法主要适用于中位直肠癌患者。相比 CRC-NOSES Ⅱ式 A 法，CRC-NOSES Ⅱ式 B 法需要先将直肠标本完全离断，然后再经肛门将标本完全取出体外（图 3-8-1）。此操作可以完全避免取标本过程中肛门挤压肿瘤导致的肿瘤血行转移风险。根据拟定的乙状结肠预切除线进行解剖，需要游离更多的肠壁，评估游离后乙状结肠的长度，以确定其是否可以经肛门取出。因此，该操作更符合无瘤原则。

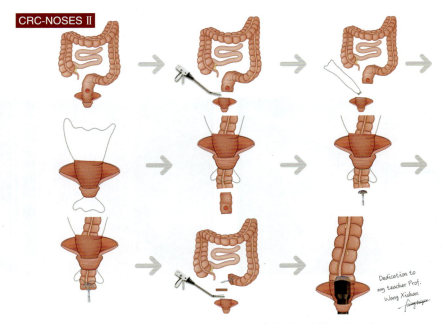

图 3-8-1　CRC-NOSES Ⅱ式 B 法标本取出及消化道重建的主要手术步骤

Figure 3-8-1　The main surgical procedures of specimen extraction and digestive tract reconstruction in CRC-NOSES ⅡB

## 一、适应证与禁忌证

【适应证】

1. 中位直肠癌或良性肿瘤。
2. 肿瘤环周直径 <3cm 为宜。
3. 肿瘤不侵出浆膜为宜。

【禁忌证】

1. 肿瘤体积过大，无法经肛门拉出。
2. 乙状结肠及系膜长度无法满足经肛门拉出。
3. 直肠系膜过于肥厚无法经肛门拉出。

4. 过于肥胖者（BMI>35kg/m²）。

## 二、手术操作步骤、技巧与要点

【戳卡位置】

1. 腹腔镜镜头戳卡孔（10mm 戳卡）　脐窗中。
2. 术者主戳卡孔（12mm 戳卡）　麦氏点。
3. 术者辅助戳卡孔（5mm 戳卡）　脐右旁正中线上 5cm。
4. 助手辅助戳卡孔（5mm 戳卡）　反麦氏点。
5. 助手主戳卡孔（5mm 戳卡）　脐水平左腹直肌外缘（图 3-8-2）。

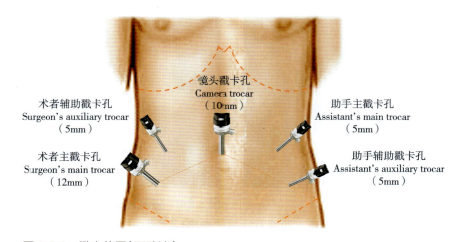

图 3-8-2　戳卡位置（五孔法）

Figure 3-8-2　Trocar placement（five-port method）

**【探查】**

1. 常规探查　观察各脏器及腹膜表面有无种植转移等病变。

2. 肿瘤探查　根据肿瘤的位置、大小、侵犯深度确定手术的可行性。

3. 解剖结构的判定　判定乙状结肠及其系膜血管长度，判定中段直肠系膜肥厚程度，评估能否经直肠拖出标本。

**【解剖与分离】**

1. 第一刀切入点　在骶骨岬下方 3~5cm 通常有一菲薄处，用超声刀从此处开始操作，易于进入 Toldt's 间隙。

2. 肠系膜下血管根部游离与离断　逐层分离裸化肠系膜下血管，充分裸化后进行结扎并切断，系膜根部淋巴结清扫应采用整块切除，注意保护下腹下丛。

3. 游离直肠系膜　打开乙状结肠系膜无血管区，向下向外游离至左侧髂总动脉分叉处，沿骶前间隙向下方分离至肿瘤下方 5cm 左右，注意保护左侧输尿管和左侧生殖血管。

4. 游离直肠右侧　横行游离右侧腹膜反折，一般在肿瘤下方 5cm 即可。

5. 游离乙状结肠及直肠左侧　切断乙状结肠外侧粘连，沿 Toldt's 筋膜向内侧游离，打开系膜向上继续分离；向下游离直肠左侧至腹膜反折处与右侧会合。

6. 裸化肿瘤下方肠管　在肿瘤下方 5cm 内进行肠壁裸化，约 3cm 范围。因此处直肠壁需进行两次切割，直肠系膜裸化范围应尽量充分。

7. 乙状结肠系膜裁剪　确定吻合预切除线，将系膜提起，沿肠系膜下血管走行进行裁剪，向预切除线分离至肠壁，裸化 2cm 范围，预判其游离长度是否满

足经肛门拉出标本。

**【标本切除与消化道重建】**

1. 标本切除　用直线切割闭合器在肿瘤下方 2cm 处横断远端直肠壁（图 3-8-3），用碘附纱条消毒直肠两侧断端，再用直线切割闭合器在肿瘤上方预切除线处横断乙状结肠远端（图 3-8-4），并用碘附纱条消毒断端（图 3-8-5），至此完成了标本的游离与切除。

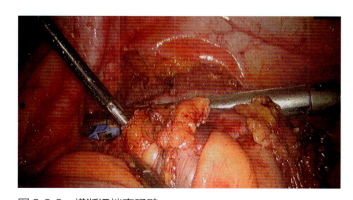

图 3-8-3　横断远端直肠壁

Figure 3-8-3　Transection of the distal rectum wall

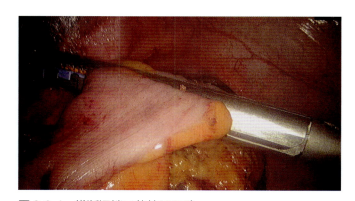

图 3-8-4　横断远端乙状结肠肠壁

Figure 3-8-4　Transection of the distal sigmoid cclon

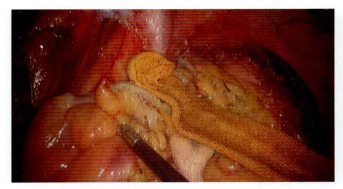

图 3-8-5　碘附纱条消毒肠管断端

Figure 3-8-5　Disinfection of the stumps using the iodoform gauze

　　术者经主操作戳卡孔置入保护套（图 3-8-6），在助手体外指引下切开远端直肠残端（图 3-8-7），助手将保护套一端经肛门拉出体外（图 3-8-8），将切除直肠标本置入保护套内（图 3-8-9），然后经肛门用卵圆钳夹住直肠标本断端，缓慢经肛门拉出（图 3-8-10）。

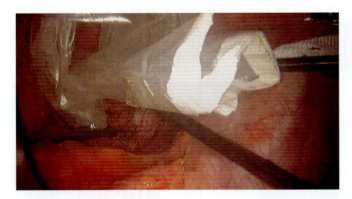

图 3-8-6　经主戳卡孔置入保护套

Figure 3-8-6　Insertion of the protective sleeve through the main trocar

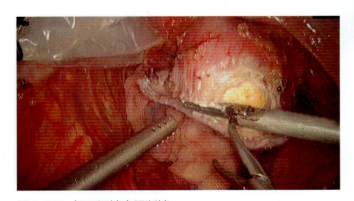

图 3-8-7　切开远端直肠断端

Figure 3-8-7　Incision of the distal rectal stump

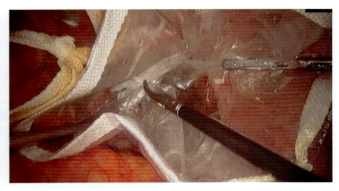

图 3-8-8　将保护套一端经肛门拉出体外

Figure 3-8-8　Transanal extraction of one end of the protective sleeve

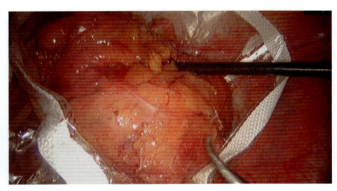

图 3-8-9　将直肠标本置入保护套内

Figure 3-8-9　Resected rectal specimen is placed into the protective sleeve

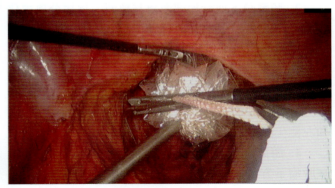

图 3-8-10　将标本经肛门拉出

Figure 3-8-10　Transanal extraction of specimen

　　2. 消化道重建　再次经术者主戳卡孔置入保护套，将乙状结肠断端拉出肛门（图 3-8-11），在肛门外乙状结肠预切除线处上荷包钳（图 3-8-12）。将抵钉座置入乙状结肠断端（图 3-8-13），收紧荷包，冲洗消毒后，用卵圆钳将其送回腹腔。向腹腔内注入 1 000ml 碘附盐水冲洗盆腔并扩肛。

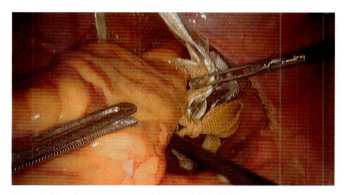

图 3-8-11 经肛门将乙状结肠断端拉出体外

Figure 3-8-11 The sigmoid colon stump is pulled through the anus

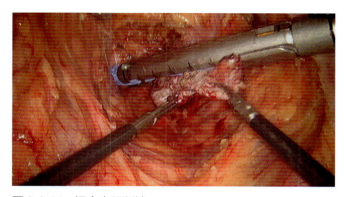

图 3-8-14 闭合直肠断端

Figure 3-8-14 Closing of the rectal stump

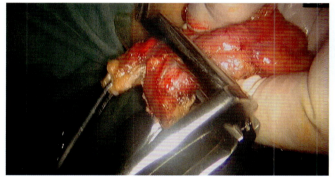

图 3-8-12 于乙状结肠预切除线置入荷包钳

Figure 3-8-12 Applying the purse string clamp at the pre-cut line on the sigmoid colon

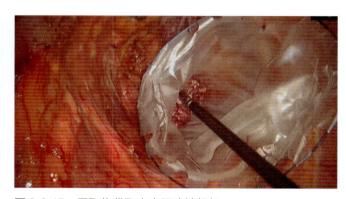

图 3-8-15 用取物袋取出直肠残端组织

Figure 3-8-15 Removal of the rectal stump tissues with the retrieval retrieval bag

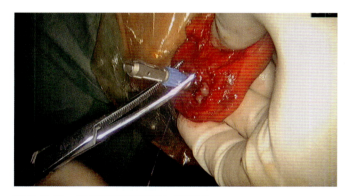

图 3-8-13 乙状结肠残端置入抵钉座

Figure 3-8-13 Inserting the anvil into the sigmoid colon stump

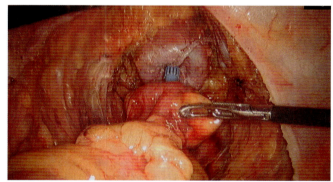

图 3-8-16 乙状结肠 - 直肠端端吻合

Figure 3-8-16 End-to-end anastomosis between the sigmoid colon and rectum

用直线切割闭合器闭合直肠残端（图 3-8-14），并用保护套将直肠残端组织取出（图 3-8-15）。经肛门置入环形吻合器，将抵钉座与机身对接，完成端端吻合（图 3-8-16）。

吻合口"危险三角区"行"8"字缝合（图 3-8-17）。注水注气试验检查吻合口有无出血、渗漏，是否通畅确切（图 3-8-18）。于盆腔放置两根引流管（图 3-8-19）。

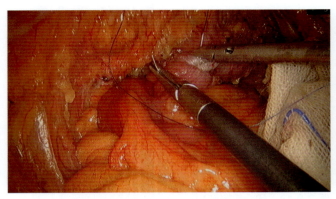

图 3-8-17　吻合口进行"8"字缝合

Figure 3-8-17　Anastomosis reinforcement with a figure-of-8 suture

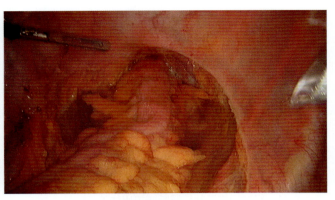

图 3-8-18　注水注气试验

Figure 3-8-18　Air and water injection tests

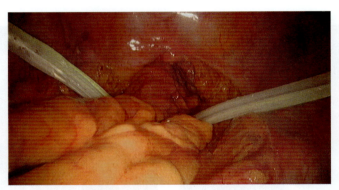

图 3-8-19　盆腔置入引流管

Figure 3-8-19　Two drainage tubes are placed in the pelvic cavity

## 第九节　腹部无辅助切口经阴道拉出标本的腹腔镜下中位直肠癌根治术

### （CRC-NOSES Ⅲ式A法）

【简介】

CRC-NOSES Ⅲ式A法主要适用于肿瘤略大的中位直肠癌女性患者，该术式的操作特点：经阴道将直肠拉至体外，在体外切除直肠标本后，再进行腹腔镜下乙状结肠 - 直肠端端吻合（图3-9-1，视频3-9）。与CRC-NOSES Ⅱ式的区别在于：①不需要在腹腔内剖开肠管，更符合无菌原则；②对阴道的术前准备要求更加严格；③阴道具有很强的延展性，因此，CRC-NOSES Ⅲ式A法的适应证更为宽泛，但仅局限于女性患者。

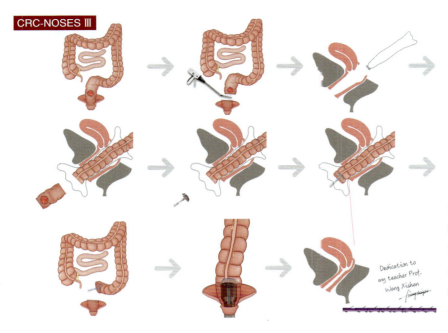

图 3-9-1 CRC-NOSES Ⅲ式 A 法标本取出及消化道重建的主要手术步骤
Figure 3-9-1 The main surgical procedures of specimen extraction and digestive tract reconstruction in CRC-NOSES ⅢA

视频 3-9 CRC-NOSES Ⅲ式 A 法
Video 3-9 CRC-NOSES ⅢA

## 一、适应证与禁忌证

### 【适应证】

1. 女性中段直肠癌或良性肿瘤。
2. 肿瘤环周直径为 3~5cm。
3. 肿瘤不侵出浆膜为宜。
4. 乙状结肠及系膜长度适合拉出者。

### 【禁忌证】

1. 肿瘤体积过大,取出有困难者。

2. 乙状结肠及系膜长度较短,无法经阴道拉出者。
3. 过于肥胖者(BMI>35kg/m$^2$)。

## 二、手术操作步骤、技巧与要点

### 【戳卡位置】

1. 腹腔镜镜头戳卡孔(10mm 戳卡) 脐窗中。
2. 术者主戳卡孔(12mm 戳卡) 麦氏点。
3. 术者辅助戳卡孔(5mm 戳卡) 平脐右侧 10cm 处。
4. 助手主戳卡孔(5mm 戳卡) 脐水平左上方腹直肌外缘。
5. 助手辅助戳卡孔(5mm 戳卡) 反麦氏点,该钳孔靠外侧便于兼顾放置引流管(图 3-9-2)。

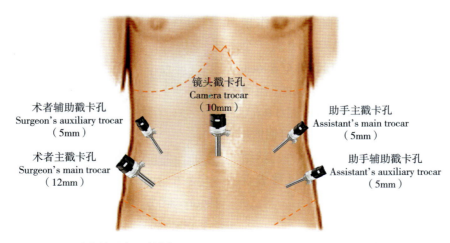

图 3-9-2 戳卡位置(五孔法)
Figure 3-9-2 Trocar placement(five-port method)

049

## 【探查】

1. 常规探查　观察各脏器及腹膜表面有无种植转移等病变。

2. 肿瘤探查　根据肿瘤的位置、大小、侵犯深度，确定手术的可行性。

3. 解剖结构的判定　判定乙状结肠及其系膜长度、系膜肥厚程度是否适合经阴道取出标本。

## 【解剖与分离】

1. 第一刀切入点　在骶骨岬下方 3~5cm 通常有一菲薄处，用超声刀从此处开始操作，易于进入 Toldt's 间隙。

2. 离断肠系膜下血管　依次结扎肠系膜下血管，注意保护下腹下丛。

3. 游离直肠系膜　游离范围依据肿瘤位置而定，一般在肿瘤下方 3~5cm 即可。

4. 游离乙状结肠外侧　切开乙状结肠外侧粘连，注意保护输尿管及生殖血管。

5. 裸化及离断肿瘤远端肠管　可在肿瘤下方 3~5cm 处横行切割直肠系膜，不用裸化过多，大约 2cm 即可。

6. 乙状结肠系膜裁剪　裁剪系膜时，保留侧血管用血管夹夹闭，另外一侧直接用超声刀离断。标本拉出拖出时，此举可避免标本上残留的血管夹损伤血管及直肠黏膜。

## 【标本切除与消化道重建】

1. 标本切除　用直线切割闭合器在肿瘤下方 4~5cm 处切断肠管（图 3-9-3）。助手再次消毒阴道后，将小膀胱拉钩置于阴道后穹隆起指示作用（图 3-9-4）。术者用超声刀在阴道后穹隆上做一个 3cm 的横向切口，并通过纵向拉伸将切口延伸至 5~6cm（图 3-9-5），经主戳卡孔将保护套送入腹腔。助手用卵圆钳夹持保护套一端，将其经阴道拉出体外（图 3-9-6）。术者将标本置入保护套内，助手经阴道用卵圆钳夹持直肠断端，将其拉出体外（图 3-9-7），在体外乙状结肠预切除线上放置荷包钳（图 3-9-8），切断并移去直肠 - 标本。

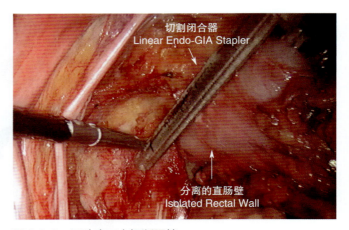

图 3-9-3　于肿瘤下方切断肠管

Figure 3-9-3　Transection of rectum below the tumor

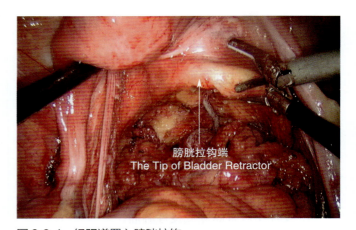

图 3-9-4　经阴道置入膀胱拉钩

Figure 3-9-4　Transvaginal placement of the bladder retractor for indication

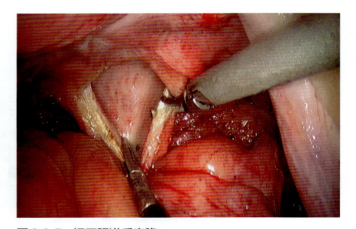

图 3-9-5　切开阴道后穹隆

Figure 3-9-5　Opening the posterior vaginal fornix

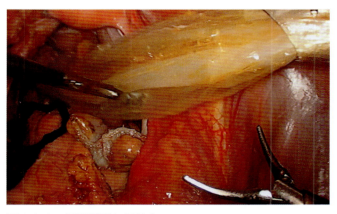

图 3-9-6　经阴道置入保护套

Figure 3-9-6　Placement of the protective sleeve via the vagina

2. 消化道重建　将吻合器抵钉座置入乙状结肠残端（图 3-9-9），收紧荷包（图 3-9-10）。冲洗消毒后，用卵圆钳将乙状结肠送回腹腔。经肛门置入环形吻合器，完成抵钉座与穿刺针连接后，行乙状结肠 - 直肠端端吻合（图 3-9-11~ 图 3-9-13）。注水注气试验检查吻合口完整性。用可吸收线在"危险三角区"行"8"字缝合。

3. 关闭戳卡孔缝合阴道切口　排出腹腔气体，腹腔镜下缝合阴道切口（图 3-9-14）。再次用生理盐水或蒸馏水冲洗盆腔，留置引流管（图 3-9-15、图 3-9-16）。关闭戳卡孔，清点纱布器械确切无误，术毕。

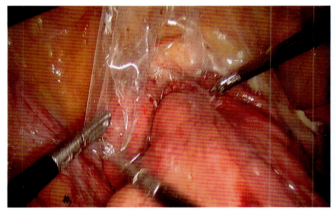

图 3-9-7　经阴道将直肠标本拉出体外

Figure 3-9-7　Transvaginal extraction of the rectal specimen

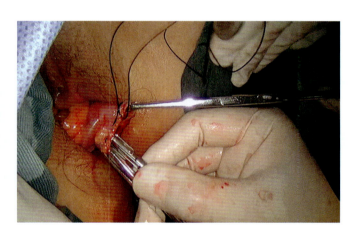

图 3-9-9　将抵钉座置入乙状结肠断端

Figure 3-9-9　The anvil is introduced into the sigmoid colon stump

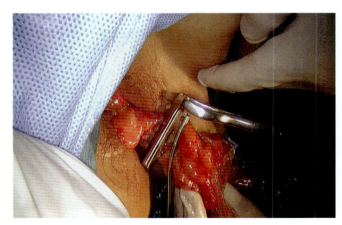

图 3-9-8　于肿瘤近端预切除线处切断肠管

Figure 3-9-8　Transection of the bowel at the pre-cut line proximal to the tumor

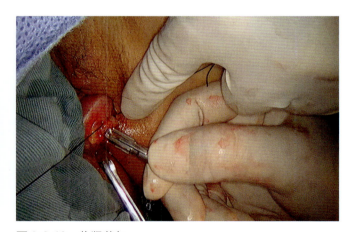

图 3-9-10　收紧荷包

Figure 3-9-10　The purse-string suture

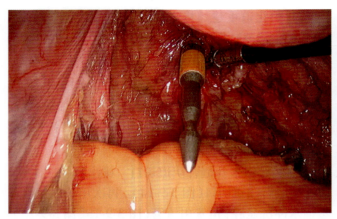

图 3-9-11　经肛门置入环形吻合器并旋出穿刺针

Figure 3-9-11　Inserting a circular stapler through the anus and extending trocar to pierce the stump

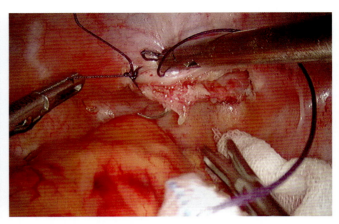

图 3-9-14　腹腔镜下缝合阴道切口

Figure 3-9-14　Suturing of vaginal incision under laparoscopy

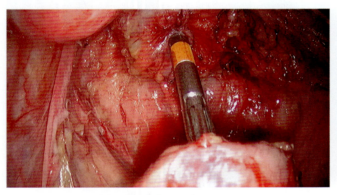

图 3-9-12　乙状结肠 - 直肠端端吻合

Figure 3-9-12　End-to-end anastomosis between the sigmoid colon and rectum

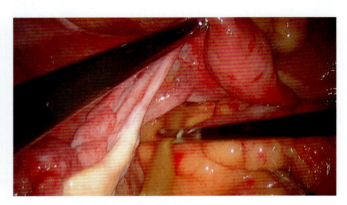

图 3-9-15　盆腔左侧置入引流管

Figure 3-9-15　One drainage tube is placed on the left side of the pelvic cavity

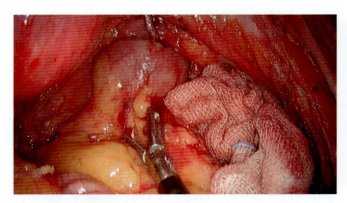

图 3-9-13　完成吻合

Figure 3-9-13　Complete the anastomosis

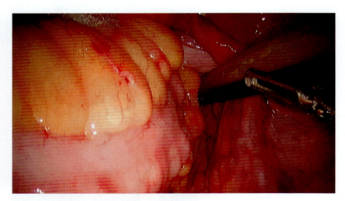

图 3-9-16　盆腔右侧置入引流管

Figure 3-9-16　One drainage tube is placed on the right side of the pelvic cavity

## 第十节　腹部无辅助切口改良式经阴道拖出标本的腹腔镜下中位直肠癌根治术

### （CRC-NOSES Ⅲ式B法）

### 【简介】

CRC-NOSES Ⅲ式B法与 CRC-NOSES Ⅲ式A法略有不同，主要适用于肿瘤略大的中位直肠癌女性患者

（图 3-10-1）。最新研究表明，经阴道取标本不会增加患者近期并发症发生率或降低远期生存。此外，阴道切口对女性术后性生活的影响有限。

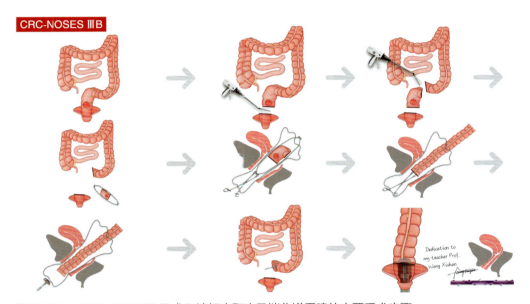

图 3-10-1　CRC-NOSES Ⅲ式B法标本取出及消化道重建的主要手术步骤

Figure 3-10-1　The main surgical procedures of specimen extraction and digestive tract reconstruction in CRC-NOSES ⅢB

### 一、适应证与禁忌证

#### 【适应证】

1. 女性直肠中段恶性或良性肿瘤。
2. 肿瘤环周直径为 3~5cm。
3. 肿瘤不侵出浆膜为宜。
4. 乙状结肠及系膜长度适合拉出者。

#### 【禁忌证】

1. 肿瘤体积过大，取出有困难者。
2. 乙状结肠及系膜长度较短，无法经阴道拉出者。
3. 过于肥胖者（BMI>35kg/m²）。

### 二、手术操作步骤、技巧与要点

#### 【戳卡位置】

1. 腹腔镜镜头戳卡孔（10mm 戳卡）　脐窗正中或脐上 1cm 处。
2. 术者主戳卡孔（12mm 戳卡）　麦氏点。
3. 术者辅助戳卡孔（5mm 戳卡）　平脐右侧 10cm 处。
4. 助手主戳卡孔（5mm 戳卡）　脐水平左上方腹直肌外缘。
5. 助手辅助戳卡孔（5mm 戳卡）　反麦氏点。此孔位置靠外侧更便于放置引流管（图 3-10-2）。

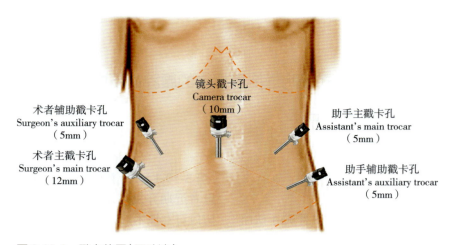

图 3-10-2 戳卡位置（五孔法）

Figure 3-10-2 Trocar placement（five-port method）

## 【探查】

1. 常规探查 观察各脏器及腹膜表面有无种植转移等病变。

2. 肿瘤探查 根据肿瘤的位置、大小、侵犯深度，确定手术的可行性。

3. 解剖结构的判定 判定乙状结肠及其系膜长度、系膜肥厚程度是否适合经阴道取出标本。

## 【解剖与分离】

1. 第一刀切入点 在骶骨岬下方 3~5cm 通常有一菲薄处，用超声刀从此处开始操作，易于进入 Toldt's 间隙。

2. 肠系膜下血管的离断 依次结扎肠系膜下血管，注意保护下腹下丛。

3. 直肠系膜的游离 游离范围依据肿瘤位置而定，一般在肿瘤下方 3~5cm 即可。

4. 乙状结肠外侧的游离 切开乙状结肠外侧粘连，注意保护输尿管及生殖血管。

5. 裸化肿瘤远端肠管 可在肿瘤下方 3~5cm 处横行切割直肠系膜，不用裸化过多，大约 2cm 即可。

6. 乙状结肠系膜裁剪 结扎切割 2~3 支乙状结肠动静脉，向肠管预切除线切割分离系膜。乙状结肠肠管裸化 2cm 即可，不宜裸化过多。

## 【标本切除与消化道重建】

1. 标本切除 用直线切割闭合器在肿瘤下方 4~5cm 处切断直肠（图 3-10-3），随后在肿瘤上方 5~10cm 处切断乙状结肠（图 3-10-4）。助手再次消毒阴道后，将膀胱拉钩置于阴道后穹隆起指示作用（图 3-10-5），术者用电凝钩或超声刀横行切开阴道

后穹隆，长 3~4cm（图 3-10-6），经 10mm 戳卡孔将保护套送入腹腔（图 3-10-7）。术者将标本置入保护套内，助手经阴道用卵圆钳夹持保护套，将其拉出体外（图 3-10-8），在体外乙状结肠预切除线上放置荷包钳（图 3-10-9）。

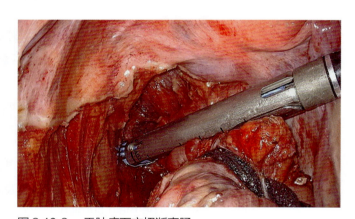

图 3-10-3 于肿瘤下方切断直肠

Figure 3-10-3 The rectum is transected at a region inferior to the tumor

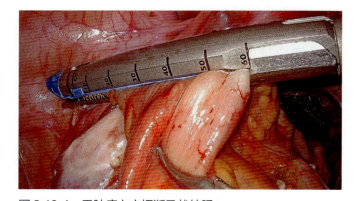

图 3-10-4 于肿瘤上方切断乙状结肠

Figure 3-10-4 The sigmoid colon is transected at a region superior to the tumor

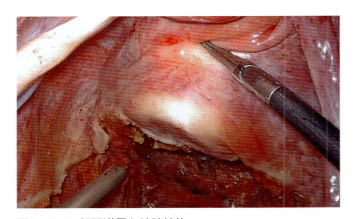

图 3-10-5　经阴道置入膀胱拉钩

Figure 3-10-5　Transvaginal placement of the bladder retractor to indicate the posterior fornix

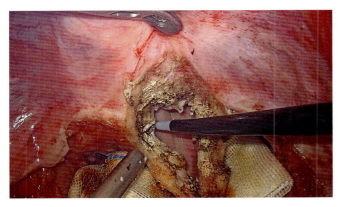

图 3-10-6　切开阴道后穹隆

Figure 3-10-6　Incision at the posterior vaginal fornix

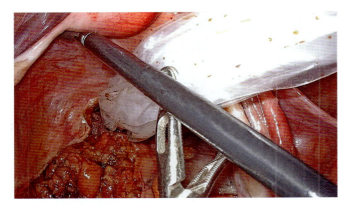

图 3-10-7　经戳卡孔置入保护套

Figure 3-10-7　Placement of the protective sleeve via the trocar

2. 消化道重建　将吻合器抵钉座置入乙状结肠残端（图 3-10-10），收紧荷包。冲洗消毒后，用卵圆钳将乙状结肠送回腹腔。经肛门置入环形吻合器，完成抵钉座与吻合器穿刺针连接后，行乙状结肠 - 直肠

端端吻合（图 3-10-11~ 图 3-10-13）。检查吻合口完整性。用可吸收线在"危险三角区"行"8"字缝合。注水注气试验检查吻合口是否通畅，有无出血及渗漏（图 3-10-14、图 3-10-15）。

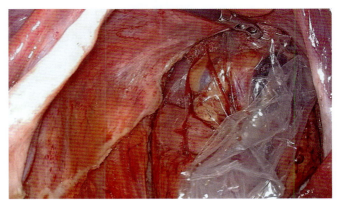

图 3-10-8　经阴道将标本拉出体外

Figure 3-10-8　Transvaginal extraction of the rectal specimen

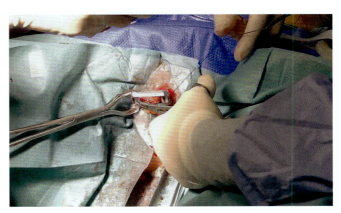

图 3-10-9　在预切除线上放置荷包钳

Figure 3-10-9　Placement of purse string forceps at the pre-cut line

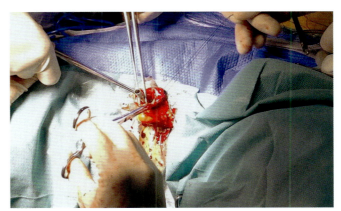

图 3-10-10　将抵钉座置入乙状结肠断端

Figure 3-10-10　Insertion of the anvil into the sigmoid colon stump

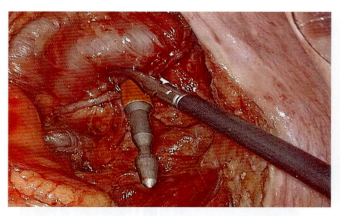

图 3-10-11　经肛门置入环形吻合器并旋出吻合器穿刺针
Figure 3-10-11　Transanal insertion of the circular stapler and extension of the stapler trocar

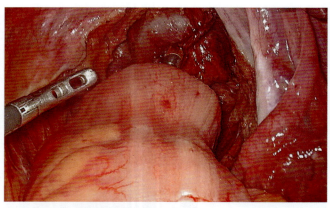

图 3-10-12　乙状结肠 - 直肠端端吻合
Figure 3-10-12　End-to-end anastomosis between the sigmoid colon and rectum

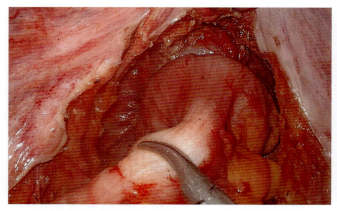

图 3-10-13　完成吻合
Figure 3-10-13　Completed anastomosis

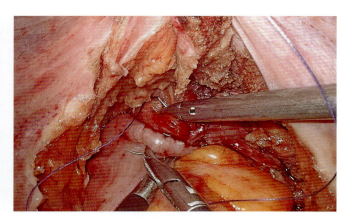

图 3-10-14　在"危险三角区"行"8"字缝合
Figure 3-10-14　8-figure suture on the "danger triangle"

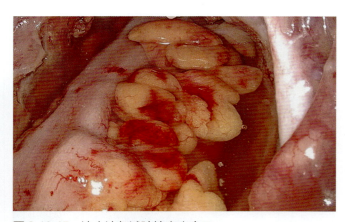

图 3-10-15　注水注气试验检查吻合口
Figure 3-10-15　Air and water injection tests

3. 关闭戳卡孔缝合阴道切口　在腹腔镜下使用倒刺线连续缝合阴道切口（图 3-10-16）。再次用生理盐水或蒸馏水冲洗盆腔，留置引流管（图 3-10-17、图 3-10-18）。关闭戳卡孔，清点纱布器械确切无误，术毕。

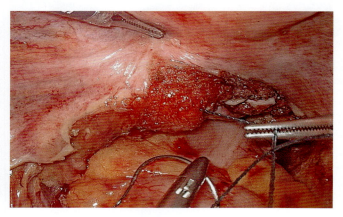

图 3-10-16　腹腔镜下连续缝合阴道切口
Figure 3-10-16　Continuous sutures on the vaginal incision under laparoscopy

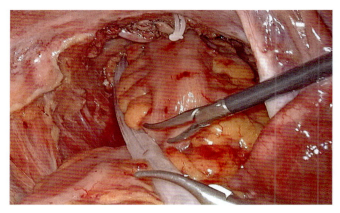

图 3-10-17　盆腔左侧置入引流管

Figure 3-10-17　Placement of a drainage tube on the left side of the pelvic cavity

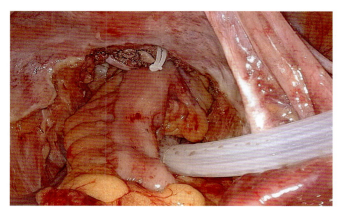

图 3-10-18　盆腔右侧置入引流管

Figure 3-10-18　Placement of a drainage tube on the right side of the pelvic cavity

## 第十一节　腹部无辅助切口经肛门取标本的腹腔镜下高位直肠癌根治术

### （CRC-NOSES Ⅳ式）

【简介】

CRC-NOSES Ⅳ式主要适用于肿瘤较小的高位直肠癌、直肠乙状结肠交界癌及远端乙状结肠癌。该术式的操作特点：在腹腔内完全游离切断直肠，经肛门将标本取出，再进行全腹腔镜下乙状结肠-直肠端端吻合（图 3-11-1，视频 3-10）。本术式难点为：在严格的无菌无瘤条件下，完成将抵钉座经肛门置入腹腔并在肿瘤上方置入近端肠腔的操作。

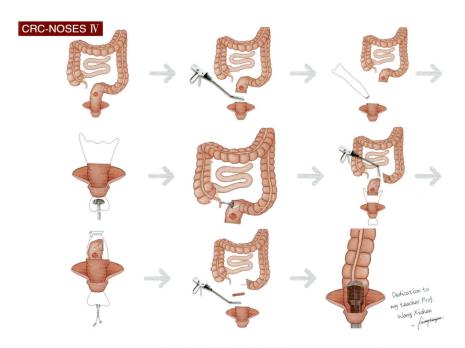

图 3-11-1　CRC-NOSES Ⅳ式标本取出及消化道重建的主要手术步骤

Figure 3-11-1　The main surgical procedures of specimen extraction and digestive tract reconstruction in CRC-NOSES Ⅳ

视频 3-10　CRC-NOSES Ⅳ式
Video 3-10　CRC-NOSES Ⅳ

# 一、适应证与禁忌证

## 【适应证】

1. 高位直肠癌（距齿状线至少 10cm）、直肠乙状结肠交界癌或远端乙状结肠癌。
2. 肿瘤环周直径 <3cm 为宜。
3. 肿瘤不侵出浆膜为宜。

## 【禁忌证】

1. 肿瘤位置或分期不符者。

2. 肿瘤过大或乙状结肠系膜过于肥厚，判定经肛门拖出困难者。
3. 过于肥胖者（BMI>35kg/m²）。

# 二、手术操作步骤、技巧与要点

## 【戳卡位置】

1. 腹腔镜镜头戳卡孔（10mm 戳卡）　脐上 3~5cm 处。
2. 术者主戳卡孔（12mm 戳卡）　麦氏点上方。
3. 术者辅助戳卡孔（5mm 戳卡）　右腹直肌旁平脐处。
4. 助手主戳卡孔（5mm 戳卡）　左腹直肌旁平脐处。
5. 助手辅助戳卡孔（5mm 戳卡）　反麦氏点，便于放置引流管充分引流（图 3-11-2）。

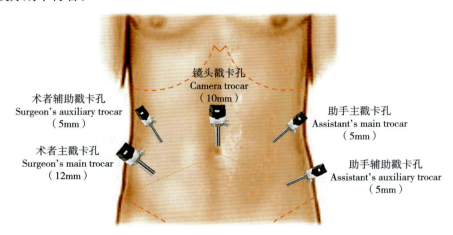

镜头戳卡孔
Camera trocar
（10mm）

术者辅助戳卡孔
Surgeon's auxiliary trocar
（5mm）

助手主戳卡孔
Assistant's main trocar
（5mm）

术者主戳卡孔
Surgeon's main trocar
（12mm）

助手辅助戳卡孔
Assistant's auxiliary trocar
（5mm）

图 3-11-2　戳卡位置（五孔法）
Figure 3-11-2　Trocar placement（five-port method）

## 【探查】

1. 常规探查　观察各脏器及腹膜表面有无种植转移等病变。
2. 肿瘤探查　根据肿瘤的位置、大小、侵犯深度，确定手术的可行性。
3. 解剖结构的判定　根据肿瘤位置决定是否保留左结肠动脉及直肠上动脉。根据乙状结肠长度、系膜血管弓的长度、系膜肥厚程度，估计标本能否经肛门取出。

## 【解剖与分离】

1. 第一刀切入点　在骶骨岬下方 3~5cm 通常有一菲薄处，用超声刀从此处开始操作，易于进入 Toldt's 间隙。
2. 离断肠系膜下血管　依次结扎肠系膜下血管，注意保护下腹下丛。

3. 游离直肠上段系膜　注意直肠系膜远端需游离至肿瘤下方 5cm 处。
4. 游离乙状结肠外侧　切开乙状结肠外侧粘连，注意保护输尿管及生殖血管。
5. 裸化及离断肿瘤远端肠管　由于需要对肿瘤远端的肠管分别进行两次离断，建议肠管裸化范围比常规更宽一些，为 3~5cm。
6. 乙状结肠系膜裁剪　裁剪系膜时，保留侧血管用血管夹夹闭，另外一侧直接用超声刀离断。标本拖出时，此举可避免标本上残留的血管夹损伤血管及直肠黏膜。

## 【标本切除与消化道重建】

1. 标本切除　术者将保护套经主戳卡孔置入腹腔（图 3-11-3），用超声刀将直肠闭合端切开，经肛门置入卵圆钳，将保护套拉出至肛门外（图 3-11-4），用卵圆钳将抵钉座经保护套送入腹腔（图 3-11-5）。

切割闭合（图 3-11-9），并用碘附纱团消毒乙状结肠断端（图 3-11-10），至此标本完全游离于保护套中（图 3-11-11）。

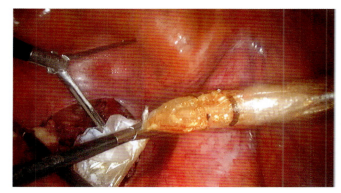

图 3-11-3　经主戳卡孔放入保护套

Figure 3-11-3　Insertion of the protective sleeve through the main trocar

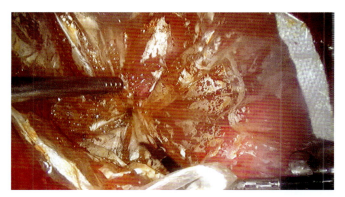

图 3-11-4　经肛门拉出保护套

Figure 3-11-4　Transanal extraction of the protective sleeve

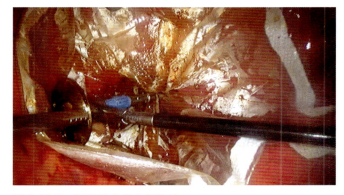

图 3-11-5　经保护套置入抵钉座

Figure 3-11-5　Inserting the anvil through the protective sleeve

将远端肠管断端置入保护套里，并在肿瘤上方肠壁纵行切开一小口（图 3-11-6），将碘附纱条经纵行切口探入乙状结肠腔，以对肠腔进行消毒（图 3-11-7），将抵钉座经纵行切口置入乙状结肠腔内（图 3-11-8），在纵行切口上方，用直线切割闭合器将肠管裸化区

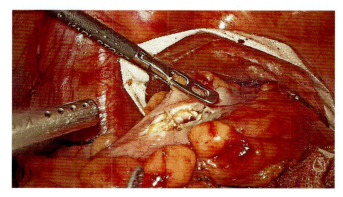

图 3-11-6　将远端肠管断端置入保护套里，并在肿瘤上方肠壁纵行切开一小口

Figure 3-11-6　Placing the distal bowel stump in the protective sleeve and making a small longitudinal incision on the bowel wall above the tumor

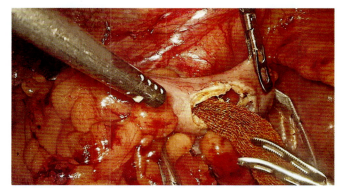

图 3-11-7　乙状结肠肠腔内消毒

Figure 3-11-7　Disinfection in the sigmoid colon lumen

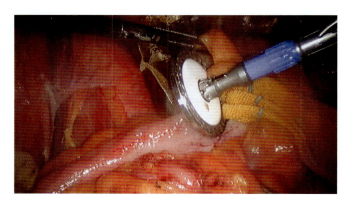

图 3-11-8　将抵钉座置入乙状结肠

Figure 3-11-8　Inserting the anvil into the sigmoid colon

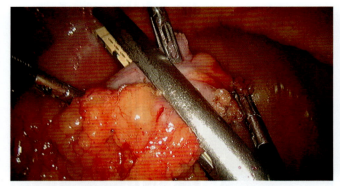

图 3-11-9　用直线切割闭合器将肠管裸化区切割闭合
Figure 3-11-9　Transection of the sigmoid colon with a linear cutting stapler

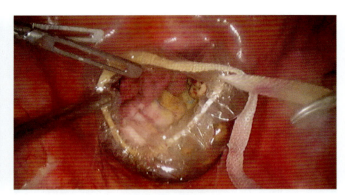

图 3-11-12　将小纱布及标本一起置入保护套内
Figure 3-11-12　Placing the gauze and specimen in the protective sleeve

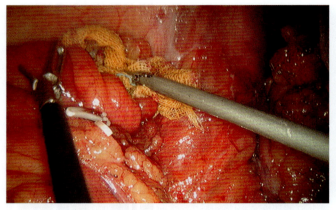

图 3-11-10　乙状结肠断端消毒
Figure 3-11-10　Disinfection of the sigmoid colon stump

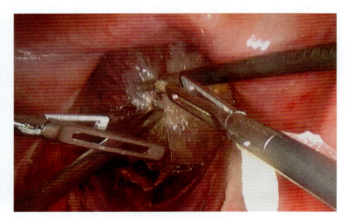

图 3-11-13　经肛门将装有标本的保护套拖出体外
Figure 3-11-13　Transanal extraction of the protective sleeve containing the specimen

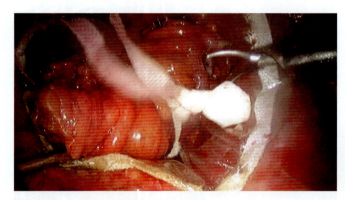

图 3-11-11　标本游离于保护套中
Figure 3-11-11　Resected specimen is placed into the protective sleeve

　　将用过的小纱布和标本一起置入保护套内（图 3-11-12）。术者收紧保护套抽绳后，经肛门将装有标本的保护套缓慢拖出体外（图 3-11-13）。

　　2. 消化道重建　用直线切割闭合器闭合直肠断端（图 3-11-14）。将切下的直肠残端置入取物袋或者自制指套（以橡胶手套制作）中，经 12mm 戳卡取出（图 3-11-15）。

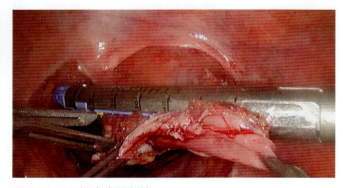

图 3-11-14　闭合直肠断端
Figure 3-11-14　Closing of the rectal stump

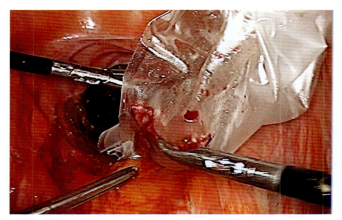

图 3-11-15　经取物袋取出直肠断端

Figure 3-11-15　Removal of the resected rectal stump with the retrieval bag

术者从肠腔外夹持、固定抵钉座,并在乙状结肠断端一角取出抵钉座连接杆(图 3-11-16、图 3-11-17),助手将环形吻合器经肛门置入,靠近直肠断端的左侧角旋出吻合器穿刺针(图 3-11-18)。完成对接,调整结肠系膜方向,完成乙状结肠 - 直肠端端吻合(图 3-11-19)。

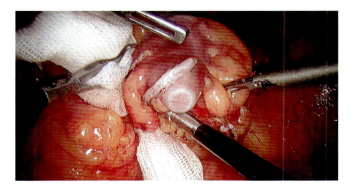

图 3-11-16　从肠腔外固定抵钉座

Figure 3-11-16　Grab the anvil from the outside of the bowel

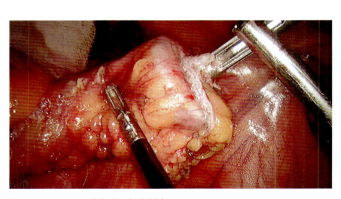

图 3-11-17　取出抵钉座连接杆

Figure 3-11-17　Taking out the anvil shaft

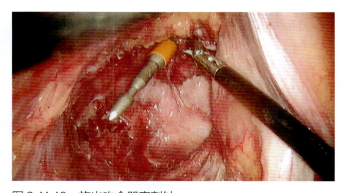

图 3-11-18　旋出吻合器穿刺针

Figure 3-11-18　Rotating out the piercing needle

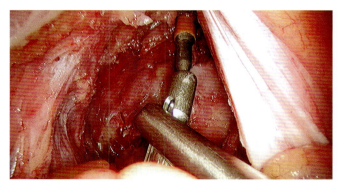

图 3-11-19　乙状结肠 - 直肠端端吻合

Figure 3-11-19　End-to-end anastomosis between the sigmoid colon and rectum

取出吻合器,检查吻合口整性。必要时腹腔镜下加固缝合"危险三角区"(图 3-11-20、图 3-11-21)。经肛门行注水注气试验检查吻合口完整性,有无渗漏及出血。冲洗腹腔,检查无误后,在左、右下腹部各放置一根引流管。

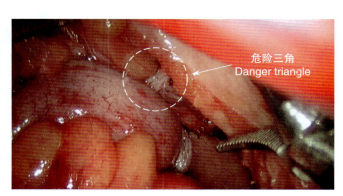

图 3-11-20　"危险三角区"

Figure 3-11-20　"Danger triangle"

危险三角
Danger triangle

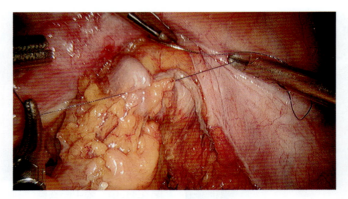

图 3-11-21　"危险三角区"加固缝合

Figure 3-11-21　Suture to reinforce the "danger triangle"

## 第十二节　腹部无辅助切口经阴道取标本的腹腔镜下高位直肠癌根治术

### （CRC-NOSES V式）

【简介】

CRC-NOSES V式主要适用于肿瘤较大的高位直肠癌、直肠乙状结肠交界癌及远端乙状结肠癌的女性患者。该术式的操作特点：在腹腔内完全游离切断直肠，经阴道将标本取出体外，再进行腹腔镜下乙状结肠 - 直肠端端吻合（图 3-12-1，视频 3-11）。本术式与 CRC-NOSES Ⅳ式的区别在于：①经由延展性很强的阴道取出标本，适用于体积偏大的肿瘤，但仅局限于女性患者；②只需在肿瘤上方肠壁开一小口置入抵钉座，因此腹腔污染机会更少，无菌操作更易掌握。

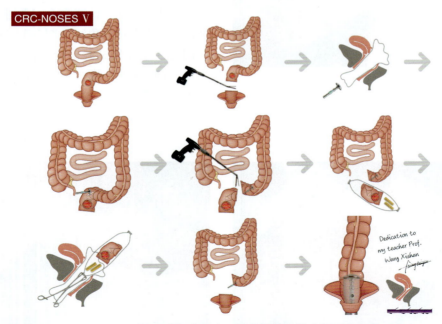

图 3-12-1　CRC-NOSES V式标本取出及消化道重建的主要手术步骤

Figure 3-12-1　The main surgical procedures of specimen extraction and digestive tract reconstruction in CRC-NOSES V

视频 3-11　CRC-NOSES Ⅴ式

Video 3-11　CRC-NOSES Ⅴ

# 一、适应证与禁忌证

## 【适应证】

1. 高位直肠癌（距齿状线至少 10cm）、直肠乙状结肠交界癌或远端乙状结肠癌。

2. 肿瘤环周径为 3~5cm。

3. 肿瘤不侵出浆膜为宜。

## 【禁忌证】

1. 肿瘤位置或分期不符者。

2. 肿瘤过大或乙状结肠系膜过于肥厚，判定经阴道拖出困难者。

3. 过于肥胖者（BMI>35kg/m$^2$）。

# 二、手术操作步骤、技巧与要点

## 【戳卡位置】

1. 腹腔镜镜头戳卡孔（10mm 戳卡）　脐上 3~5cm 处。

2. 术者主戳卡孔（12mm 戳卡）　麦氏点上方。

3. 术者辅助戳卡孔（5mm 戳卡）　右腹直肌旁平脐处。

4. 助手主戳卡孔（5mm 戳卡）　左腹直肌旁平脐处。

5. 助手辅助戳卡孔（5mm 戳卡）　反麦氏点，便于放置引流管充分引流（图 3-12-2）。

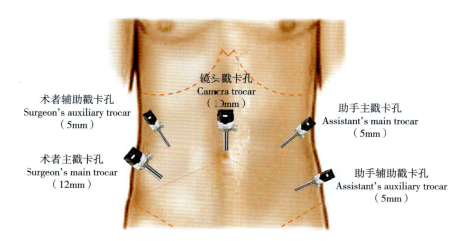

图 3-12-2　戳卡位置（五孔法）

Figure 3-12-2　Trocar placement（five-port method）

## 【探查】

1. 常规探查　观察各脏器及腹膜表面有无种植转移等病变。

2. 肿瘤探查　根据肿瘤的位置、大小、侵犯深度，评估手术的可行性。

3. 解剖结构的判定　根据肿瘤位置决定是否保留左结肠动脉及直肠上动脉。根据乙状结肠长度、系膜血管弓的长度、系膜肥厚程度，估计标本能否经阴道取出。

## 【解剖与分离】

1. 第一刀切入点　在骶骨岬下方 3~5cm 通常有一菲薄处，用超声刀从此处开始操作，易于进入 Toldt's 间隙。

2. 离断肠系膜下血管　依次结扎肠系膜下血管，注意保护下腹下丛。

3. 游离直肠上段系膜　注意直肠系膜远端需游离至肿瘤下方 5cm 处。

4. 游离乙状结肠外侧　切开乙状结肠外侧粘连，注意保护输尿管及生殖血管。

5. 裸化及离断肿瘤远端肠管　肠管裸化范围一般约为 2cm。

6. 乙状结肠系膜裁剪　裁剪系膜时，保留侧血管用血管夹夹闭，另外一侧直接用超声刀离断。标本拖出时，此举可避免标本上残留的血管夹损伤血管及阴道。

## 【标本切除与消化道重建】

1. 标本切除　术者将保护套经主戳卡孔置入腹腔（图 3-12-3），助手经阴道用膀胱拉钩将阴道后穹隆抬起（图 3-12-4），术者用超声刀横行切开阴道约 3cm，再纵行牵拉切口，扩大至 5~6cm（图 3-12-5）。助手经阴道置入卵圆钳将保护套拉出体外并打开（图 3-12-6），再经保护套内将抵钉座送入腹腔（图 3-12-7）。

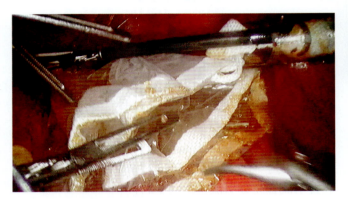

图 3-12-3　经主戳卡孔置入保护套

Figure 3-12-3　Insertion of the protective sleeve through the main trocar

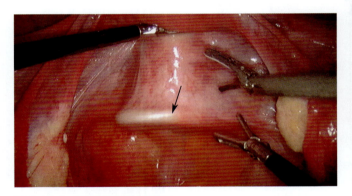

图 3-12-4　膀胱拉钩体外指示

Figure 3-12-4　Indication of the bladder retractor

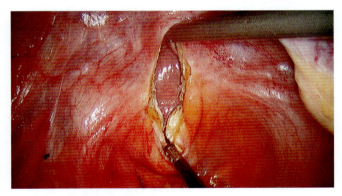

图 3-12-5　切开阴道后穹隆

Figure 3-12-5　Opening the posterior vaginal fornix

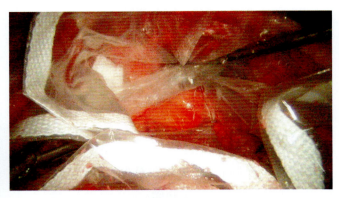

图 3-12-6　经阴道将保护套拉出体外

Figure 3-12-6　Transvaginal extraction of the protective sleeve

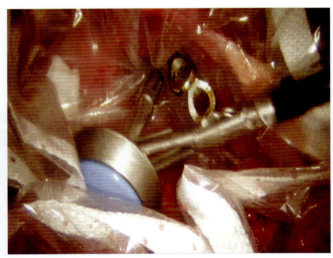

图 3-12-7　经保护套置入抵钉座

Figure 3-12-7　Inserting the anvil through the protective sleeve

在肿瘤上方乙状结肠预切除线下方 1cm 纵行切开肠壁（图 3-12-8）。术者将一碘附纱条经该切口塞入肠腔内，以消毒和润滑；助手用吸引器及时吸引肠内容物，并将纱条推入远端肠腔内（图 3-12-9、图 3-12-10）。将抵钉座置入乙状结肠近端肠腔内（图 3-12-11），用直线切割闭合器横断近端乙状结肠（图 3-12-12）。随后，再用直线切割闭合器在肿瘤下方肠管裸化区横行切断直肠（图 3-12-13）。至此，直肠肿瘤及肠段完全游离于腹腔。

术者与助手将标本及用过的小纱布置入保护套内，另一助手用卵圆钳在保护套内夹持住肿瘤下方肠壁断端，拉紧保护套，缓慢将保护套、标本及纱布拖出体外（图 3-12-14）。

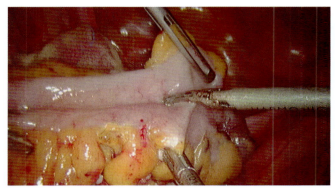

图 3-12-8　在肿瘤上方肠壁切开一小口

Figure 3-12-8　Making a small incision on the bowel wall above the tumor

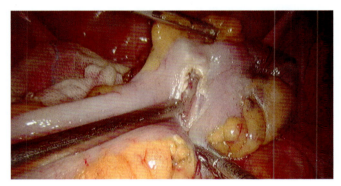

图 3-12-9　及时吸引肠内容物

Figure 3-12-9　Timely suction of bowel contents

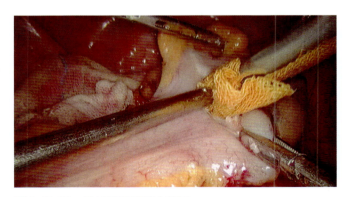

图 3-12-10　乙状结肠肠腔内消毒

Figure 3-12-10　Disinfection of the sigmoid colon lumen

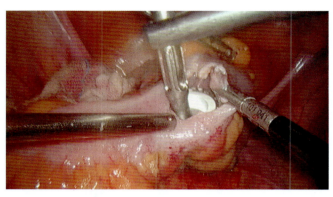

图 3-12-11　将抵钉座置入乙状结肠近端

Figure 3-12-11　Inserting the anvil into the proximal sigmoid colon

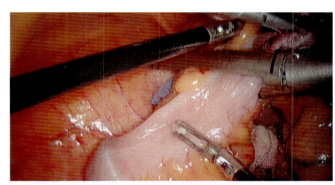

图 3-12-12　用直线切割闭合器横断近端乙状结肠

Figure 3-12-12　Transection of the proximal bowel of the sigmoid colon with the linear cutting stapler

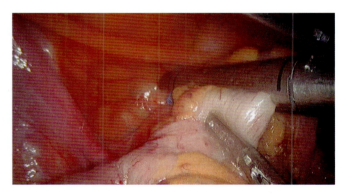

图 3-12-13　切断闭合肿瘤下方直肠

Figure 3-12-13　Transection of the rectal bowel below the tumor

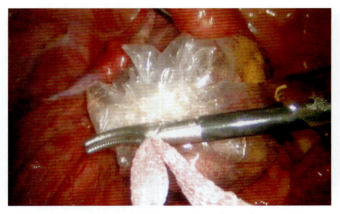

图 3-12-14　经阴道将直肠标本及小纱布拖出体外

Figure 3-12-14　Transvaginal extraction of the rectal specimen and the gauze

2. 消化道重建　在乙状结肠近端一角取出抵钉座连接杆（图 3-12-15），助手经肛门置入环形吻合器并旋出吻合器穿刺针（图 3-12-16），将抵钉座与吻合器机身对接（图 3-12-17），确认结肠系膜方向，完成乙状结肠 - 直肠端端吻合（图 3-12-18）。

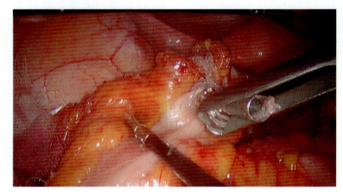

图 3-12-15　取出抵钉座连接杆

Figure 3-12-15　Taking out the anvil shaft

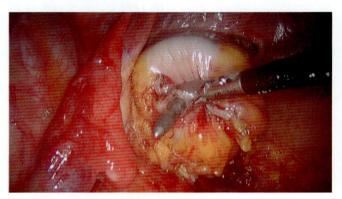

图 3-12-16　旋出吻合器穿刺针

Figure 3-12-16　Extend trocar to pierce the rectal stump

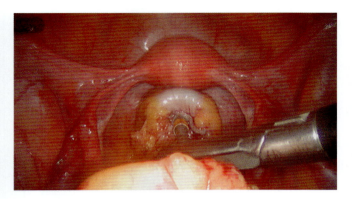

图 3-12-17　连接吻合器穿刺针

Figure 3-12-17　Connecting the anvil and trocar

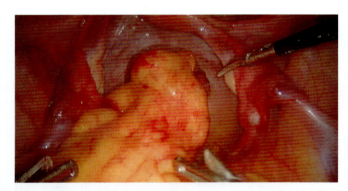

图 3-12-18　乙状结肠 - 直肠端端吻合

Figure 3-12-18　End-to-end anastomosis between the sigmoid colon and rectum

取出吻合器，检查吻合口完整性，必要时腹腔镜下加固缝合"危险三角区"（图 3-12-19）。经肛门行注水注气试验检查吻合口完整性（图 3-12-20）。冲洗腹腔，检查无误后，经腹或经阴道放置腹腔引流管（图 3-12-21）。

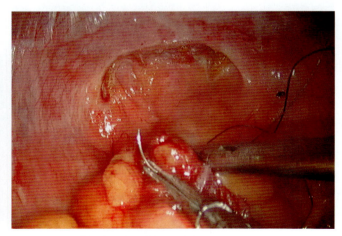

图 3-12-19　"危险三角区"加固缝合

Figure 3-12-19　Suture to reinforce "danger triangle"

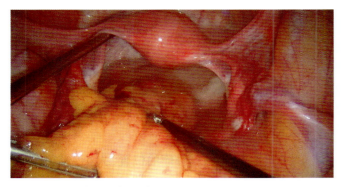

图 3-12-20  注水注气试验
Figure 3-12-20  air and water injection test

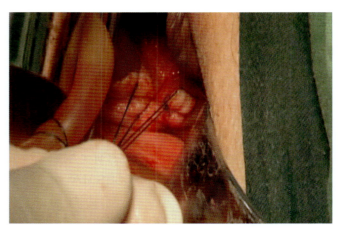

图 3-12-21  经阴道置入引流管
Figure 3-12-21  Transvaginal placement of drainage tubes

3. 缝合阴道切口  摆放好引流管后，排出腹腔气体。充分显露阴道切口，用两把 Allis 钳提起切口的前后壁，用可吸收线间断缝合即可。也可经腹腔以倒刺线连续缝合阴道切口。

## 第十三节  腹部无辅助切口经直肠拖出标本的腹腔镜下左半结肠癌根治术
### （CRC-NOSES Ⅵ式 A 法）

【简介】

CRC-NOSES Ⅵ式 A 法的操作特点：腹腔内完全游离切断左半结肠，经直肠 - 肛门将标本取出体外，再进行腹腔镜下横结肠 - 直肠端端吻合（图 3-13-1，视频 3-12）。从腹腔镜技术角度而言，CRC-NOSES Ⅵ式 A

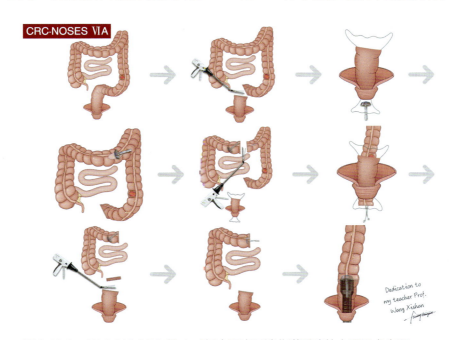

图 3-13-1  CRC-NOSES Ⅵ A 式标本取出及消化道重建的主要手术步骤
Figure 3-13-1  The main surgical procedures of specimen extraction and digestive tract reconstruction in CRC-NOSES Ⅵ A

法的操作难点包括左半结肠系膜的完整切除、系膜根部淋巴结清扫,以及结肠脾曲的游离。从 NOSES 技术角度而言,CRC-NOSES Ⅵ式 A 法的操作难点包括标本经直肠 - 肛门拖出,腹腔镜下消化道重建,无菌术、无瘤操作的精准运用等。

视频 3-12　CRC-NOSES Ⅵ式 A 法
Video 3-12　CRC-NOSES ⅥA

## 一、适应证及禁忌证

### 【适应证】

1. 肿瘤位于降结肠、乙状结肠近端。
2. 肿瘤环周径 <3cm 为宜。
3. 肿瘤未侵出浆膜为宜。

### 【禁忌证】

1. 肿瘤位于结肠脾曲和横结肠近结肠脾曲处。
2. 肿瘤环周径 >3cm。
3. 肿瘤侵出浆膜。
4. 过于肥胖者(BMI>35kg/m²)。

## 二、手术操作步骤、技巧与要点

### 【戳卡位置】

1. 腹腔镜镜头戳卡孔(10mm 戳卡)　脐下 2~3cm 处。
2. 术者主戳卡孔(12mm 戳卡)　麦氏点。
3. 术者辅助戳卡孔(5mm 戳卡)　脐上方 10cm 水平与右腹直肌外缘交叉处的横结肠投影区。
4. 助手主戳卡孔(5mm 戳卡)　脐上方 10cm 水平

与左锁骨中线交叉处。
5. 助手辅助戳卡孔(5mm 戳卡)　反麦氏点,便于放置引流管(图 3-13-2)。

### 【探查】

1. 常规探查　观察各脏器及腹膜表面有无种植转移等病变。
2. 肿瘤探查　根据肿瘤的位置、大小、侵犯深度,确定手术的可行性。
3. 解剖结构的判定　首先,判定结肠及系膜的结构特点,即肠管游离后,下拉的长度和血管弓的走行是否有利于腹腔镜下吻合;其次,判定肠系膜肥厚程度及肿瘤环周直径情况是否适合经直肠拖出。

### 【解剖与分离】

1. 肠系膜下血管根部的处理　裸化肠系膜下动脉根部,双重结扎并切断。提起根部向外侧游离,向上游离至屈氏韧带外侧,在胰腺下缘横断肠系膜下静脉。
2. 内侧入路的左半结肠系膜游离　提起肠系膜下静脉断端和肠系膜下动脉断端,用超声刀分别向外、向下、向上以锐性和钝性分离相结合的方式游离 Toldt's 筋膜。
3. 乙状结肠及直肠系膜的处理　沿肠系膜下动脉走行提起系膜,向下分离至骶骨岬水平,注意保护腹主动脉前神经。
4. 左半横结肠和结肠脾曲的处理　将横结肠提起,在屈氏韧带外侧肠系膜下静脉断端开始切割分离横结肠系膜,与网膜囊贯通,沿胰腺下缘向左侧切割分离至脾下极。
5. 游离左结肠旁沟　将乙状结肠翻向右侧,在直肠左侧预切除线沿 Toldt's 筋膜向上分离,借助纱布条

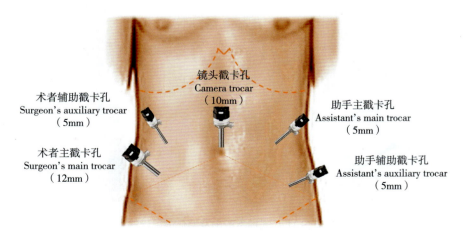

图 3-13-2　戳卡位置(五孔法)
Figure 3-13-2　Trocar placement(five-port method)

指示向上打开左结肠旁沟至脾下极。

6. 肿瘤上方结肠系膜的裁剪与裸化　游离横结肠系膜至边缘血管弓，切断结扎边缘血管弓，游离至肠壁，裸化肠管 2cm 备用。

### 【标本切除与消化道重建】

1. 标本切除　在肿瘤下方，乙状结肠肠管裸化区横行切一小口（图 3-13-3），助手用卵圆钳夹持抵钉座经保护套送入腹腔（图 3-13-4）。在肿瘤上方裸化区的远端开一纵行小口（图 3-13-5），将抵钉座置入近端结肠内（图 3-13-6），并用直线切割闭合器切断结肠（图 3-13-7），将抵钉座封闭于近端肠管，并用碘附纱布消毒肠管断端（图 3-13-8）。在肿瘤下方横行切口的基础上继续横断直肠（图 3-13-9），至此左半结肠完全游离于腹腔。经主戳卡孔将保护套置入腹腔。术者与助手配合将标本顺畅置入保护套中，助手于体外用卵圆钳夹持住肠管一端，缓慢经直肠 - 肛门拖出标本（图 3-13-10）。

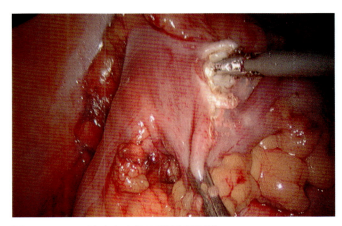

图 3-13-5　于肿瘤上方切开横结肠肠壁

Figure 3-13-5　Incision of the transverse colon wall above the tumor

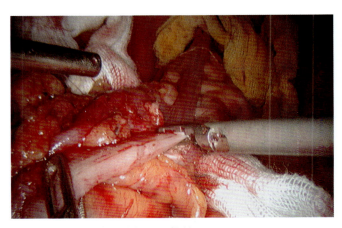

图 3-13-3　于肿瘤下方切开乙状结肠

Figure 3-13-3　Incision of the sigmoid colon below the tumor

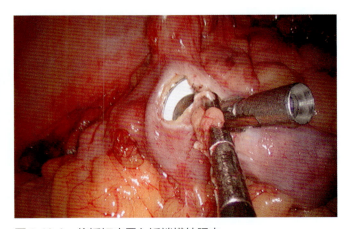

图 3-13-6　将抵钉座置入近端横结肠内

Figure 3-13-6　Inserting the anvil into the proximal transverse colon

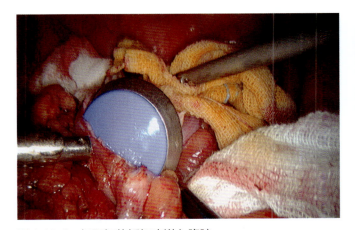

图 3-13-4　经肛门将抵钉座送入腹腔

Figure 3-13-4　Insertion of the anvil into the abdominal cavity through anus

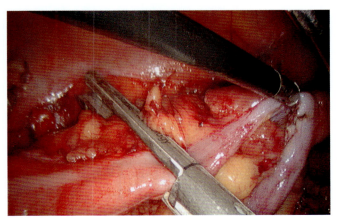

图 3-13-7　闭合切断横结肠肠管

Figure 3-13-7　Close and transect the transverse colon

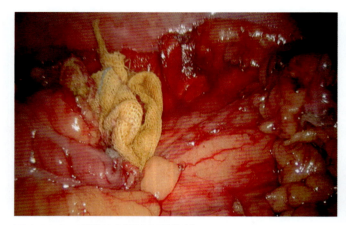

图 3-13-8 碘附纱布消毒肠管断端
Figure 3-13-8 Broken stump of enteric tube disinfected with iodoform gauze

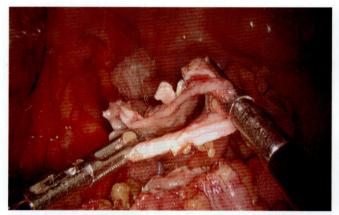

图 3-13-9 横断肿瘤下方肠管
Figure 3-13-9 Transection of the bowel below the tumor

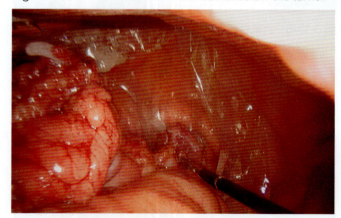

图 3-13-10 经直肠 - 肛门将左半结肠标本拖出体外
Figure 3-13-10 The left half colon specimen was pulled out of the body through the rectum and anus

2. 消化道重建 此时直肠断端是开放的，用直线切割闭合器闭合直肠断端（图 3-13-11），将切割下的残端置入标本袋后经 12mm 戳卡孔取出。用生理盐水或蒸馏水冲洗腹腔，以减少腹腔感染的可能性。将抵钉座连接杆从近端结肠闭合线一角取出（图 3-13-12）。助手经肛门置入环形吻合器，在直肠断端左侧角旋

出吻合器穿刺针（图 3-13-13），完成吻合器连接，调整结肠系膜方向（图 3-13-14）。旋紧击发，完成吻合（图 3-13-15）。术者检查吻合口是否完整。"危险三角区"行"8"字缝合（图 3-13-16）。通过注水注气试验，检查吻合口是否通畅，吻合是否确切（图 3-13-17）。冲洗腹腔、检查无误后，于吻合口旁留置两根引流管（图 3-13-18、图 3-13-19）。排出腹腔气体，关闭戳卡孔。

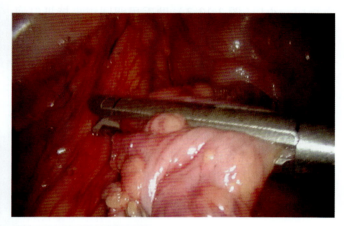

图 3-13-11 闭合直肠断端
Figure 3-13-11 Closing the rectal stump

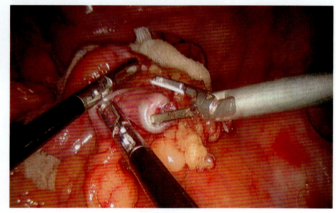

图 3-13-12 取出抵钉座连接杆
Figure 3-13-12 Taking out the anvil shaft

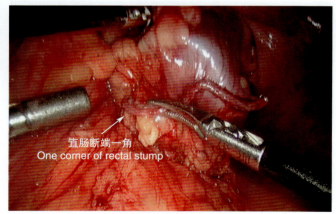

直肠断端一角
One corner of rectal stump

图 3-13-13 于直肠断端左侧角旋出吻合器穿刺针
Figure 3-13-13 Unscrew the stapler pierce rod at the left corner of the rectal stump

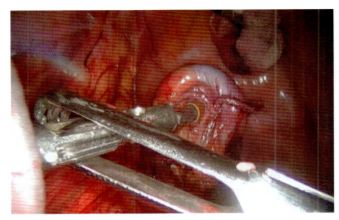

图 3-13-14　完成吻合器连接

Figure 3-13-14　Complete connecting of the danvil and the stapler

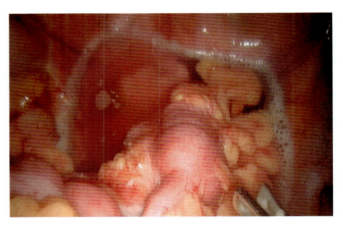

图 3-13-17　注水注气试验

Figure 3-13-17　Air and water injection test

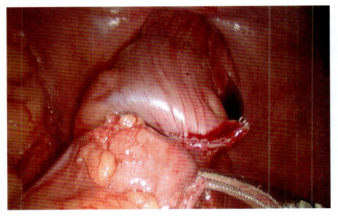

图 3-13-15　行横结肠 - 直肠端端吻合

Figure 3-13-15　End-to-end anastomosis between transverse colon and rectum

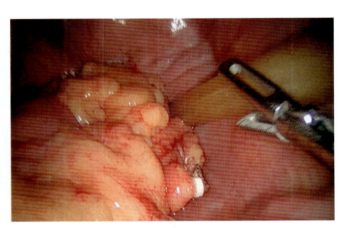

图 3-13-18　于右侧盆腔置入引流管

Figure 3-13-18　Insertion of right pelvic drainage tube

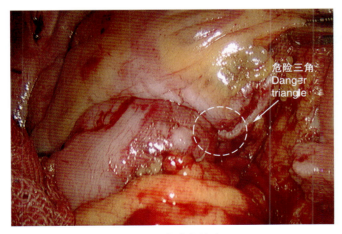

图 3-13-16　"危险三角区"行"8"字缝合

Figure 3-13-16　Suture the "danger triangle" with 8-figure suture

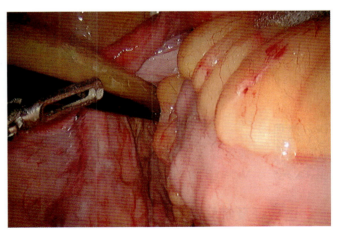

图 3-13-19　于左侧盆腔置入引流管

Figure 3-13-19　Insertion of left pelvic drainage tube

# 第十四节  腹部无辅助切口经直肠取标本的腹腔镜下左半结肠癌根治术

## （CRC-NOSES Ⅵ式 B 法）

### 【简介】

CRC-NOSES Ⅵ式 B 法的特点表现在它适用于肿瘤位置相对更高，离腹膜反折更远的病例；标本经直肠前壁切口拖出，而非经直肠断端；消化道重建适合采用全腹腔镜下功能性侧侧吻合（图 3-14-1，视频 3-13）。CRC-NOSES Ⅵ式 B 法的操作难点主要涉及两方面：从腹腔镜技术角度而言，操作难点包括左半结肠系膜的完整切除、系膜根部淋巴结清扫，以及结肠脾曲的游离。从 NOSES 技术角度而言，难点包括经直肠 - 肛门标本取出，全腹腔镜下消化道重建，无菌术、无瘤操作的精准运用等，这些都是术者需要面对和克服的主要困难。

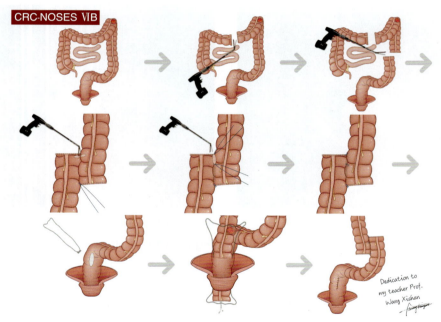

图 3-14-1　CRC-NOSES Ⅵ式 B 法标本取出及消化道重建的主要手术步骤

Figure 3-14-1　The main surgical procedures of specimen extraction and digestive tract reconstruction in CRC-NOSES ⅥB

视频 3-13　CRC-NOSES Ⅵ式 B 法
Video 3-13　CRC-NOSES ⅥB

## 一、适应证及禁忌证

### 【适应证】

1. 肿瘤位于横结肠近脾曲、结肠脾曲、降结肠和乙状结肠近端。

2. 肿瘤环周径 <3cm 为宜。

3. 肿瘤未侵出浆膜为宜。

### 【禁忌证】

1. 肿瘤环周径 >3cm。

2. 肿瘤侵出浆膜。

3. 过于肥胖者（BMI>35kg/m$^2$）。

## 二、手术操作步骤、技巧与要点

### 【戳卡位置】

1. 腹腔镜镜头戳卡孔（10mm 戳卡）　脐下 2~3cm 处。
2. 术者主戳卡孔（12mm 戳卡）　麦氏点。
3. 术者辅助戳卡孔（5mm 戳卡）　脐上方 10cm 水平与右腹直肌外缘交叉处的横结肠投影区。
4. 助手主戳卡孔（5mm 戳卡）　脐上方 10cm 水平与左锁骨中线交叉处。
5. 助手辅助戳卡孔（5mm 戳卡）　反麦氏点，便于放置引流管（图 3-14-2）。

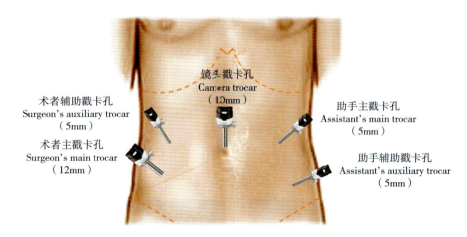

图 3-14-2　戳卡位置（五孔法）
Figure 3-14-2　Trocar placement（five-port method）

### 【探查】

1. 常规探查　观察各脏器及腹膜表面有无种植转移等病变。
2. 肿瘤探查　根据肿瘤的位置、大小、侵犯深度，确定手术的可行性。
3. 解剖结构的判定　首先，判定结肠及系膜的结构特点，即肠管游离后，下拉的长度和血管弓的走行是否有利于腹腔镜下吻合；其次，判定肠系膜肥厚程度及肿瘤环周直径情况是否适合经直肠拖出。

### 【解剖与分离】

1. 肠系膜下血管根部的处理　裸化肠系膜下动脉根部，双重结扎并切断。向上游离至屈氏韧带外侧，在胰腺下缘横断肠系膜下静脉。
2. 内侧入路的左半结肠系膜游离　提起肠系膜下静脉断端和肠系膜下动脉断端，用超声刀分别向外、向下、向上以锐性和钝性分离相结合的方式游离 Toldt's 筋膜。
3. 乙状结肠系膜的处理　提起乙状结肠系膜，沿预切除线分离至边缘血管弓，然后结扎并横断边缘血管。继续分离至肠壁，裸化出 3~4cm 长的肠管备用。

4. 左侧横结肠及结肠脾曲的处理　抬起横结肠时，术者从位于屈氏韧带外侧的肠系膜下静脉断端横断结肠系膜，以便直接进入网膜囊。然后沿胰腺下缘向左侧解剖至脾下极。
5. 游离左结肠旁沟　将乙状结肠翻向右侧，在直肠左侧切割线沿 Toldt's 筋膜向上分离，借助纱布条指示向上打开左结肠旁沟至脾下极。
6. 肿瘤上方结肠系膜的裁剪与裸化　下拉结肠脾曲，判定预切除线。游离横结肠系膜至边缘血管弓，切断结扎边缘血管弓，游离至肠壁，裸化肠管 2cm 备用。

### 【标本切除与消化道重建】

1. 标本切除　在横结肠裸化处离断横结肠（图 3-14-3），在乙状结肠裸化处离断乙状结肠（图 3-14-4），完成病变肠管的游离，至此完成标本切除。
2. 消化道重建　将两侧断端拉近，平行放置，判断拟吻合的张力，可吸收线缝合固定断端（图 3-14-5）。切开预吻合的两侧断端对系膜侧肠壁（图 3-14-6），进行功能性侧侧吻合（图 3-14-7），检查吻合口内有无活动性出血，闭合公共开口（图 3-14-8），间断缝合加固吻合口（图 3-14-9），完成横结肠 - 乙状结肠吻合（图 3-14-10）。

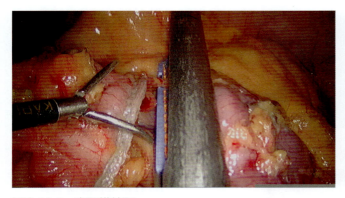

图 3-14-3 离断横结肠

Figure 3-14-3 Dissecting the transverse colon

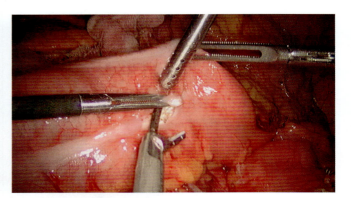

图 3-14-6 切开对系膜侧肠壁

Figure 3-14-6 Lateral dissection of the bowel wall against the mesentery

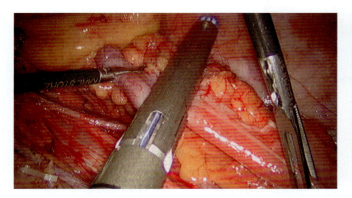

图 3-14-4 裸化、离断乙状结肠

Figure 3-14-4 Isolating and dissecting the sigmoid colon

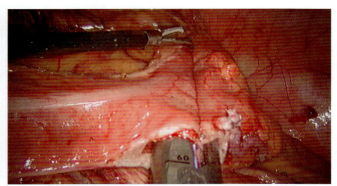

图 3-14-7 功能性侧侧吻合

Figure 3-14-7 Functional side-to-side anastomosis

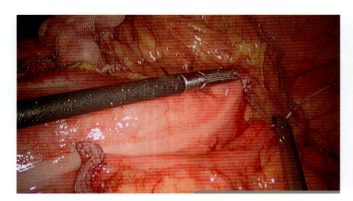

图 3-14-5 判断拟吻合的张力，缝合固定两断端

Figure 3-14-5 Judging the tension of the proposed anastomosis and fixing the two severed ends with sutures

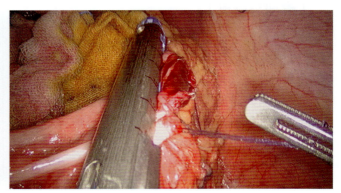

图 3-14-8 闭合公共开口

Figure 3-14-8 Closure of the common opening

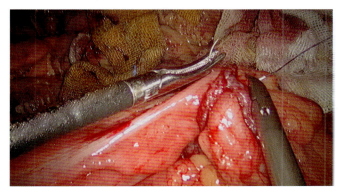

图 3-14-9　间断缝合加固吻合口

Figure 3-14-9　Interrupted sutures to reinforce the anastomosis

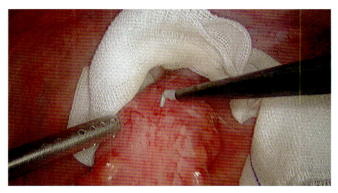

图 3-14-11　在直肠上部切开直肠前壁

Figure 3-14-11　Incision of the anterior rectal wall in the upper rectum

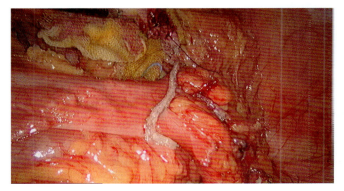

图 3-14-10　横结肠 - 乙状结肠吻合

Figure 3-14-10　Transverse-sigmoid anastomosis

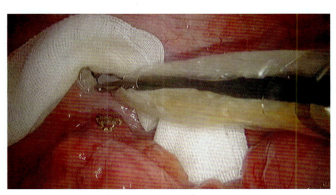

图 3-14-12　从主戳卡孔置入保护套

Figure 3-14-12　Insert the protective sleeve through the main trocar

3. 标本取出　助手经肛门注入稀碘附溶液进行冲洗，并放置碘附纱布。然后，在碘附纱布的位置打开直肠壁，在直肠上部纵行切开一个约 5cm 的切口（图 3-14-11）。通过 12mm 戳卡孔置入保护套（图 3-14-12），然后助手通过直肠上部切口使用卵圆钳将保护套末端从肛门拖出（图 3-14-13）。将腹腔中所有用过的纱布放入保护套中，然后通过保护套取出。在术者和助手的配合下，将标本一端缓慢放入保护套。助手用卵圆钳夹住标本一端，经直肠和肛门将标本慢慢拖出（图 3-14-14、图 3-14-15）。在腹腔镜下纵行连续缝合直肠切口（图 3-14-16），然后缝合包埋浆肌层（图 3-14-17）。用蒸馏水冲洗腹腔（图 3-14-18），经 5mm 戳卡孔置入腹腔引流管（图 3-14-19）。排出腹腔气体，关闭戳卡孔。

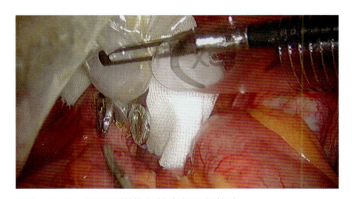

图 3-14-13　用卵圆钳将保护套经肛门拖出

Figure 3-14-13　Dragging the protective sleeve through through the anus

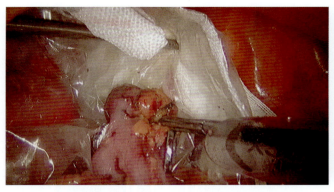

图 3-14-14　卵圆钳夹持住标本一端，经直肠 - 肛门拖出标本
Figure 3-14-14　Oval forceps hold one end of the specimen and drag the specimen through the rectum and anus

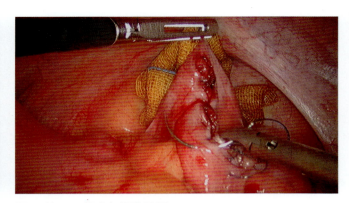

图 3-14-17　缝合包埋浆肌层
Figure 3-14-17　Plasma muscle layer suture embedding

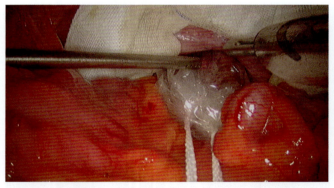

图 3-14-15　助手协助拖出标本
Figure 3-14-15　Assistant assists in dragging out the specimen

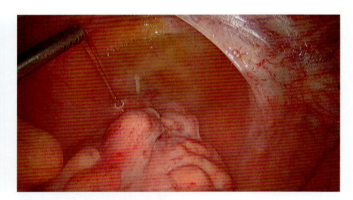

图 3-14-18　注水注气试验
Figure 3-14-18　Air and water injection test

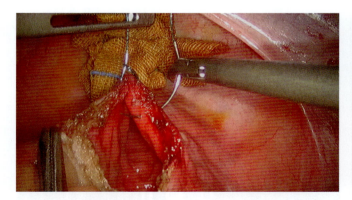

图 3-14-16　缝合直肠前壁切口
Figure 3-14-16　Suturing the anterior rectal wall incision

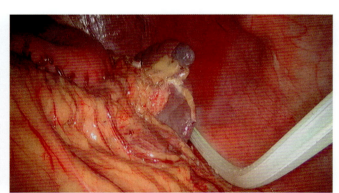

图 3-14-19　置入腹腔引流管
Figure 3-14-19　Placement of abdominal drainage tube

# 第十五节　腹部无辅助切口经阴道取标本的腹腔镜下左半结肠癌根治术

## （CRC-NOSES Ⅶ式）

### 【简介】

　　CRC-NOSES Ⅶ式主要适用于左半结肠肿瘤略大的女性患者。该术式的操作特点：腹腔镜下完全游离切断左半结肠，经阴道将标本取出体外，再进行全腹腔镜下横结肠 - 直肠端端吻合（图 3-15-1，视频 3-14）。与 CRC-NOSES Ⅵ相比，该术式经阴道取标本，由于阴道具有很好的延展性，更容易完成标本取出这一步骤，故适应证略为宽泛，但需要确切地缝合阴道切口。从腹腔镜技术角度而言，CRC-NOSES Ⅶ式的操作难点包括左半结肠系膜的完整游离，系膜根部淋巴结清扫，以及结肠脾曲的游离。从 NOSES 技术角度而言，CRC-NOSES Ⅶ式的操作难点包括经阴道取出标本，全腹腔镜下消化道重建，阴道切口缝合，以及无菌术、无瘤操作的严格把控等。

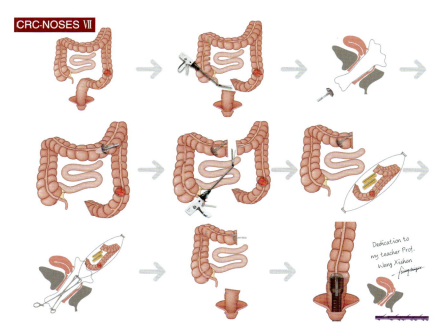

图 3-15-1　CRC-NOSES Ⅶ式标本取出及消化道重建的主要手术步骤

Figure 3-15-1　The main surgical procedures of specimen extraction and digestive tract reconstruction in CRC-NOSES Ⅶ

视频 3-14　CRC-NOSES Ⅶ式
Video 3-14　CRC-NOSES Ⅶ

## 一、适应证与禁忌证

### 【适应证】

　　1. 肿瘤位于横结肠近脾曲、结肠脾曲、降结肠和乙状结肠近端。

　　2. 肿瘤环周直径 <5cm 为宜。

　　3. 肿瘤未侵出浆膜为宜。

### 【禁忌证】

　　1. 肿瘤环周直径 >5cm 者。

　　2. 肿瘤侵出浆膜。

　　3. 过于肥胖者（BMI>35kg/m$^2$）。

## 二、手术操作步骤、技巧与要点

### 【戳卡位置】

1. 腹腔镜镜头戳卡孔（10mm 戳卡）　脐下 2~3cm 处。
2. 术者主戳卡孔（12mm 戳卡）　麦氏点。

3. 术者辅助戳卡孔（5mm 戳卡）　脐上方 10cm 水平与右腹直肌外缘交叉处的横结肠体表投影区。
4. 助手主戳卡孔（5mm 戳卡）　脐上方 10cm 水平与左锁骨中线交叉处。
5. 助手辅助戳卡孔（5mm 戳卡）　反麦氏点（图 3-15-2）。

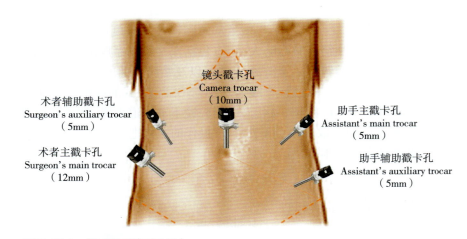

图 3-15-2　戳卡位置（五孔法）

Figure 3-15-2　Trocar placement（five-port method）

### 【探查】

1. 常规探查　观察各脏器及腹膜表面有无种植转移等病变。
2. 肿瘤探查　根据肿瘤的位置、大小、侵犯深度，确定手术的可行性。
3. 解剖结构的判定　①结肠解剖结构，即结肠脾曲游离后，结肠脾曲下拉的长度，根据其系膜血管弓的情况，判断能否有足够的长度进行镜下吻合；②经阴道行指诊，了解阴道后穹隆的状态是否适合切开并取标本。

### 【解剖与分离】

1. 肠系膜下血管根部的处理　在肠系膜下动脉的上方、下方、左侧分离出一定空间，双重结扎并切断肠系膜下动脉。
2. 内侧入路的左半结肠系膜游离　提起肠系膜下静脉断端和肠系膜下动脉断端，沿着 Toldt's 筋膜向上、向下、向外游离。
3. 乙状结肠及直肠系膜的处理　横断乙状结肠或直肠系膜，用血管夹夹闭直肠上动静脉远端。

4. 横结肠左侧及结肠脾曲的处理　将横结肠提起，在屈氏韧带外侧肠系膜下静脉断端，裁剪横结肠系膜至肠壁，向左侧分离切断系膜至左结肠旁沟。
5. 打开左结肠旁沟　沿 Toldt's 筋膜，沿着纱布条指示向上打开左结肠旁沟。
6. 肿瘤上方结肠系膜的裁剪与裸化　进一步裁剪系膜，处理边缘血管弓，切断分离至肠壁，裸化肠管 2cm 备用。

### 【标本切除与消化道重建】

1. 标本切除　经术者主戳卡孔置入保护套（图 3-15-3），助手于体外经阴道用膀胱拉钩指示阴道后穹隆（图 3-15-4）。术者用超声刀横行切开阴道后穹隆约 3cm，纵行牵拉扩大切口至 5~6cm（图 3-15-5）。助手经阴道置入卵圆钳将保护套远端拉出，并经保护套置入抵钉座（图 3-15-6）。术者在肿瘤上方预切除线远端纵行切开一小口，用 1/4 碘附纱布对结肠腔内消毒和润滑（图 3-15-7、图 3-15-8），随后助手用吸引器将碘附纱布推入远端肠腔。术者将抵钉座经切口置入近端肠腔（图 3-15-9），并用直线切割闭合器切断近端肠管

（图 3-15-10），至此左半结肠游离于腹腔。助手用卵圆钳夹住标本一端，缓慢将标本经阴道拖出体外（图 3-15-11）。

2. 消化道重建　将抵钉座连接杆从近端结肠断端一角取出（图 3-15-12）。助手经肛门直肠置入环形吻合器，在直肠断端左侧角旋出吻合器穿刺针（图 3-15-13），完成结肠 - 直肠端端吻合（图 3-15-14）。检查吻合口上下切缘完整性，"危险三角区"（图 3-15-15）行 "8" 字缝合。注水注气试验检查吻合口通畅确实（图 3-15-16）。腹腔冲洗后，经腹壁放置两根引流管（图 3-15-17）。

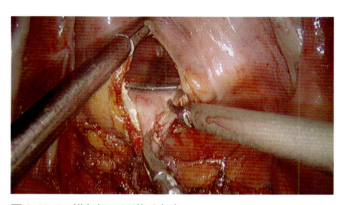

图 3-15-5　横行切开阴道后穹隆

Figure 3-15-5　Transverse incision of the posterior vaginal fornix

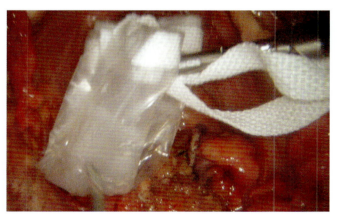

图 3-15-3　经主戳卡孔置入保护套

Figure 3-15-3　Placement of a protective sleeve through the surgeon's main trocar

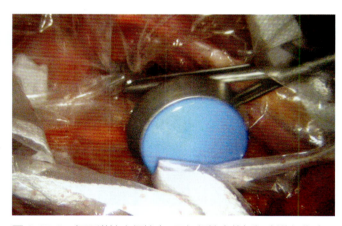

图 3-15-6　经阴道拉出保护套，再经保护套将抵钉座送入盆腔

Figure 3-15-6　Transvaginal pull-out of the protective sleeve and transvaginal delivery of the anvil into the pelvic cavity

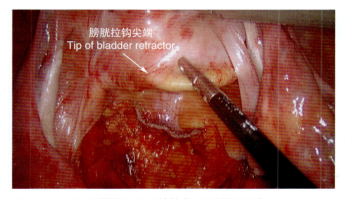

图 3-15-4　经阴道置入膀胱拉钩指示阴道后穹隆

Figure 3-15-4　Transvaginal placement of a bladder hook to indicate the posterior vaginal fornix

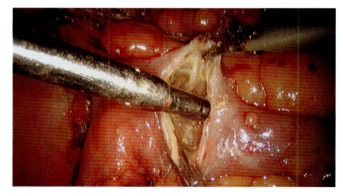

图 3-15-7　及时吸引肠腔内容物

Figure 3-15-7　Timely suction of the bowel contents

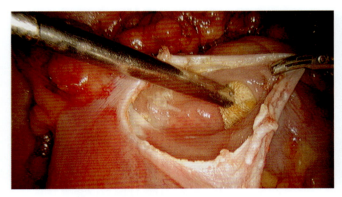

图 3-15-8　碘附纱布进行肠腔内消毒

Figure 3-15-8　Sterilisation of the intestinal lumen with the iodoform gauze

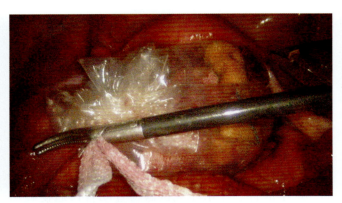

图 3-15-11　经阴道将纱布及拖出体外

Figure 3-15-11　Transvaginal pulling of gauze and specimen out of the body

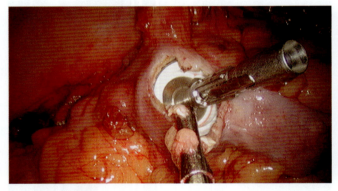

图 3-15-9　将抵钉座送入近端横结肠内

Figure 3-15-9　Delivery of the anvil into the proximal transverse colon

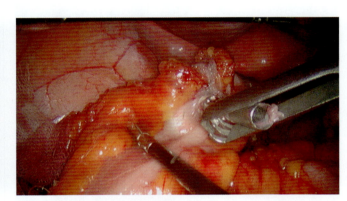

图 3-15-12　取出抵钉座连接杆

Figure 3-15-12　Removing the Nail Seat Attachment Bar

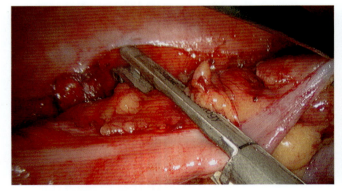

图 3-15-10　闭合切断横结肠肠管

Figure 3-15-10　Closure and severing of the transverse colon tube

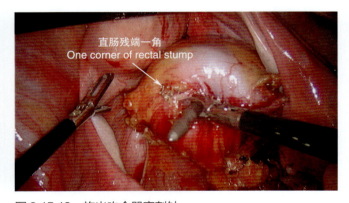

图 3-15-13　旋出吻合器穿刺针

Figure 3-15-13　Threading the anastomotic needle

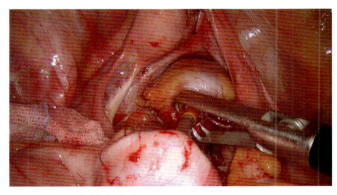

图 3-15-14　连接吻合器

Figure 3-15-14　Connecting the staple

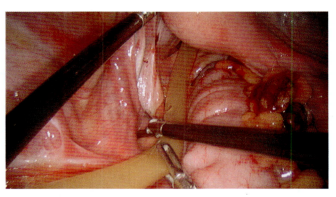

图 3-15-17　置入引流管

Figure 3-15-17　Placing drainage tubes

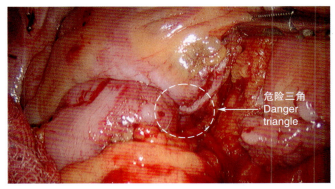

危险三角
Danger
triangle

图 3-15-15　"危险三角区"

Figure 3-15-15　"Danger triangle"

3. 关闭戳卡孔,缝合阴道切口　摆放好引流管,排出腹腔内气体,关闭戳卡孔,腹腔镜下或体外缝合阴道切口。体外缝合的步骤是:拉开阴道切口,用两把 Allis 钳提起切口的前后壁,用可吸收线间断缝合即可(图 3-15-18)。

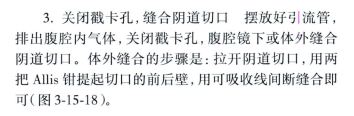

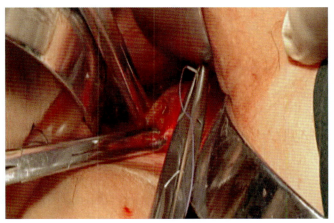

图 3-15-18　体外间断缝合阴道切口

Figure 3-15-18　In vitro interrupted suture closure of the vaginal incision

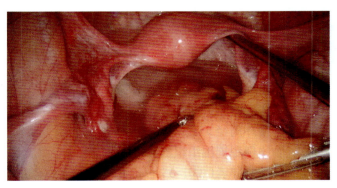

图 3-15-16　注水注气试验检查吻合口

Figure 3-15-16　Air and water injection test

## 第十六节　腹部无辅助切口经阴道拖出标本的腹腔镜下右半结肠癌根治术

### （CRC-NOSES Ⅷ式A法）

### 【简介】

右半结肠毗邻脏器多、血管关系复杂，解剖变异大，因此 CRC-NOSES Ⅷ式也是 NOSES 系列中难度较大的一种术式。右半结肠标本多经阴道拖出，CRC-NOSES Ⅷ式A法的操作特点：在腹腔内完全游离切断右半结肠，经阴道将标本取出体外，再进行腹腔镜下末端回肠 - 横结肠功能性端端吻合（图 3-16-1，视频 3-15）。CRC-NOSES Ⅷ式A法在腹腔镜下进行消化道重建，重建难度超过其他术式，对术者和助手的要求较高，在标本经阴道取出的过程中，无菌术、无瘤操作的精准运用至关重要。

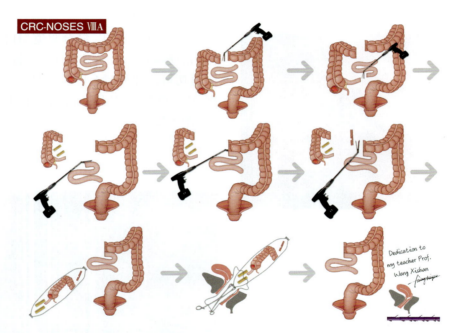

图 3-16-1　CRC-NOSES Ⅷ式A法标本取出及消化道重建的主要手术步骤

Figure 3-16-1　The main surgical procedures of specimen extraction and digestive tract reconstruction in CRC-NOSES ⅧA

视频 3-15　CRC-NOSES Ⅷ式A法
Video 3-15　CRC-NOSES ⅧA

## 一、适应证和禁忌证

### 【适应证】

1. 女性右半结肠肿瘤。
2. 肿瘤环周径 <5cm 为宜。
3. 肿瘤未侵出浆膜为宜。

### 【禁忌证】

1. 肿瘤环周径 >5cm。
2. 肿瘤侵犯周围组织器官。
3. 过于肥胖者（BMI>35kg/m$^2$）。
4. 男性右半结肠癌。

## 二、手术操作步骤、技巧与要点

### 【戳卡位置】

1. 腹腔镜镜头戳卡孔（10mm 戳卡）　脐至脐下方

5cm 的范围内均可。

2. 术者主戳卡孔（12mm 戳卡）　左上腹中部，腹直肌外缘。

3. 术者辅助戳卡孔（5mm 戳卡）　左下腹，与腹腔镜镜头戳卡孔不在同一水平线。

4. 助手主戳卡孔（12mm 戳卡）　麦氏点，便于消化道重建时放入直线切割闭合器。

5. 助手辅助戳卡孔（5mm 戳卡）　右上腹，右锁骨中线与横结肠投影区交叉处（图 3-16-2）。

【探查】

1. 常规探查　腹腔镜下常规探查肝脏、胆囊、胃、脾脏、结肠、小肠、大网膜和盆腔有无肿瘤种植和腹水。

2. 肿瘤探查　肿瘤位于右半结肠，未侵出浆膜，肿瘤环周直径 <5cm 为宜。

3. 解剖结构的判定　右半结肠切除术较为复杂，毗邻脏器较多，需判定回结肠动静脉、右结肠动静脉、中结肠动静脉的解剖位置及分支关系，尤其中结肠动静脉，血管分支较多，如果处理困难，建议在中结肠动静脉根部结扎并切断。此外，还需判定横结肠游离后可否行腹腔镜下回肠 - 横结肠功能性端端吻合。因为目前设备、技术条件无法在腹腔镜下应用环形吻合器完成回肠 - 横结肠端端或侧端吻合，若横结肠系膜过短，勿实施 CRC-NOSES Ⅷ式 A 法手术。

【解剖与分离】

1. 回结肠动静脉根部的处理　术者左手持钳，沿肠系膜上静脉充分显露系膜表面。此时可见回结肠动静脉与肠系膜上静脉夹角有一凹陷薄弱处，用超声刀打开此处系膜，慢慢分离裸化血管。沿 Toldt's 间隙向上、向外分离，呈洞穴状，向上游离可见十二指肠，表明间隙正确。在回结肠动静脉根部尽量打开肠系膜上静脉鞘，向上分离，在其右侧与后方相贯通。裸化回结肠动静脉根部，清扫纤维结缔组织，用血管夹双重结扎并切断。

2. 右结肠动静脉根部的处理　术者沿着 Toldt's 筋膜在十二指肠表面游离，仔细分离后可见右结肠静脉、胃网膜右静脉、Henle 干（胃结肠干）共同汇合进入肠系膜上静脉，结扎并切断右结肠静脉，沿肠系膜上静脉向上分离可见右结肠动脉，在根部双重结扎并切断。

3. 中结肠动静脉根部的处理　在分离右结肠动静脉之后，继续向上分离。在胰颈表面透过一层薄膜可见胃窦后壁即停止分离，随即垫一块小纱布。沿肠系膜上静脉向上分离，于胰腺下缘双重结扎并切断中结肠动静脉。至此，供应右半结肠的血管均离断。

4. 结肠系膜的游离　继续沿 Toldt's 间隙进一步向外、向上及向下分离，可见整个游离的表面光滑、平整、干净。

5. 回肠系膜的处理　当盲肠下部腹膜贯穿后，尽量打开其根部附着的筋膜，使回肠的游离度变大一些，便于腹腔镜下肠管吻合。助手提起末端回肠，术者用超声刀裁剪回肠系膜，注意系膜的血运走行与方向。切割至末端回肠壁，向近端裸化 2cm 肠管。

6. 大网膜及第 6 组淋巴结的处理　判断横结肠预切除线，游离大网膜。用超声刀裁剪右侧大网膜至横结肠肠壁。将其拉向右侧腹腔，助手左手持钳提起胃壁，可见胃网膜右动静脉走行。从横结肠向其分离切断胃结肠韧带进入网膜腔。沿胃网膜右动静脉血管

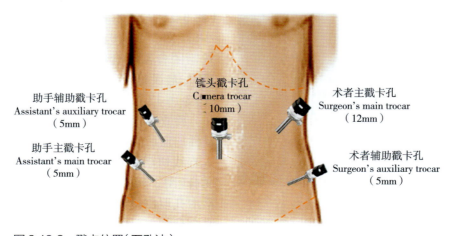

图 3-16-2　戳卡位置（五孔法）
Figure 3-16-2　Trocar placemert（five-port method）

弓外缘向右侧分离切断，分离至胰头可见胃网膜右静脉与 Henle 干，同时与下方游离间隙贯通。

7. 横结肠系膜的处理　胃窦十二指肠胰头区离断后，可见垫于系膜后方的纱布，将系膜横行切开，向横结肠系膜无血管方向分离。结扎离断边缘血管，进一步向横结肠预切除线分离，裸化肠壁 1cm。

**【标本切除与消化道重建】**

1. 标本切除　用直线闭合切割器在横结肠预切除线处缝合切割肠管（图 3-16-3），将近端翻向右下腹，此时横结肠在右结肠旁沟及肝下的附着处清晰可见，并可见后方垫的纱布。用超声刀在纱布的指示和保护下沿右结肠旁沟向右髂窝分离，直至与下方贯通（图 3-16-4）。在回肠裸化区，可见清晰血运分界线（图 3-16-5），用直线切割闭合器在血运分界线内侧横断回肠（图 3-16-6）。至此，完成右半结肠切除，将标本置于盆腔。

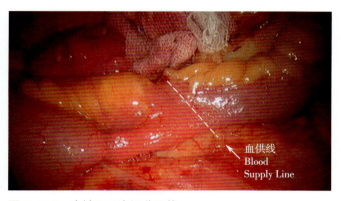

图 3-16-5　末端回肠血运分界线
Figure 3-16-5　Blood supply line of the terminal ileum

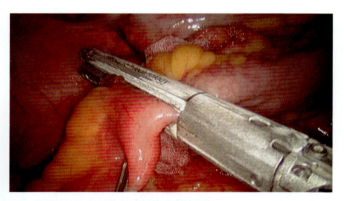

图 3-16-6　在血运分界线内侧横断回肠
Figure 3-16-6　Transects the ileum medial to the blood supply line

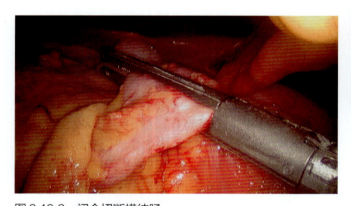

图 3-16-3　闭合切断横结肠
Figure 3-16-3　Closure and transection of the transverse colon

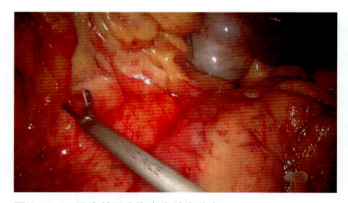

图 3-16-4　沿右结肠旁沟向右髂窝分离
Figure 3-16-4　Dissection along the right paracolic sulcus to the right iliac fossa

2. 消化道重建　术者将横结肠拉直摆放，并将末端回肠拉至上腹部与横结肠平行摆放（图 3-16-7）。用剪刀将回肠末端一角沿吻合钉剪开 5mm 小口（图 3-16-8）。助手经右下腹 12mm 戳卡孔置入 60mm 直线切割闭合器，将抵钉座置入回肠肠腔内并含住（图 3-16-9）。术者在横结肠断端一角剪开约 10mm 小口（图 3-16-10），助手和术者将结肠提起，将直线切割闭合器钉仓侧置入结肠肠腔内（图 3-16-11），确认无误后击发，完成回肠 - 横结肠侧侧吻合（图 3-16-12）。

检查吻合口有无明显出血（图 3-16-13），确认无活动性出血后，提起断端，术者经左上腹 12mm 戳卡孔置入直线切割闭合器，横行闭合残端，完成功能性端端吻合（图 3-16-14），切下的残端组织用保护套经 12mm 戳卡孔取出。浆肌层缝合回肠横结肠吻合处，以减轻吻合口张力（图 3-16-15）。至此完成右半结肠切除后的消化道重建。

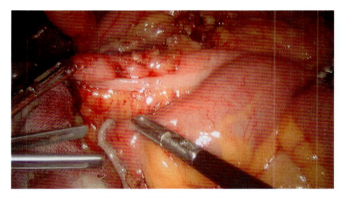

图 3-16-7　将末端回肠与横结肠平行摆放

Figure 3-16-7　Placing the transverse colon parallel to the ileum

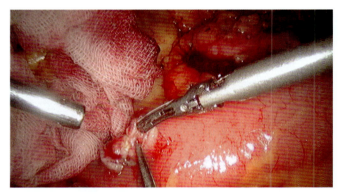

图 3-16-8　剪开末端回肠

Figure 3-16-8　Making an incision at the terminal ileum

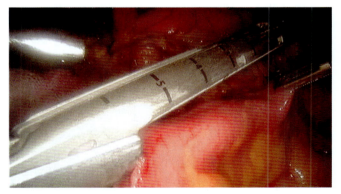

图 3-16-9　将直线切割闭合器抵钉座置入回肠

Figure 3-16-9　Placing the anvil into the ileum lumen

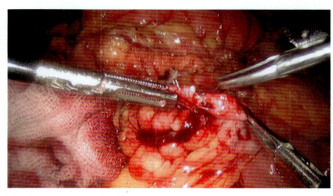

图 3-16-10　剪开横结肠

Figure 3-16-10　Making an incision of the transverse colon

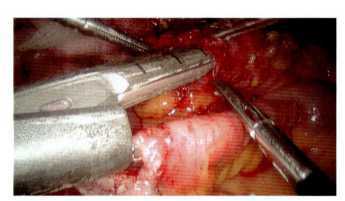

图 3-16-11　将直线切割闭合器钉仓侧置入横结肠

Figure 3-16-11　Placing the cartridge jaw into the colon lumen

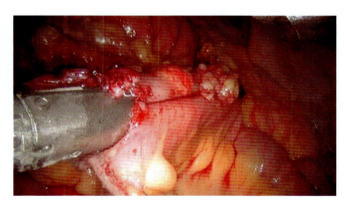

图 3-16-12　回肠 - 横结肠侧侧吻合

Figure 3-16-12　End-to-end anastomosis between the ileum and the transverse colon

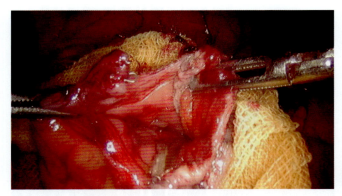

图 3-16-13 检查吻合口有无出血

Figure 3-16-13 Checking the anastomotic bleeding

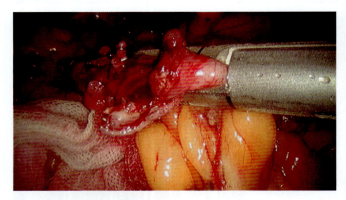

图 3-16-14 横行闭合残端

Figure 3-16-14 Closing the stump transversely

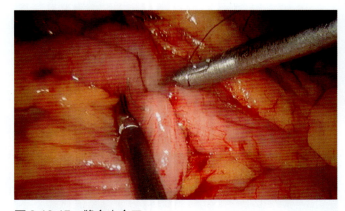

图 3-16-15 缝合吻合口

Figure 3-16-15 Suturing of the anastomosis

3. 标本取出 经左上腹 12mm 戳卡孔置入保护套（图 3-16-16），术者与助手配合，撑开保护套，将腹腔内的纱布及标本置于保护套内（图 3-16-17），扎紧袋口后以 Hem-Lock 夹紧（图 3-16-18）。在切开阴道之前，术者需换位置于患者右侧，同时转换腹腔镜显示器位置，患者体位由头高足低位改为足高头低位。助手于体外用举宫器将子宫抬起，进而充分显露阴道后穹隆（图 3-16-19）。术者用超声刀横行切开阴道 3cm（图 3-16-20），纵行牵拉将切口扩展至 5~6cm。助手于体外用卵圆钳夹持

住标本一端慢慢向外牵拉（图 3-16-21），术者与助手配合将标本和保护套缓缓从阴道拖出，至此标本移出体外（图 3-16-22）。

4. 缝合阴道切口，关闭戳卡孔 助手在阴道后穹隆切口前壁和后壁各置一根 Allis 钳牵拉，切口清晰可见，用可吸收线间断缝合（图 3-16-23、图 3-16-24）。利用右侧两个戳卡孔置入两根引流管于右上腹。

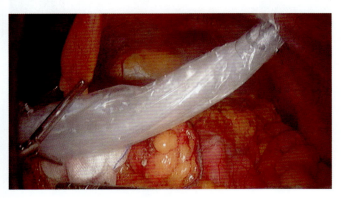

图 3-16-16 经主戳卡孔置入保护套

Figure 3-16-16 Insertion of protective sleeve through the main trocar

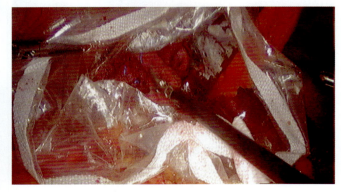

图 3-16-17 纱布及标本置于保护套内

Figure 3-16-17 Placing the gauze and specimen into the protective sleeve

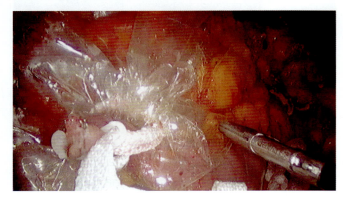

图 3-16-18 扎紧袋口后以 Hem-Lock 夹紧

Figure 3-16-18 After tying the bag opening tightly, clamp it with Hem-Lock

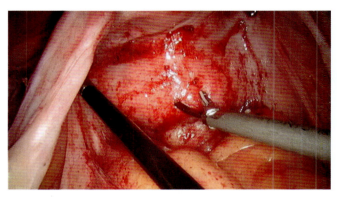

图 3-16-19　显露阴道后穹隆

Figure 3-16-19　Exposing the posterior vaginal fornix

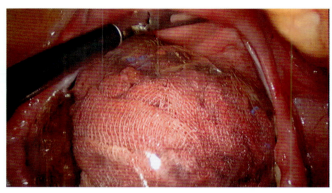

图 3-16-22　经阴道将标本拖出体外

Figure 3-16-22　Pulling the specimen and the protective sleeve out of the body

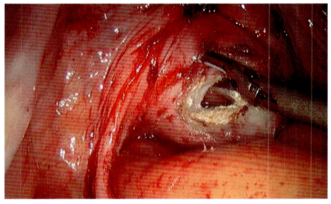

图 3-16-20　切开阴道后穹隆

Figure 3-16-20　Opening the posterior vaginal fornix

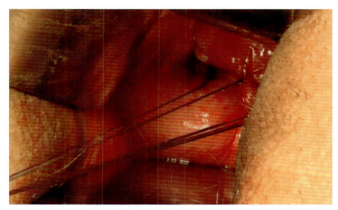

图 3-16-23　充分显露并缝合阴道切口

Figure 3-16-23　Exposing and suturing the vaginal incision

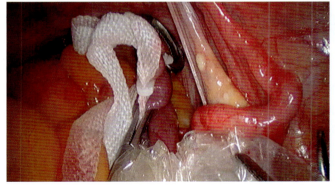

图 3-16-21　经阴道置入卵圆钳夹持内含标本的保护套

Figure 3-16-21　Transvaginal placement of oval forceps to hold a protective sleeve containing a specimen

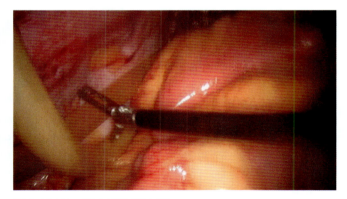

图 3-16-24　置入腹腔引流管

Figure 3-16-24　Placing two drainage tubes in the right upper quadrant

# 第十七节 腹部无辅助切口经直肠切口拖出标本的腹腔镜下右半结肠癌根治术

## （CRC-NOSES Ⅷ式B法）

【简介】

对于女性右半结肠癌患者，可选择 CRC-NOSES Ⅷ式 A 法，但对于男性右半结肠癌患者则可选择 CRC-NOSES Ⅷ式 B 法（图 3-17-1，视频 3-16）。由于右半结肠毗邻脏器多、血管关系复杂、解剖变异大，且需要自直肠上段另开切口取标本，并于腹腔镜下完成该切口的闭合，因此，该术式是 NOSES 系列中难度较

大、风险大、损伤效益比大的一种术式。该术式的操作特点：腹腔内完全游离切断右半结肠，在腹腔镜下进行末端回肠与横结肠的消化道重建，再经直肠切口拖出标本。在标本经直肠取出的过程中，无菌术、无瘤操作的精准运用及该术式适应证的精准把握至关重要。与 CRC-NOSES Ⅷ式 A 法相比，该术式需要更严格地把握适应证，具有清晰的手术思路，以及娴熟的操作技巧。

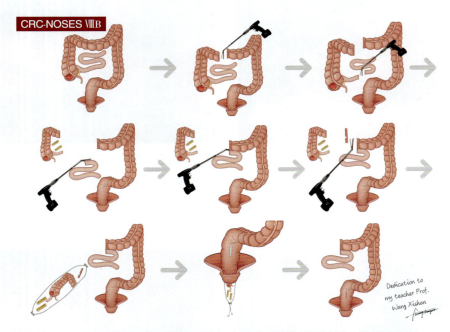

图 3-17-1　CRC-NOSES Ⅷ式 B 法标本取出及消化道重建的主要手术步骤

Figure 3-17-1　The main surgical procedures of specimen extraction and digestive tract reconstruction in CRC-NOSES ⅧB

视频 3-16　CRC-NOSES Ⅷ式 B 法
Video 3-16　CRC-NOSES ⅧB

## 一、适应证与禁忌证

### 【适应证】

1. 男性右半结肠癌或良性肿瘤。

2. 肿瘤环周直径 <3cm 为宜。

3. 肿瘤不侵出浆膜为宜。

### 【禁忌证】

1. 肿瘤环周直径 >3cm。

2. 肿瘤侵犯周围组织器官。

3. 曾行直肠、肛门手术或因直肠肛门疾病导致直肠中下段及肛门狭窄者。

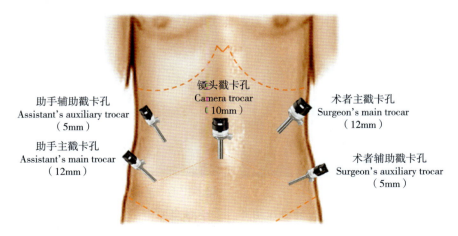

图 3-17-2　戳卡位置（五孔法）

Figure 3-17-2　Trocar placement( five-port method )

血管方向分离、切断胃结肠韧带，进入网膜腔。沿胃网膜右动静脉血管弓外缘向右侧分离切断，分离至胰头可见胃网膜右静脉与 Henle 干，同时与下方游离间隙贯通。

7. 横结肠系膜的处理　在胃窦十二指肠胰头区离断系膜后，将系膜横行切开，向横结肠系膜无血管方向分离。结扎离断边缘血管，进一步向横结肠预切除线分离，裸化肠壁1cm。

**【标本切除与消化道重建】**

1. 标本切除　用直线切割闭合器在横结肠预定线处切割闭合肠管（图 3-17-3），将近端翻向右下腹，此时横结肠在右结肠旁沟及肝下的附着处清晰可见。用超声刀沿右结肠旁沟向右髂窝分离，直至与下方贯通。在回肠裸化区，可见清晰血运分界线（图 3-17-4），用直线切割闭合器在血运分界线内侧横断回肠（图 3-17-5）。至此，完成右半结肠切除，将标本置于标本袋中，置于盆腔。

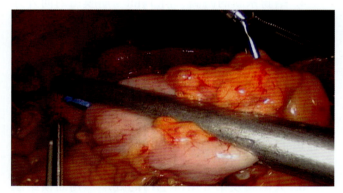

图 3-17-3　切割闭合横结肠
Figure 3-17-3　Cutting and closing transverse colon

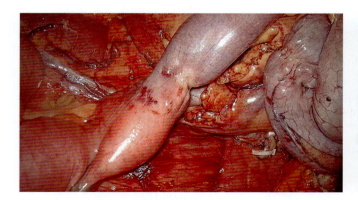

图 3-17-4　末端回肠血运分界线
Figure 3-17-4　Tie the specimen bag tightly and hold it with oval pliers to pull it out of the body

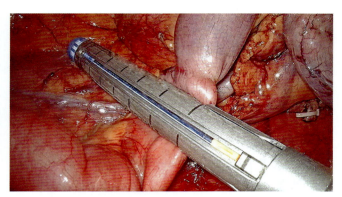

图 3-17-5　切割闭合回肠
Figure 3-17-5　Cutting and closing the ileum

2. 消化道重建　将横结肠拉直摆放，并将末端回肠拉至上腹部与横结肠重叠摆放（图 3-17-6）。检查两侧肠管血运，估计吻合口两侧张力。分别于末端回肠断端对系膜侧肠壁与相应位置的横结肠对系膜侧肠壁做 1cm 切口（图 3-17-7、图 3-17-8），碘附纱布消毒肠腔。右下腹戳卡孔更换为 12mm 戳卡孔，并置入直线切割闭合器，于一侧肠腔内置入直线切割闭合器钉仓，暂时关闭钳口，术者和助手抓取另一侧肠腔，松开钳口，将肠管套上抵钉座，进行必要的调整，确认无误后击发，完成回肠 - 横结肠功能性端端吻合（图 3-17-9）。

碘附纱布擦拭肠腔，检查吻合口完整性。确认无出血后，术者和助手分别牵拉缝线尾端，使肠管断端远离对侧肠壁，并呈直线，用直线切割闭合器闭合两侧肠管共同开口，完成回肠 - 横结肠功能性端端吻合（图 3-17-10）。使用可吸收线加固缝合吻合口。

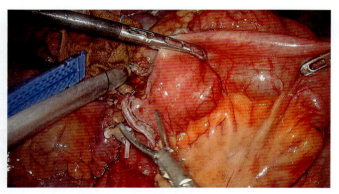

图 3-17-6　末端回肠与横结肠重叠摆放
Figure 3-17-6　Placing the transverse colon overlapping with the ileum

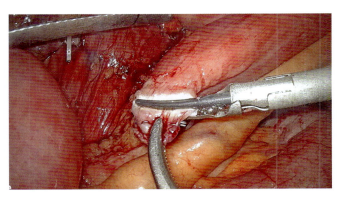

图 3-17-7　末端回肠断端对系膜侧肠壁做 1cm 切口

Figure 3-17-7　Making a 1cm incision at the antimesenteric border of the terminal ileum

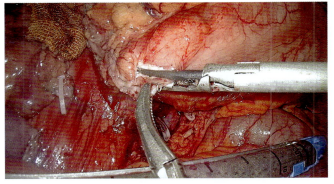

图 3-17-8　相应位置的横结肠对系膜侧肠壁做 1cm 切口

Figure 3-17-8　Making a 1cm incision at the antimesenteric border of the transverse colon

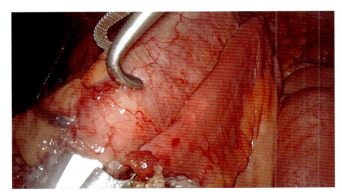

图 3-17-9　完成回肠 - 横结肠端端吻合

Figure 3-17-9　End-to-end anastomosis between the ileum and transverse colon

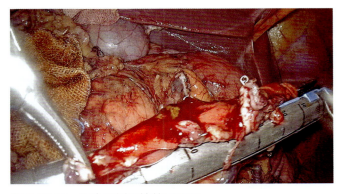

图 3-17-10　闭合两侧肠管共同开口

Figure 3-17-10　Closure of the common opening of the intestinal canal on both sides

3. 标本取出　经 12mm 戳卡孔将保护套置入腹腔（图 3-17-11），将标本置入保护套中并收紧（图 3-17-12）。在切开直肠壁之前，术者需换位置于患者右侧，同时转换腹腔镜显示器位置，患者体位由头高足低位改为足高头低位。助手经肛门用稀碘附溶液充分冲洗直肠后，选择直肠上段长约 3cm 纵行开口（图 3-17-13），第二助手经肛门至直肠上段开口，用卵圆钳将保护套及标本经肛门拖出（图 3-17-14 ~ 图 3-17-16）。

碘附纱布擦拭肠腔，检查吻合口内腔有无活动性出血，确认无出血后，使用可吸收线在腹腔镜下全层缝合切口。腹腔镜下浆肌层缝合包埋吻合口（图 3-17-17）。蒸馏水冲洗腹腔，经右侧 12mm 戳卡孔留置腹腔引流管一根。停止气腹，排出腹腔气体，关闭戳卡孔。

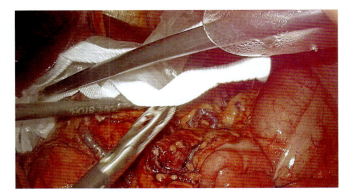

图 3-17-11　经 12mm 戳卡孔将保护套置入腹腔

Figure 3-17-11　Insertion of protective sleeve through 12mm trocar port

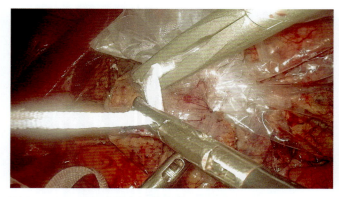

图 3-17-12　将标本置入保护套中

Figure 3-17-12　Placing the specimen into the protective sleeve

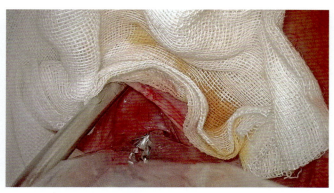

图 3-17-15　将标本缓慢拖出

Figure 3-17-15　Dragging the specimen out slowly

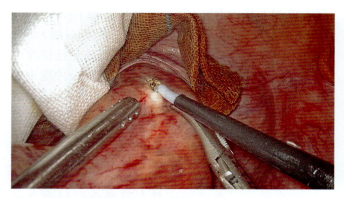

图 3-17-13　卵圆钳经肛门至直肠上段开口

Figure 3-17-13　Inserting oval forceps through the anus to the opening of the upper rectum

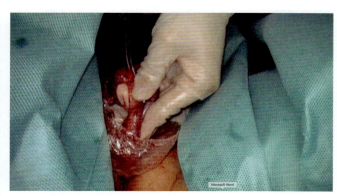

图 3-17-16　标本移出体外

Figure 3-17-16　Removing the specimen out of the body

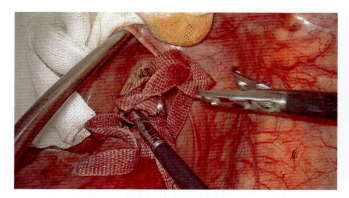

图 3-17-14　将标本袋束紧并用卵圆钳夹持拉出体外

Figure 3-17-14　Tightening the specimen bag and extracting it out of the body with an oval forceps

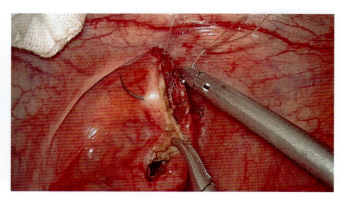

图 3-17-17　缝合直肠切口

Figure 3-17-17　Suturing the rectal incision

## 第十八节　腹部无辅助切口经结肠拖出标本的腹腔镜下右半结肠癌根治术

### （CRC-NOSES Ⅷ式C法）

【简介】

CRC-NOSES Ⅷ式C法主要适用于肿瘤不大的右半结肠切除术患者。CRC-NOSES Ⅷ式C法的操作特点：①腹腔镜右半结肠根治性切除；②结肠镜辅助下经左半横结肠、结肠脾曲、降结肠、乙状结肠、直肠、肛门取出标本；③腹腔镜下行横结肠 - 回肠功能性侧侧顺行吻合（图 3-18-1，视频 3-17）。对于严格筛选的右半结肠肿瘤患者，腹部无辅助切口经结肠 - 直肠 - 肛门取出标本的腹腔镜下右半结肠癌根治术 CRC-NOSES Ⅷ式C法是安全可行的。

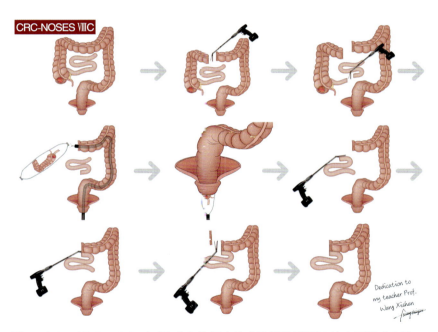

图 3-18-1　CRC-NOSES Ⅷ式C法标本取出及消化道重建的主要手术步骤
Figure 3-18-1　9 CRC-NOSES ⅧC

视频 3-17　CRC-NOSES Ⅷ式C法
Video 3-17　CRC-NOSES ⅧC

## 一、适应证与禁忌证

【适应证】

1. 回盲部、升结肠、结肠肝曲及右半横结肠的早期肿瘤。

2. 肿瘤环周直径不超过 5cm。

3. 肿瘤未侵出浆膜为宜。

【禁忌证】

1. 肿瘤体积过大，取出有困难者。

2. 肿瘤侵出浆膜外并侵犯邻近器官和组织。

3. 过于肥胖者（BMI>30kg/m²）。

## 二、手术操作步骤、技巧与要点

【戳卡位置】

1. 腹腔镜镜头戳卡孔（10mm 戳卡）　脐至脐下方 5cm 的范围均可。

2. 术者主戳卡孔（12mm 戳卡）　左上腹中部，腹直肌外缘。

3. 术者辅助戳卡孔（5mm 戳卡）　左下腹，与腹腔镜镜头戳卡孔不在同一水平线处。

4. 助手主戳卡孔（10mm 戳卡）　麦氏点，兼顾术毕放置引流管。

5. 助手辅助戳卡孔（5mm 戳卡）　右上腹，右锁骨中线与横结肠投影区交叉处（图 3-18-2）。

### 【手术团队站位】

右半结肠切除时，术者站位于患者左侧，助手站位于患者右侧，扶镜手站位于患者两腿之间。标本取出与消化道重建时，术者站位于患者右侧，助手站位于患者左侧，扶镜手站位于术者同侧，内镜医生与助手站位于患者两腿之间。

### 【探查】

1. 常规探查　进镜至腹腔，探查肝脏、胆囊、胃、脾脏、结肠、小肠、大网膜和盆腔有无肿瘤种植。

2. 肿瘤探查　肿瘤的具体位置、大小。

3. 解剖结构的判定　探查右半结肠系膜、大网膜和肠脂垂肥厚程度及结肠肠管粗细，判定是否适合经结肠、直肠、肛门拖出体外。

### 【解剖与分离】

1. 标记右半结肠的切除范围　提起回结肠动静脉系膜，可见其与肠系膜上静脉夹角下方有一凹陷薄弱处，用超声刀在该薄弱处行第一刀切割，向回肠末端切开系膜表层至回肠预切除线（距离回盲部约 15cm），向上切开系膜表层至横结肠中点拟切断处，依此标记右半结肠切除的范围。

2. 回结肠动静脉根部的解剖与离断　用超声刀沿 Toldt's 间隙向上、向外分离，向上游离可见十二指肠，清除回结肠动静脉根部周围的脂肪、结缔组织和淋巴结，然后 Hem-Lock 夹分别结扎，并离断回结肠动脉和静脉。

3. 解剖右结肠动静脉和中结肠动静脉　继续沿肠系膜上静脉前壁向头侧分离。清除中结肠动静脉根部周围的脂肪和淋巴结后，分别结扎并离断中结肠动脉和静脉的右支。Helen 干由胃网膜右静脉和右结肠静脉汇合而成。结扎和离断右结肠静脉。右结肠动脉起源多样，41% 的患者起源于肠系膜上动脉，18% 的患者没有右结肠动脉。

4. 解剖右结肠系膜和横结肠系膜　根据 CME 原则，从内侧向外侧游离右结肠系膜，并沿十二指肠和胰腺头部表面分离。助手用肠钳将横结肠挑起，在横结肠系膜显露清楚的情况下，术者切开横结肠中段系膜无血管区，离断朝向横结肠中段肠壁的血管。裸化横结肠长度 2～3cm。

5. 解剖大网膜和肝结肠韧带　用超声刀沿横结肠中点边缘切开大网膜。助手从腹侧抬起胃前壁。这样，胃结肠韧带被置于张力之下，可以更容易地分开。最初分离胃结肠韧带始于横结肠中部，随后进入网膜囊。沿胃网膜右动脉外缘从中间向右继续分离，继续向外侧切开肝结肠韧带和右半结肠外侧韧带。

6. 裁剪回结肠系膜和游离回盲部腹膜　助手用肠钳提起回肠末端，沿手术开始标记的切除范围，裁剪肠系膜，直到距离回盲部约 15cm 的末端回肠肠壁，裸化回肠 1～2cm。提起回盲部，向左、向上切开回盲部下外侧腹膜，并沿升结肠外侧向上、向内游离，与上方、内侧汇合，至此，右半结肠完全游离。

7. 离断回肠末端与右半结肠　经 12mm 戳卡孔将保护套置入腹腔。右半结肠完全游离后，可见回肠末端明显的缺血线，使用 60mm 直线切割闭合器于缺血线近端拟切除处切断闭合末段回肠。用碘溶液小纱布消毒末端回肠断端，然后，将小纱布放入保护套中。内镜医生经肛门伸入结肠镜，到达升结肠确认升结肠病变

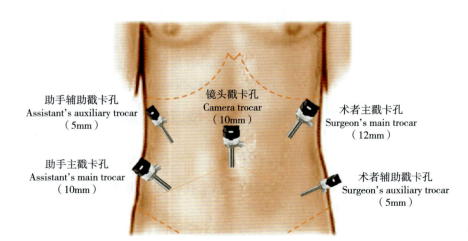

助手辅助戳卡孔
Assistant's auxiliary trocar
（5mm）

镜头戳卡孔
Camera trocar
（10mm）

术者主戳卡孔
Surgeon's main trocar
（12mm）

助手主戳卡孔
Assistant's main trocar
（10mm）

术者辅助戳卡孔
Surgeon's auxiliary trocar
（5mm）

图 3-18-2　戳卡位置（五孔法）

Figure 3-18-2　Trocar placement（five-port method）

后,使用 60mm 直线切割闭合器于缺血线内侧切断闭合横结肠中部,用碘溶液小纱布消毒横结肠残端。

【标本取出与消化道重建】

1. 标本取出　将右半结肠切除标本置入保护套内(图 3-18-3)。内镜医生将结肠镜通过肛门送达横结肠闭合端(图 3-18-4)。结肠镜灌肠后,用超声刀切开横结肠残端,用碘溶液小纱布消毒。伸出结肠镜的前端,再次用碘溶液小纱布消毒(图 3-18-5),同时抽吸溢出的肠液,内镜医生张开异物钳夹住装有标本的保护套(图 3-18-6),在腹腔镜无损伤钳的帮助下,将装有右半结肠的保护套移入左半结肠,缓慢通过横结肠左半部、结肠脾曲、降结肠、乙状结肠、直肠,最后经肛门取出(图 3-18-7 ~ 图 3-18-11)。

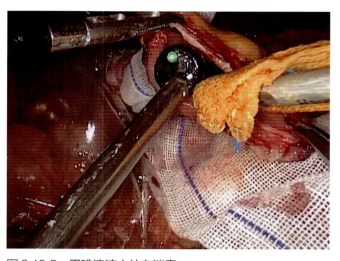

图 3-18-5　用碘溶液小纱布消毒
Figure 3-18-5　Disinfection with the povidone gauze

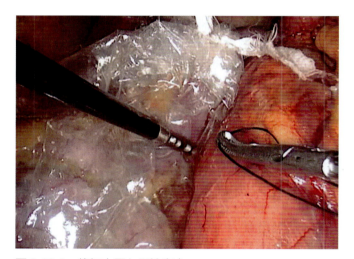

图 3-18-3　将标本置入保护套中
Figure 3-18-3　Placing the specimen into the protective sleeve

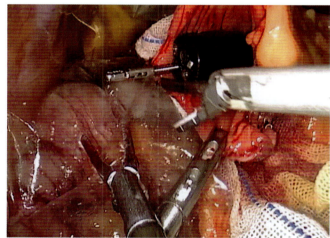

图 3-18-6　伸出结肠镜异物钳,钳夹住保护套
Figure 3-18-6　Clamping the protective sleeve with endoscopic foreign body forceps

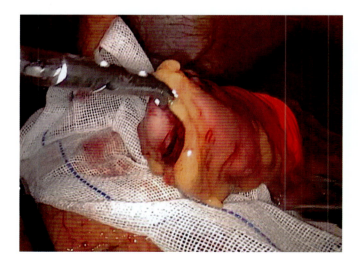

图 3-18-4　将结肠镜从肛门送入横结肠
Figure 3-18-4　The colonoscopy reaches the closed transverse colon through the anus

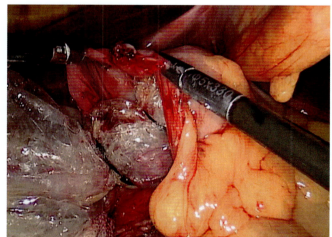

图 3-18-7　将标本拖入左半结肠
Figure 3-18-7　Dragging the specimen into the left-sided colon

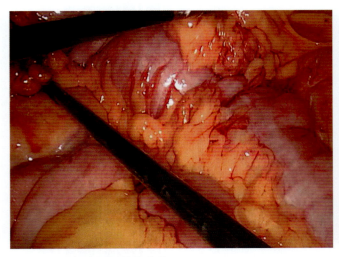

图 3-18-8　标本通过结肠脾曲

Figure 3-18-8　Passing the splenic flexure of the colon

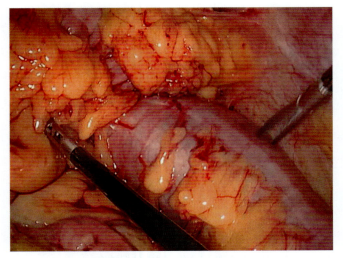

图 3-18-9　标本到达降结肠

Figure 3-18-9　Arriving at the descending colon

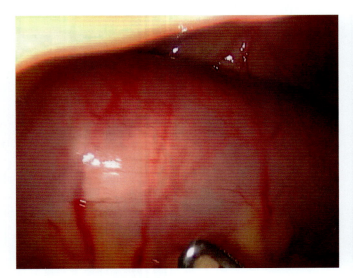

图 3-18-10　标本进入乙状结肠

Figure 3-18-10　Entering the sigmoid colon

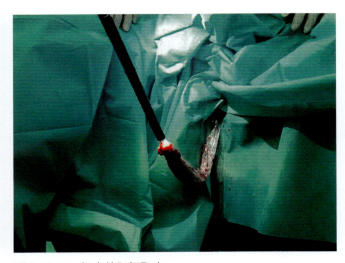

图 3-18-11　标本从肛门取出

Figure 3-18-11　Removing the specimen from the anus

2. 消化道重建　将打开的横结肠残端用 60mm 直线切割闭合器切断闭合（图 3-18-12），切除的残端组织放入保护套中。将末段回肠提拉到上腹部，使其与横结肠断端处肠管平行放置。用超声刀在末端回肠断端的对系膜侧肠壁切开一小口，并用碘溶液小纱布消毒（图 3-18-13）。同样，在距断端约 6cm 的横结肠对系膜侧肠壁切开一小切口（图 3-18-14），将碘溶液小纱布放入打开的肠腔内进行消毒（图 3-18-15）。采用 60mm 直线切割闭合器对末段回肠与横结肠进行功能性侧侧顺行吻合（图 3-18-16）。仔细检查肠腔共同开口，确认无出血，再次用碘溶液小纱布消毒肠腔共同开口（图 3-18-17），用可吸收线缝合共同开口并加固吻合口浆肌层（图 3-18-18），以减少吻合口张力。最后，缝合关闭系膜裂孔，以避免腹内疝（图 3-18-19）。

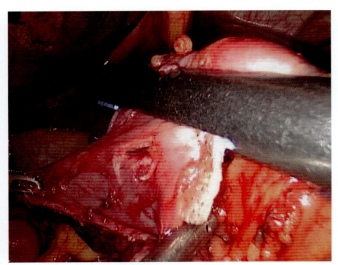

图 3-18-12　闭合横结肠断端

Figure 3-18-12　Closing the opening of the transverse colon

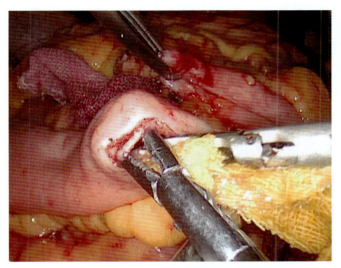

图 3-18-13　在末端回肠断端对系膜侧肠壁切开一小口

Figure 3-18-13　Making a little incision at the antime-senteric border of the terminal ileum stump

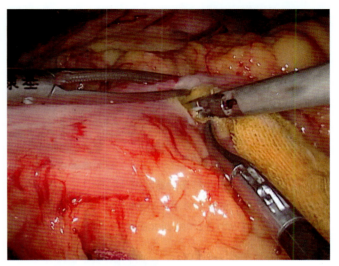

图 3-18-15　用碘溶液小纱布消毒结肠肠腔

Figure 3-18-15　Disinfecting the bowel lumen with a small piece of povidone gauze

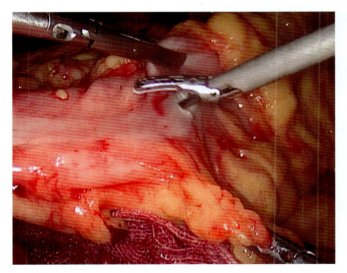

图 3-18-14　在横结肠对系膜侧肠壁切开一小口

Figure 3-18-14　Making a little incision at the antime-senteric border of the transverse colon

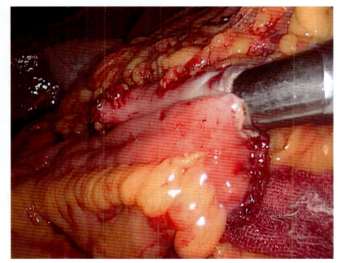

图 3-18-16　直线切割闭合器行侧侧吻合

Figure 3-18-16　Side-to-side anastomosed with a linear cutting stapler

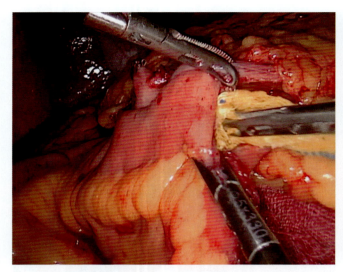

图 3-18-17　用碘溶液小纱布消毒肠腔共同开口
Figure 3-18-17　Sterilize the common opening of the intestinal lumen with a small piece of povidone gauze

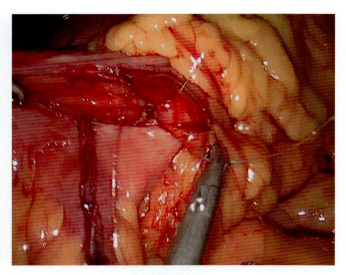

图 3-18-18　用可吸收线关闭吻合口
Figure 3-18-18　Closing the anastomosis with an absorbable suture

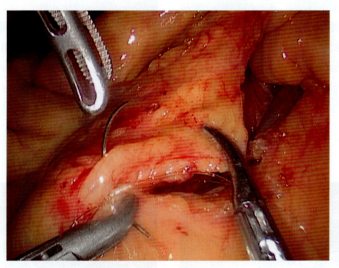

图 3-18-19　缝合关闭系膜裂孔
Figure 3-18-19　Suturing the ileocolic mesentery

## 第十九节　腹部无辅助切口经肛门拖出标本的腹腔镜下全结肠切除术

### （CRC-NOSES Ⅸ式）

**【简介】**

　　CRC-NOSES Ⅸ式是在腹腔镜全结肠切除术的基础上，结合独特的消化道重建和经肛门取标本方式完成的。该术式的操作特点：腹腔镜下完全游离全结肠及其系膜，经肛门将全结肠标本取出，再进行全腹腔镜下末端回肠 - 直肠侧端吻合（图 3-19-1、图 3-19-2，视频 3-18）。从技术角度而言，全结肠切除术是结直肠手术中难度最大、操作最复杂的术式之一，手术范围广泛，右半结肠、左半结肠，以及直肠切除术的技术要点和难点在该术式中均会涉及，这些因素对外科医生，尤其是青年外科医生提出了很高的技术要求。从

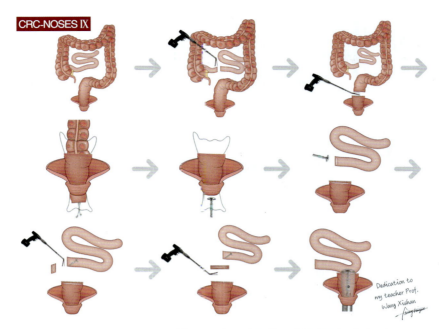

图 3-19-1　CRC-NOSES Ⅸ 式标本取出及消化道重建的主要手术步骤

Figure 3-19-1　The main surgical procedures of specimen extraction and digestive tract reconstruction in CRC-NOSES Ⅸ

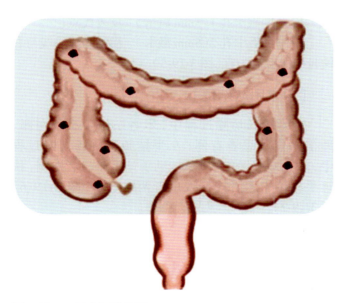

图 3-19-2　手术切除范围

Figure 3-19-2　Surgical resection area

视频 3-18　CRC-NOSES Ⅸ 式

Video 3-18　CRC-NOSES Ⅸ

理念角度而言,多数外科医生认为经肛门将全结肠标本取出的难度极大,甚至是无法实现的。这也导致经肛门取标本的全结肠切除术在外科领域极为罕见。我

们提出将保留大网膜的结肠癌根治术理念运用到该术式中,从而降低经肛门取标本的难度。只要严格掌握该术式的适应证,具备清晰缜密的手术思路和适当的手术技巧,这一技术是完全可以实现的。

## 一、适应证与禁忌证

### 【适应证】（图 3-19-3）

1. 家族性腺瘤性息肉病。
2. 林奇综合征相关结直肠癌。
3. 结肠多原发癌,且最大病灶环周直径 <3cm 为宜。
4. 溃疡性结肠炎经内科治疗无效者。
5. 便秘等良性疾病需全结肠切除者。

### 【禁忌证】

1. 结肠多原发癌,且最大病灶环周直径 >3cm 者。
2. 过于肥胖者（BMI>35kg/m$^2$）,或系膜肥厚者。
3. 肿瘤侵出浆膜者。

## 二、手术操作步骤、技巧与要点

### 【麻醉方式】

全身麻醉或全身麻醉联合硬膜外麻醉。

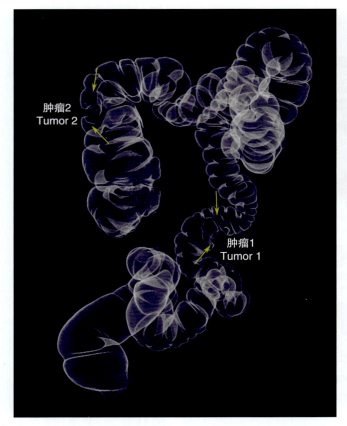

图 3-19-3 结肠三维重建 CT：肿瘤 1 位于降结肠乙状结肠交界处，肿瘤 2 位于升结肠近肝曲处

Figure 3-19-3 3D Reconstruction CT of the colon: tumor 1 located at the junction of the descending colon and sigmoid colon, tumor 2 located near the hepatic flexure of the ascending colon

## 【患者体位】

患者取功能截石位，双侧大腿尽量外展，上抬角度 <15°，以利于术者操作（图 3-19-4）。

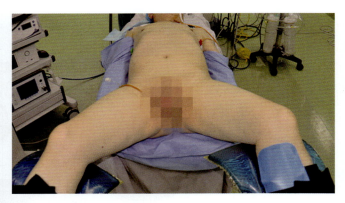

图 3-19-4 患者体位

Figure 3-19-4 Patient position

## 【戳卡位置】

1. 腹腔镜镜头戳卡孔（10mm 戳卡） 脐内，同时需兼顾右半结肠、左半结肠及直肠操作视野。

2. 术者主戳卡孔 1（12mm 戳卡） 左上腹，用于右半结肠的游离。

3. 术者主戳卡孔 2（12mm 戳卡） 麦氏点，用于左半结肠和直肠的游离。

4. 辅助戳卡孔 1（5mm 戳卡） 反麦氏点。

5. 辅助戳卡孔 2（5mm 戳卡） 横结肠投影线与右锁骨中线交点为宜（图 3-19-5）。

## 【手术团队站位】

右半结肠切除过程中，术者站位于患者左侧，助手站位于患者右侧；左半结肠及直肠切除过程中，术者站位于患者右侧，助手站位于患者左侧，扶镜手站位于术者同侧或患者两腿之间（图 3-19-6、图 3-19-7）。

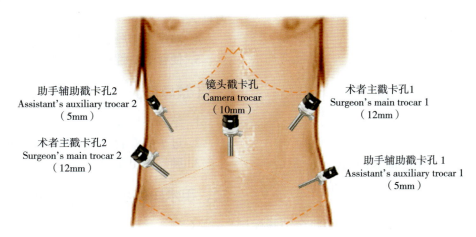

图 3-19-5 戳卡位置（五孔法）

Figure 3-19-5 Trocar placement（five-port method）

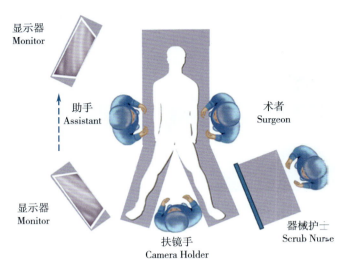

图 3-19-6　手术团队站位（右半结肠切除）

Figure 3-19-6　Surgical team position（right hemicolectomy）

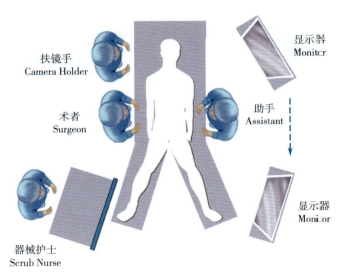

图 3-19-7　手术团队站位（左半结肠及直肠切除）

Figure 3-19-7　Surgical team position（left hemicolectomy, rectal resection）

【特殊手术器械】

超声刀、60mm 直线切割闭合器、25mm 环形吻合器、保护套。

【探查】

1. 常规探查　进镜至腹腔，常规探查肝脏、胆囊、胃、脾脏、大网膜、结肠、小肠、盆腔表面有无结节和腹水。

2. 肿瘤探查　对于多原发肿瘤或息肉病伴癌变，最大病灶的环周直径应 <3cm。

3. 解剖结构的判定　全结肠切除术难度大，脏器毗邻关系复杂，需观察全结肠结构及血管有无异常，

直肠壶腹部有无异常，系膜是否肥厚，进而综合判定采用该术式的可行性。

【解剖与分离】

1. 回结肠动静脉根部的处理　术者位于患者左侧，患者取头高足低左倾位。提起回结肠动静脉，可见回结肠动静脉与肠系膜上静脉形成一个夹角（图 3-19-8）。用超声刀于回结肠动静脉根部打开系膜，沿 Toldt's 间隙向上、向外分离，上方可看到十二指肠水平部（图 3-19-9、图 3-19-10），沿着肠系膜上静脉表面，清扫回结肠动静脉根部淋巴结，充分裸化后（图 3-19-11），在根部结扎并切断回结肠血管（图 3-19-12、图 3-19-13）。

2. 右结肠动静脉根部的处理　提起回结肠动静脉断端，继续沿着 Toldt's 筋膜在十二指肠表面分离，逐渐扩大游离范围。沿着右结肠静脉，向胰头前方和肠系膜上静脉方向小心剥离。可在右结肠静脉根部结扎并切断（图 3-19-14）。沿着肠系膜上静脉外科干向上分离，可见右结肠动脉，在根部结扎并切断（图 3-19-15）。

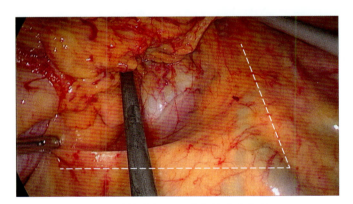

图 3-19-8　回结肠动静脉与肠系膜上静脉夹角处

Figure 3-19-8　Angle between superior mesenteric vein and ileocolic vessels

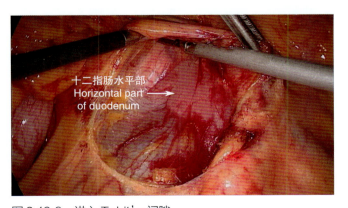

十二指肠水平部
Horizontal part
of duodenum

图 3-19-9　进入 Toldt's 间隙

Figure 3-19-9　Entering the Toldt's space

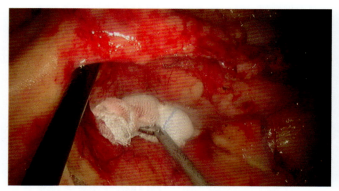

图 3-19-10　沿 Toldt's 间隙向外分离

Figure 3-19-10　Dissecting laterally along the Toldt's space

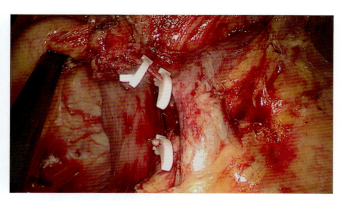

图 3-19-13　切断回结肠血管

Figure 3-19-13　Division of the ileocolic vessels

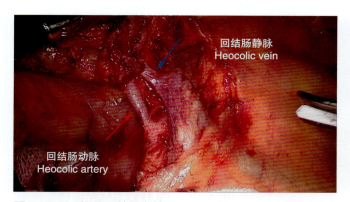

图 3-19-11　裸化回结肠血管

Figure 3-19-11　Skeletonizing the ileocolic vessels

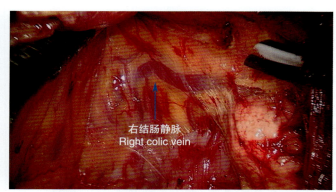

图 3-19-14　系膜内走行的右结肠静脉

Figure 3-19-14　Intramesenteric course of the right colic vein

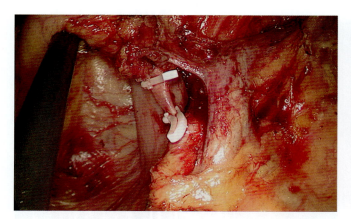

图 3-19-12　结扎回结肠血管

Figure 3-19-12　Ligation of the ileocolic vessels

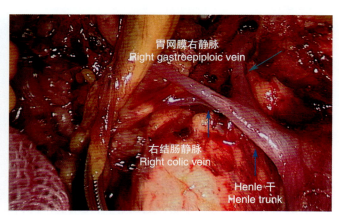

图 3-19-15　显露 Henle 干

Figure 3-19-15　Exposure of Henle's trunk

3. 中结肠血管根部的处理　处理完右结肠动静脉以后,往往可见胰腺颈部下缘及胃窦的后壁,尽量向上游离,在右结肠动脉根部上方附近,往往可见中结肠动静脉),此处小心分离,可以同时双重结扎并切断。这时可以沿胰腺颈部向左分离横结肠系膜至屈氏韧带。

4. 末段回肠的处理　在裁剪末段回肠系膜时,同时打开盲肠后方腹膜附着处,与 Toldt's 筋膜相贯通,游离回肠系膜至回肠肠壁(图 3-19-16),裸化 2cm 回肠肠壁(图 3-19-17),以便观察血运界限,确保吻合口血运良好。

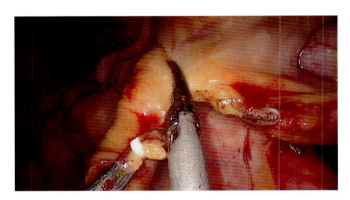

图 3-19-16　游离回肠系膜
Figure 3-19-16　Dissecting the ileal mesentery

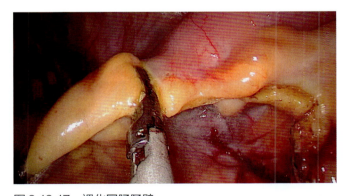

图 3-19-17　裸化回肠肠壁
Figure 3-19-17　Skeletonizing the ileal wall

5. 大网膜的处理　在横结肠中部,沿结肠带切断大网膜与横结肠肠壁粘连处,进入网膜腔(图 3-19-18),助手将大网膜翻转后,可见胰体部表面的纱布。在胃和结肠右侧,胃结肠韧带与横结肠系膜多为融合状态,但有间隙可将两者分开,沿胃网膜右动静脉向右侧游离,可于之前放置的纱布指示下,与胰

腺下缘切除系膜相贯通。分离至十二指肠表面,与之前的游离间隙相贯通,完全分离右侧大网膜。沿结肠带打开大网膜的附着处,直至结肠脾曲,可见脾下极,在胰尾表面置一纱布条以起保护和指示作用(图 3-19-19)。

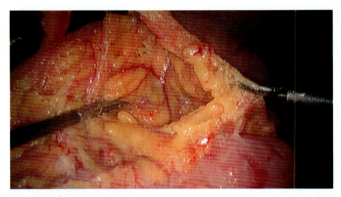

图 3-19-18　打开大网膜
Figure 3-19-18　Opening the greater omentum

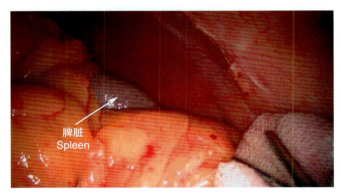

图 3-19-19　向左侧分离大网膜至脾下极
Figure 3-19-19　Separation of the greater omentum to the left side to the lower pole of the spleen

6. 右结肠旁沟及其系膜的游离　沿着十二指肠表面及 Toldt's 筋膜,从结肠肝曲向下向外逐步分离切断系膜(图 3-19-20、图 3-19-21),直至与盲肠处完全贯通,此时右半结肠完全处于游离状态。

7. 肠系膜下动脉根部的处理　术者位于患者右侧,患者取头高足低位并向右侧倾斜。在骶骨岬下方打开直肠系膜,进入骶前间隙,向上、向左分离(图 3-19-22、图 3-19-23),可见下腹下丛,向上分离肠系膜下动脉根部(图 3-19-24),裸化血管约 1cm,并在其根部双重结扎并切断肠系膜下动脉(图 3-19-25、图 3-19-26)。

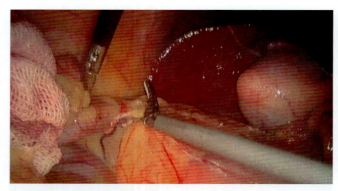

图 3-19-20　游离结肠肝曲

Figure 3-19-20　Dissecting the hepatic flexure of the colon

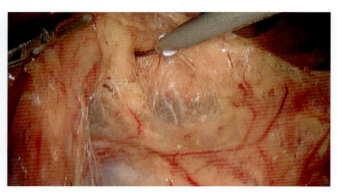

图 3-19-23　沿 Toldt's 间隙向下方游离

Figure 3-19-23　Dissecting downwards along the Toldt's space

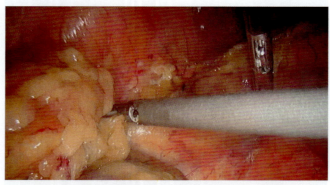

图 3-19-21　自结肠肝曲向下打开右结肠旁沟

Figure 3-19-21　Opening the right paracolic gutter from the hepatic flexure downwards

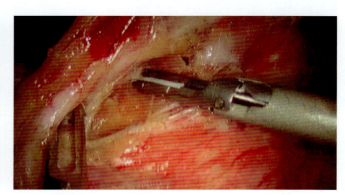

图 3-19-24　沿 Toldt's 间隙向上游离

Figure 3-19-24　Dissecting upwards along the Toldt's space

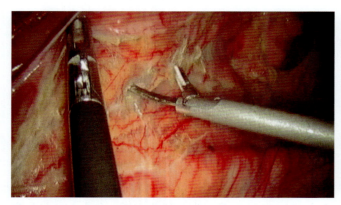

图 3-19-22　沿 Toldt's 间隙向左游离

Figure 3-19-22　Dissecting leftward along the Toldt's space

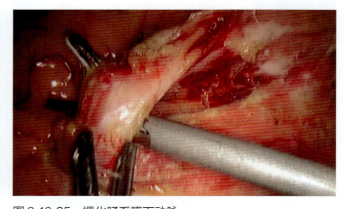

图 3-19-25　裸化肠系膜下动脉

Figure 3-19-25　Skeletonizing the inferior mesenteric artery

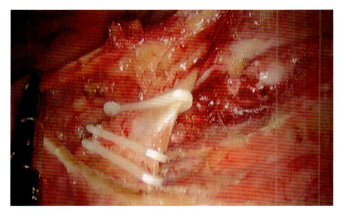

图 3-19-26　双重结扎肠系膜下动脉

Figure 3-19-26　Double ligation of the inferior mesen-teric artery

8. 肠系膜下静脉的处理　提起肠系膜下动脉根部，在腹主动脉外侧向屈氏韧带方向逐层打开后腹膜，沿 Toldt's 筋膜扩大游离范围，肠系膜下静脉的走行往往比较清晰，不难判定（图 3-19-27）。在屈氏韧带左侧、胰腺下缘，结扎并切断肠系膜下静脉（图 3-19-28）。系膜游离后，将一小纱布置于系膜后方以起保护和指示作用（图 3-19-29）。至此，左半结肠的供应血管均已离断。

9. 左半结肠系膜及左结肠旁沟的处理　将系膜提起向外侧沿 Toldt's 筋膜分离，可见左侧输尿管蠕动走行（图 3-19-30），及左侧生殖血管和左肾脂肪囊（图 3-19-31），如游离平面光滑、平整、干净，表明间隙正确。在屈氏韧带处，与右半结肠切除的横结肠系膜相遇，沿着胰腺下缘，在纱布条的指示和保护下，向左侧分离结肠脾曲系膜，分离至脾下极（图 3-19-32），沿左结肠旁沟向下游离至乙状结肠（图 3-19-33）。

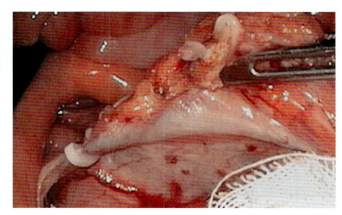

图 3-19-28　结扎肠系膜下静脉

Figure 3-19-28　Ligation of the inferior mesenteric vein

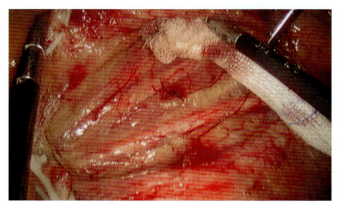

图 3-19-29　小纱布置于系膜后方

Figure 3-19-29　Placement of small gauze behind the mesentery

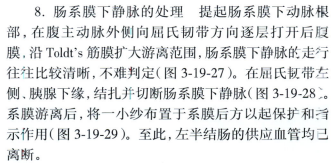

图 3-19-27　裸化肠系膜下静脉

Figure 3-19-27　Skeletonizing the inferior mesenteric vein

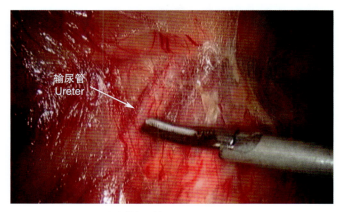

图 3-19-30　显露左侧输尿管

Figure 3-19-30　Exposure of the left ureter

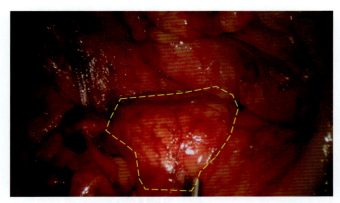

图 3-19-31　显露肾脂肪囊

Figure 3-19-31　Exposure of the adipose capsule of the kidney

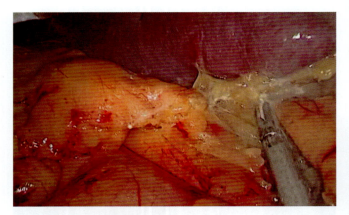

图 3-19-32　分离系膜至脾下极

Figure 3-19-32　Dissecting the mesentery to the inferior pole of the spleen

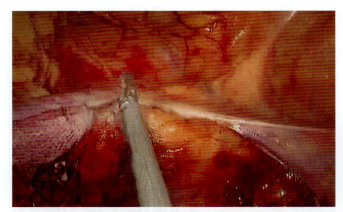

图 3-19-33　沿左结肠旁沟向结肠脾曲游离系膜

Figure 3-19-33　Dissecting the mesentery along the left paracolic gutter to the splenic flexure

　　10. 直肠系膜的游离　根据病变性质决定直肠的切除范围。如直肠病灶有恶变，切除范围可至病变下方 3 ~ 5cm。如直肠病灶为良性，可保留直肠壶腹。对于直肠上的息肉，可行肠镜下切除。按 TME 原则，沿

骶前间隙处理直肠系膜的后壁和右侧壁（图 3-19-34、图 3-19-35），具体步骤同前。切断乙状结肠与左侧腹壁粘连带（图 3-19-36），游离直肠左侧腹膜至预切除线。

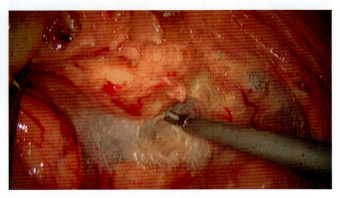

图 3-19-34　分离直肠后壁

Figure 3-19-34　Dissecting the posterior wall of the rectum

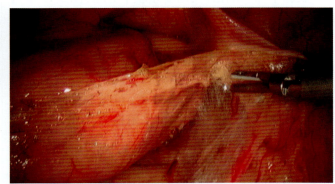

图 3-19-35　分离直肠右侧壁

Figure 3-19-35　Dissecting the right lateral wall of the rectum

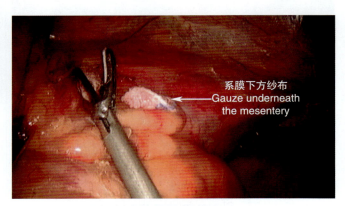

系膜下方纱布
Gauze underneath the mesentery

图 3-19-36　切断乙状结肠与左侧腹壁粘连带

Figure 3-19-36　Opening the adhesion band between the sigmoid colon and the left abdominal wall

11. 预切除线直肠的裸化　在预切除线右侧逐层裸化直肠。在直肠左侧同一水平横断直肠系膜，将直肠提起，在后方进一步裸化直肠壁使左右贯通（图 3-19-37），于腹膜反折处打开直肠前壁使左右贯通（图 3-19-38）。

肠吻合点。术者在回肠断端沿吻合钉在肠壁剪开约 2cm 切口（图 3-19-47），将抵钉座置入回肠腔内预吻合处（图 3-19-48）。再用直线切割闭合器闭合回肠断端（图 3-19-49）。在回肠预吻合处打一小孔，将抵钉座连接杆取出，确认无误后备用（图 3-19-50）。

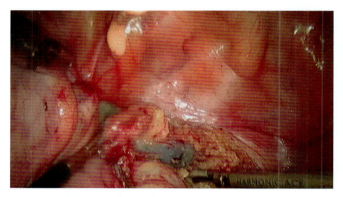

图 3-19-37　裸化直肠右侧壁

Figure 3-19-37　Skeletonizing the right lateral wall of the rectum

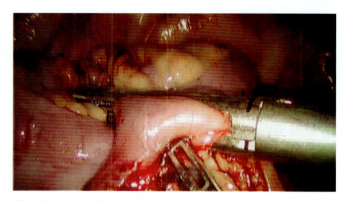

图 3-19-39　闭合切断回肠

Figure 3-19-39　Closing and dividing the ileum

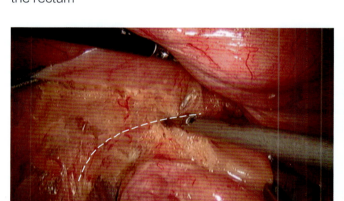

图 3-19-38　打开腹膜反折处

Figure 3-19-38　Opening the peritoneal reflection

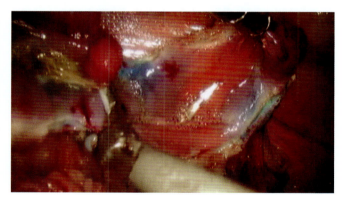

图 3-19-40　在直肠预切除线上端横行切开直肠壁

Figure 3-19-40　Transversely incising the rectal wall above the pre-cut line

### 【标本切除与消化道重建】

1. 标本切除　在回肠裸化区用直线切割闭合器切断回肠（图 3-19-39），在直肠预切除线上端横行切开直肠壁（图 3-19-40）。在确定有足够下切缘的情况下，将直肠完全横断。至此，全结肠的游离与切除全部完成。

2. 标本取出　术者将保护套经 12mm 戳卡孔送入腹腔（图 3-19-41）。助手与术者将标本置入保护套内（图 3-19-42），助手用卵圆钳夹持住直肠断端，在保护套内缓慢将全结肠标本拖出体外（图 3-19-43、图 3-19-44）。

3. 消化道重建　大量碘附盐水冲洗腹腔及盆腔（图 3-19-45）。探查腹腔及盆腔无渗血后，即可进行消化道重建。助手经肛门将吻合器抵钉座送入腹腔（图 3-19-46），检查末端回肠与直肠断端距离，选择回

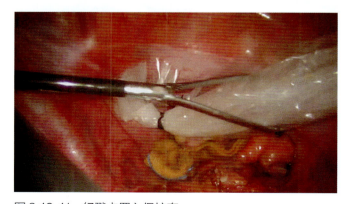

图 3-19-41　经戳卡置入保护套

Figure 3-19-41　Inserting a sterile plastic protective sleeve through the 12mm trocar port

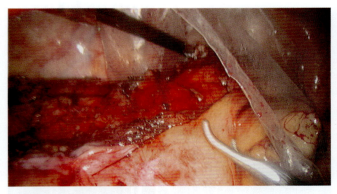

图 3-19-42　将标本置入保护套内
Figure 3-19-42　Placing the specimen into the protective sleeve

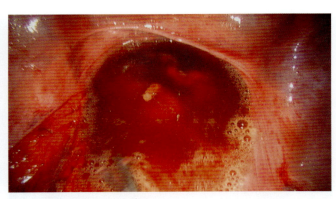

图 3-19-45　碘附盐水冲洗
Figure 3-19-45　Iodine solution irrigation

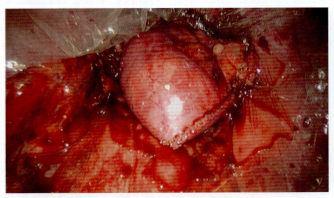

图 3-19-43　经肛门将标本拖出体外（腹腔内面观）
Figure 3-19-43　Extracting the specimen through the anus（intra-abdominal view）

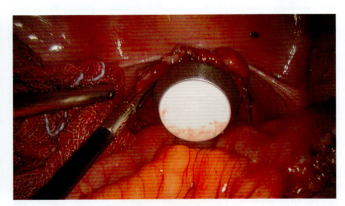

图 3-19-46　经肛门置入吻合器抵钉座
Figure 3-19-46　Inserting the anvil of the stapler through the anus

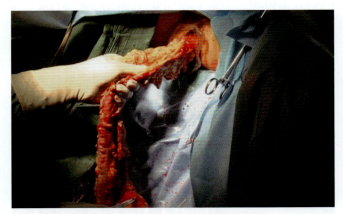

图 3-19-44　经肛门将标本拖出体外（体外观）
Figure 3-19-44　Extracting the specimen through the anus（external view）

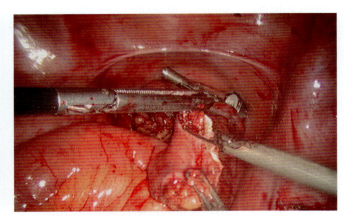

图 3-19-47　剪开回肠断端
Figure 3-19-47　Cutting open the ileal stump

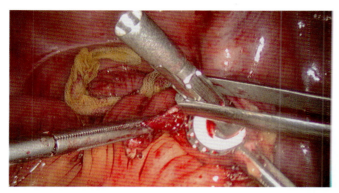

图 3-19-48　将抵钉座置入回肠

Figure 3-19-48　Placing the anvil into the ileum

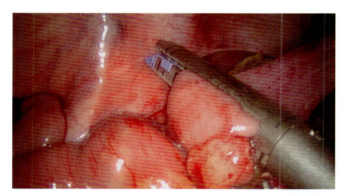

图 3-19-49　闭合回肠断端

Figure 3-19-49　Closing ileum stump

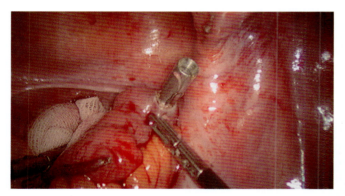

图 3-19-50　取出抵钉座连接杆

Figure 3-19-50　Removing the anvil shaft

气试验再次检查吻合口完整性（图 3-19-56）。确认无出血，在左右下腹部戳卡孔分别置入一根引流管于盆腔的两侧（图 3-19-57、图 3-19-58）。排净气腹内气体，缝合戳卡孔，术毕。

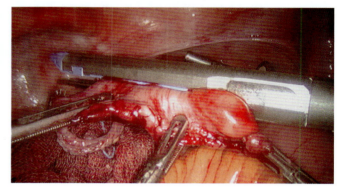

图 3-19-51　闭合切断直肠残端

Figure 3-19-51　Closing and dividing the rectal stump

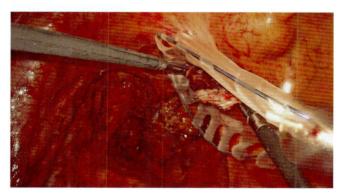

图 3-19-52　直肠残端经戳卡孔取出

Figure 3-19-52　Extracting the rectal stump through the trocar port

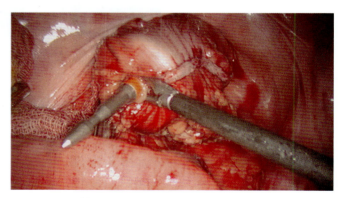

图 3-19-53　旋出吻合器穿刺针

Figure 3-19-53　Unscrewing the stapler piercing rod

用直线切割闭合器关闭直肠残端（图 3-19-51），切下的直肠残端组织经 12mm 戳卡孔取出（图 3-19-52）。助手经肛门置入环形吻合器，并于直肠断端的一角旋出吻合器穿刺针（图 3-19-53）。完成抵钉座与吻合器穿刺针对接（图 3-19-54），旋紧击发完成回肠 - 直肠侧端吻合（图 3-19-55）。

检查吻合口上下切缘是否完整。经肛门行注水注

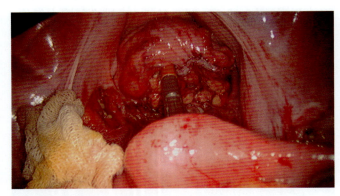

图 3-19-54 与吻合器穿刺针对接

Figure 3-19-54 Align and connect with the stapler trocar

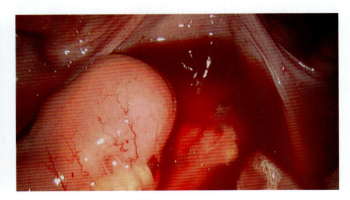

图 3-19-56 注水注气试验

Figure 3-19-56 Air and water injection test

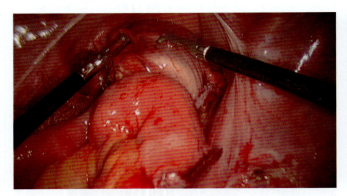

图 3-19-55 行回肠 - 直肠侧端吻合

Figure 3-19-55 Performing side-to-end anastomosis between the ileum and the rectum

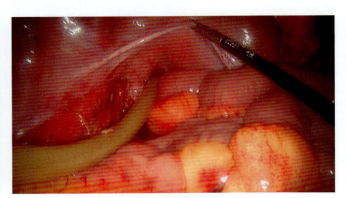

图 3-19-57 置入左侧腹腔引流管

Figure 3-19-57 Inserting left abdominal drainage tube

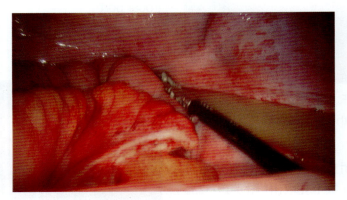

图 3-19-58 置入右侧腹腔引流管

Figure 3-19-58 Inserting right abdominal drainage tube

## 第二十节 腹部无辅助切口经阴道拖出标本的腹腔镜下全结肠切除术 （CRC-NOSES X 式）

### 【简介】

全结肠切除术手术范围广泛，操作步骤复杂，切除病变组织多，是结直肠手术中难度最大的术式之一。CRC-NOSES X 式与常规腹腔镜全结肠切除术相比，最大的区别就在于消化道重建方式和标本取出途径。该术式的操作特点：腹腔镜下完全游离全结肠及其系膜，经阴道将全结肠标本取出，再进行腹腔镜下末端回肠 - 直肠侧端吻合（图 3-20-1）。与 CRC-NOSES IX 式经肛门取标本相比，经阴道取标本可以适当放宽手术适应证。同时，减少因肠管切开污染腹腔的概率（图 3-20-2）。

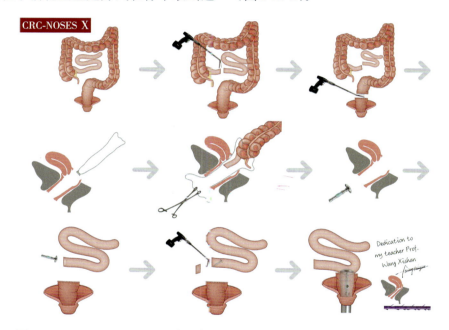

图 3-20-1　CRC-NOSES X式标本取出及消化道重建的主要手术步骤
Figure 3-20-1　The main surgical procedures of specimen extraction and digestive tract reconstruction in CRC-NOSES X

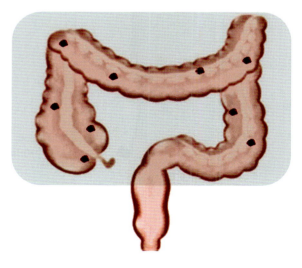

图 3-20-2　手术切除范围
Figure 3-20-2　Surgical resection area

# 一、适应证与禁忌证

## 【适应证】

1. 结肠多发恶性肿瘤，最大环周径 3~5cm 者为最佳。

2. 家族性腺瘤性息肉病，经肛门取出困难者。

3. 林奇综合征相关结直肠癌。

4. 溃疡性结肠炎内科治疗无效，局部肠段系膜肥厚，经肛门取出困难者。

5. 需要切除全部大网膜的全结肠切除术。

## 【禁忌证】

1. 结直肠多原发癌，其最大病灶环周直径 >5cm 者。

2. 过于肥胖者（BMI>35kg/m²），或系膜肥厚者。

3. 肿瘤侵出浆膜者。

# 二、手术操作步骤、技巧与要点

## 【麻醉方式】

全身麻醉或全身麻醉联合硬膜外麻醉。

## 【患者体位】

患者取功能截石位，双侧大腿上抬角度 <15°，以利于术者操作（图 3-20-3）。

## 【戳卡位置】

1. 腹腔镜镜头戳卡孔（10mm 戳卡）　脐内，同时需兼顾右半结肠、左半结肠及直肠操作视野。

2. 术者主戳卡孔 1（12mm 戳卡）　左上腹，用于右半结肠的游离。

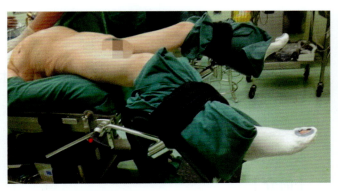

图 3-20-3　患者体位

Figure 3-20-3　Patient position

3. 术者主戳卡孔 2（12mm 戳卡）　麦氏点，用于左半结肠和直肠的游离。

4. 辅助戳卡孔 1（5mm 戳卡）　反麦氏点。

5. 辅助戳卡孔 2（5mm 戳卡）　横结肠体表投影区与右锁骨中线交点为宜（图 3-20-4）。

## 【手术团队站位】

右半结肠切除过程中，术者站位于患者左侧，助手站位于患者右侧；左半结肠及直肠切除过程中，术者站位于患者右侧，助手站位于患者左侧。扶镜手站位于术者同侧或患者两腿之间（图 3-20-5、图 3-20-6）。

## 【特殊手术器械】

超声刀、60mm 直线切割闭合器、25mm 环形吻合器、阴道缝合线、举宫器、保护套。

## 【探查】

1. 常规探查　进镜至腹腔，常规探查肝脏、胆囊、胃、脾脏、大网膜、结肠、小肠、盆腔表面有无肿瘤种植结节和腹水。

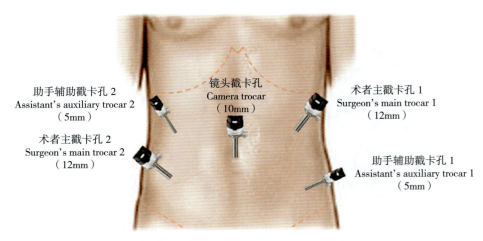

图 3-20-4　戳卡位置（五孔法）

Figure 3-20-4　Trocar placement（five-port method）

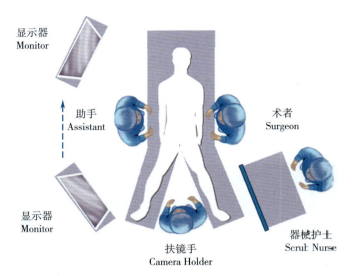

图 3-20-5　手术团队站位（右半结肠切除）

Figure 3-20-5　Surgical team position（right hemico-lectomy）

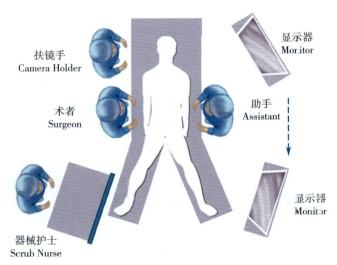

图 3-20-6　手术团队站位（左半结肠及直肠切除）

Figure 3-20-6　Surgical team position（left hemico-lectomy，rectal resection）

2. 肿瘤探查　对于多原发肿瘤而言，最大瘤灶的判定最为关键，其环周径大小是能否采用该术式最重要的参考指标。

3. 解剖结构的判定　全结肠切除术实际操作复杂，需仔细观察脏器毗邻关系，全结肠供应血管有无异常，肠系膜肥厚程度，盆腔、阴道后穹隆有无异常改变，再次评估手术可行性。

【解剖与分离】

1. 回结肠血管根部的处理　术者位于患者左侧，患者取头高足低位并向左侧倾斜。充分显露术野，术者在回结肠血管根部下方（图 3-20-7）、肠系膜上静

表面打开系膜（图 3-20-8、图 3-20-9），向上分离，以肠系膜上静脉作为标记，在其表面小心分离。回结肠动静脉多紧靠在一起，并且回结肠动脉跨过肠系膜上静脉与回结肠静脉伴行。偶尔两者分开，回结肠动脉从肠系膜上静脉后方发出。充分裸化后，于血管根部结扎并切断回结肠血管（图 3-20-10、图 3-20-11）。

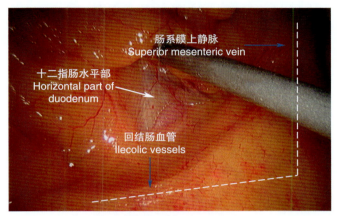

图 3-20-7　肠系膜上静脉与回结肠血管交界处

Figure 3-20-7　Junction of superior mesenteric vein and ileocolic vessels

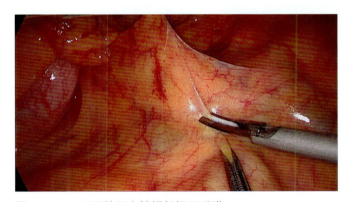

图 3-20-8　于回结肠血管根部切开系膜

Figure 3-20-8　Incising the mesentery at the root of ileocolic vessels

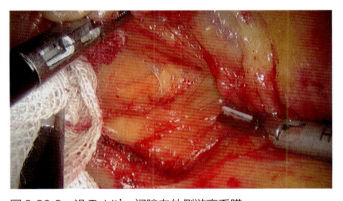

图 3-20-9　沿 Toldt's 间隙向外侧游离系膜

Figure 3-20-9　Dissecting the mesentery laterally along the Toldt's space

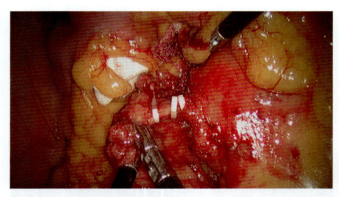

图 3-20-10　结扎回结肠血管

Figure 3-20-10　Ligation of ileocolic vessels

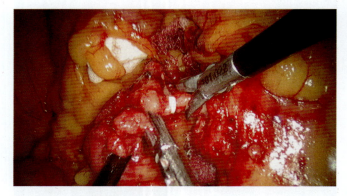

图 3-20-11　切断回结肠血管

Figure 3-20-11　Clip of ileocolic vessels

2. 右结肠动静脉根部的处理　沿肠系膜上静脉向上分离（图 3-20-12），打开血管鞘（图 3-20-13），往往先发现右结肠动脉。右结肠动静脉通常相互分离，需分别予以处理；但在少数情形下，二者会合为一束，此时可一并进行处理（图 3-20-14、图 3-20-15）。提起右结肠动脉断端，向上、向右外侧小心分离，游离过程中可见胰腺被膜，需在胰腺表面分离 Toldt's 间隙（图 3-20-16、图 3-20-17）。Henle 干一般位于胰腺表面，向右、向上分别发出两个属支，向右走行的血管为右结肠静脉，可在其根部结扎，向上分支与胃网膜右静脉相连续。

3. 中结肠动静脉根部的处理　处理完右结肠动静脉以后，可见胰腺颈部下缘，打开系膜，进一步裸化中结肠动静脉根部（图 3-20-18），用血管夹双重结扎并切断。至此，供应右结肠的血管处理完毕。

4. 右结肠系膜的游离　首先处理血管根部，提起右结肠动静脉断端，沿着 Toldt's 筋膜向下、向上、向外以锐性与钝性相结合的方式进行分离。在十二指肠表面分离，整个游离平面光滑、平整，可见右侧输尿管及右侧生殖血管，表明游离间隙正确（图 3-20-19）。

5. 末端回肠的处理　将末端回肠展开，根据血管弓的情况，仔细裁剪系膜。如全结肠标本能经阴道拖出体外，可行回肠 - 直肠端端吻合，如拖出困难，切勿勉强，可行回肠 - 直肠侧端吻合。将回肠系膜裁剪至预切除线，并裸化 3cm 肠壁，以便观察血运分界线（图 3-20-20）。

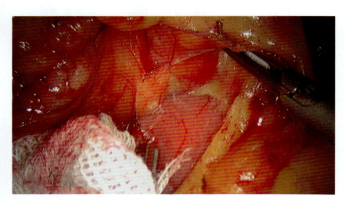

图 3-20-12　游离十二指肠表面系膜

Figure 3-20-12　Dissecting the mesentery on the surface of the duodenum

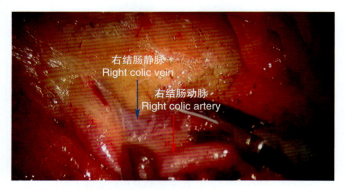

右结肠静脉 Right colic vein
右结肠动脉 Right colic artery

图 3-20-13　裸化右结肠血管

Figure 3-20-13　Skeletonizing the right colic vessels

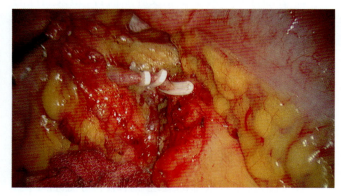

图 3-20-14　结扎右结肠血管

Figure 3-20-14　Ligation of the right colic vessels

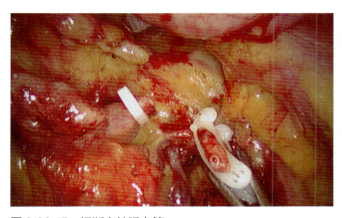

图 3-20-15　切断右结肠血管

Figure 3-20-15　Division of the right colic vessels

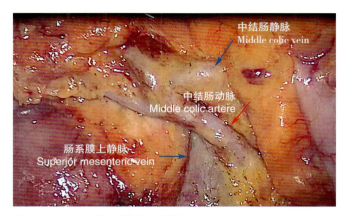

图 3-20-18　裸化中结肠血管根部

Figure 3-20-18　Skeletonizing the middle colic vessels at the root

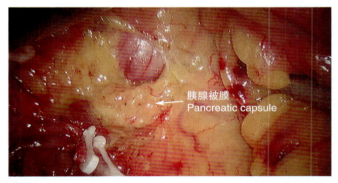

图 3-20-16　显露胰腺被膜

Figure 3-20-16　Exposure of the pancreatic capsule

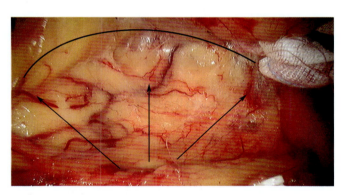

图 3-20-19　完全游离 Toldt's 间隙

Figure 3-20-19　Complete dissection of Toldt's space

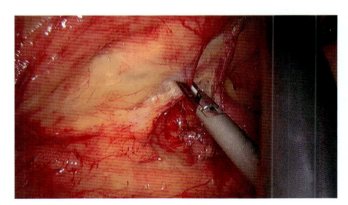

图 3-20-17　在胰腺被膜表面分离 Toldt's 间隙

Figure 3-20-17　Dissecting the Toldt's space on the surface of the pancreatic capsule

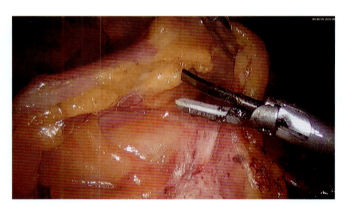

图 3-20-20　游离回肠系膜

Figure 3-20-20　Dissecting the ileal mesentery

6. 游离右结肠旁沟及大网膜　提起胃大弯，清晰可见胃网膜血管走行，在胃结肠韧带透明薄弱区，用超声刀打开胃结肠韧带进入网膜囊（图 3-20-21 ～图 3-20-23），可见胰腺走行。沿胃网膜右动静脉走行，分离切断胃结肠韧带（图 3-20-24、图 3-20-25）。向右分离至 Henle 干（图 3-20-26），同时处理胃后壁及横结肠右侧系膜，上下贯通。切断肝结肠韧带（图 3-20-27），向下沿右结肠旁沟分离至盲肠附着处（图 3-20-28），与末端回肠系膜游离处相贯通，至此完成整个右半结肠的游离。

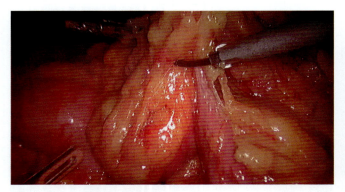

图 3-20-21　打开胃结肠韧带

Figure 3-20-21　Opening the gastrocolic ligament

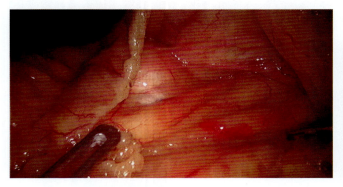

图 3-20-22　可见垫入的纱布

Figure 3-20-22　Visible inserted gauze

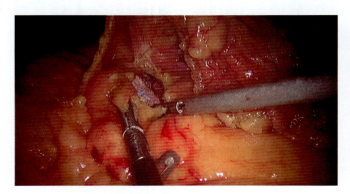

图 3-20-23　处理横结肠系膜

Figure 3-20-23　Handling the transverse mesocolon

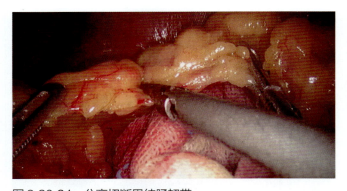

图 3-20-24　分离切断胃结肠韧带

Figure 3-20-24　Dissecting and dividing the gastrocolic ligament

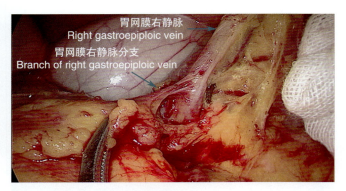

图 3-20-25　显露胃网膜右静脉分支

Figure 3-20-25　Exposure of the right gastroepiploic vein branches

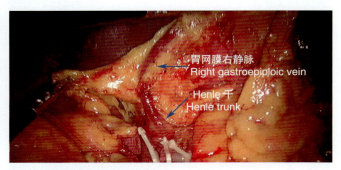

图 3-20-26　显露 Henle 干

Figure 3-20-26　Exposure of Henle's trunk

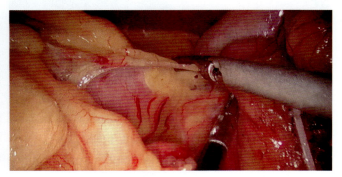

图 3-20-27　切断肝结肠韧带

Figure 3-20-27　Division of the hepatocolic ligament

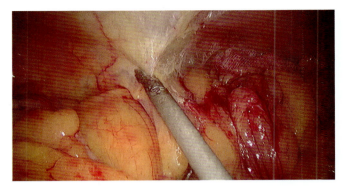

图 3-20-28　游离右结肠旁沟

Figure 3-20-28　Dissecting the right paracolic gutter

7. 肠系膜下动脉根部的处理　术者转至患者右侧，患者取头高足低并向右侧倾斜。充分显露术野，末段回肠系膜游离已经完成，此时可见腹主动脉及其分叉部（图 3-20-29）。在腹主动脉与肠系膜下动脉夹角打开后腹膜。在肠系膜下动脉根部清扫淋巴结、脂肪组织，在根部双重结扎并切断（图 3-20-30、图 3-20-31）。

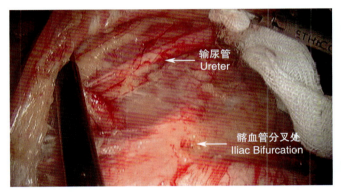

图 3-20-29　沿 Toldt's 间隙向外侧游离

Figure 3-20-29　Dissecting laterally along the Toldt's space

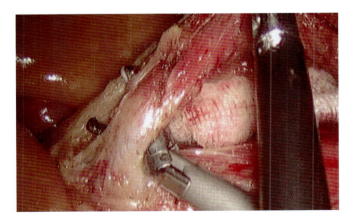

图 3-20-30　裸化肠系膜下动脉

Figure 3-20-30　Skeletonizing the inferior mesenteric artery

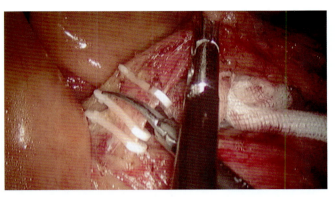

图 3-20-31　双重结扎并切断肠系膜下动脉

Figure 3-20-31　Double ligation and division of the inferior mesenteric artery

8. 肠系膜下静脉根部的处理　沿腹主动脉左侧，从肠系膜下动脉根部向屈氏韧带方向游离，同时向外游离，并将左结肠系膜掀起（图 3-20-32）。在屈氏韧带外侧胰体尾部下缘横断肠系膜下静脉（图 3-20-33）。

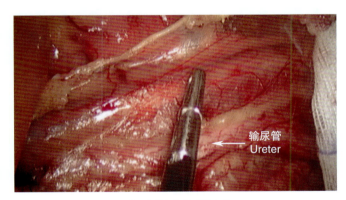

图 3-20-32　沿 Toldt's 间隙向外侧游离

Figure 3-20-32　Dissecting laterally along the Toldt's space

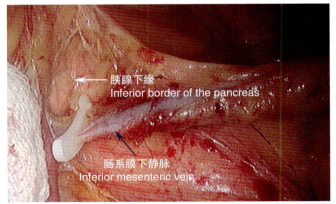

图 3-20-33　结扎肠系膜下静脉

Figure 3-20-33　Ligation of the inferior mesenteric vein

9. **左半结肠系膜的游离**　掀起左结肠系膜和肠系膜下动脉断端，向外、向下、向上尽量扩大游离的范围，可见操作平面平整、光滑、干净，此为沿 Toldt's 筋膜操作分离的最佳状态（图 3-20-34）。同时可见左侧输尿管走行及蠕动，左侧生殖血管和左肾脂肪囊完整、用纱布垫入系膜后方以起保护和指示作用（图 3-20-35）。

则处理完直肠系膜后壁和右侧壁后（图 3-20-42），切断乙状结肠生理粘连，直肠左侧系膜游离至预切除线（图 3-20-43）。在直肠预切除线的右侧横断直肠系膜。若直肠上动静脉过粗，可用血管夹闭合，避免远端出血。术者在直肠左侧同一水平横断直肠系膜，助手将直肠提起，术者在后方进一步裸化直肠壁使左右贯通。

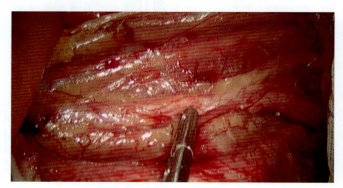

图 3-20-34　左半结肠系膜表面
Figure 3-20-34　Surface of the left hemicolon mesentery

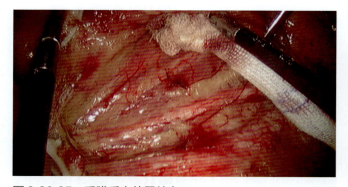

图 3-20-35　系膜后方放置纱布
Figure 3-20-35　Placing the gauze behind the mesentery

10. **左半大网膜及横结肠左半系膜的处理**　术者左手将胃网膜血管弓提起，沿胃网膜血管弓向左游离（图 3-20-36）。逐步分离至胃结肠韧带，再至脾下极（图 3-20-37）。助手将大网膜拉下，可见横结肠左半系膜与胰腺尾部，此处多数情况为无血管系膜区，偶可见空肠屈氏韧带左侧及近胰尾有血管分支走向结肠脾曲。术者用超声刀从屈氏韧带和肠系膜下静脉断端开始，沿胰腺下缘向脾及结肠脾曲外侧结肠旁沟分离（图 3-20-38～图 3-20-40），与垫于左半结肠系膜后方的纱布条会合贯通。至此，左半结肠游离完毕（图 3-20-41）。

11. **直肠系膜的游离与直肠裸化**　直肠的切除范围根据病变性质而定，力争保留直肠壶腹，因排便感受器位于直肠壶腹，保留直肠壶腹能够维持排便反射弧完整性，有利于肠道功能的保留与恢复。按 TME 原

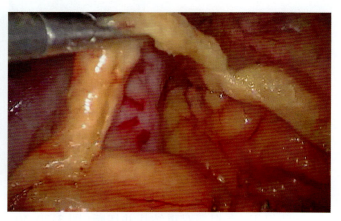

图 3-20-36　沿胃网膜血管弓向左游离
Figure 3-20-36　Dissecting leftward along the gastroepiploic vascular arch

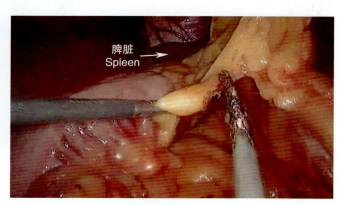

脾脏
Spleen

图 3-20-37　向左游离至脾下极
Figure 3-20-37　Dissecting leftward to the inferior pole of the spleen

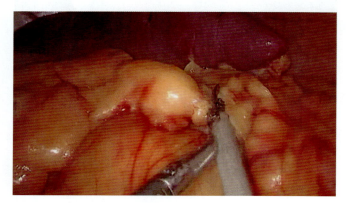

图 3-20-38　游离脾结肠韧带
Figure 3-20-38　Dissecting the splenocolic ligament

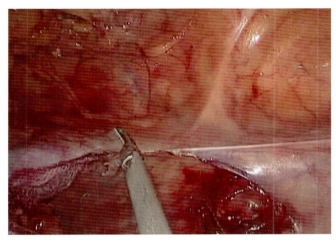

图 3-20-39　游离左结肠旁沟

Figure 3-20-39　Dissecting the left paracolic gutter

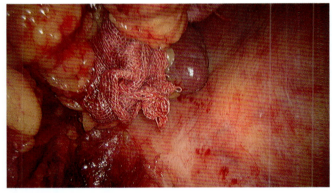

图 3-20-40　沿左结肠旁沟向上游离至结肠脾曲

Figure 3-20-40　Dissecting upward along the left paracolic gutter to the splenic flexure

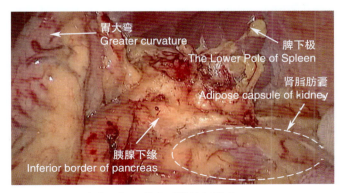

胃大弯
Greater curvature
脾下极
The Lower Pole of Spleen
肾脂肪囊
Adipose capsule of kidney
胰腺下缘
Inferior border of pancreas

图 3-20-41　胰腺下缘及游离后的结肠脾曲

Figure 3-20-41　Inferior border of the pancreas and the dissected splenic flexure of the Colon

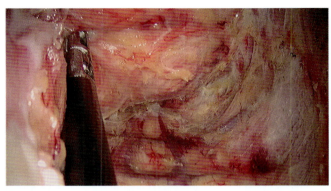

图 3-20-42　沿 Toldt's 间隙向下方游离

Figure 3-20-42　Dissecting downward along the Toldt's space

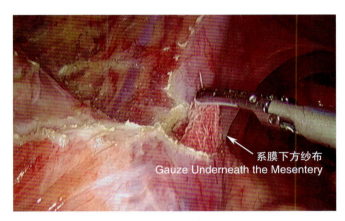

系膜下方纱布
Gauze Underneath the Mesentery

图 3-20-43　打开乙状结肠左侧系膜

Figure 3-20-43　Opening the left mesosigmoid

## 【标本切除与消化道重建】

1. 标本切除　在直肠预切除线的裸化区，用直线切割闭合器切断闭合直肠（图 3-20-44）。在回肠预切除线，用直线切割闭合器切断闭合回肠（图 3-20-45）。

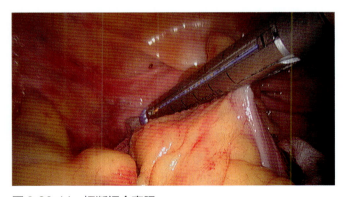

图 3-20-44　切断闭合直肠

Figure 3-20-44　Closing and dividing the rectum

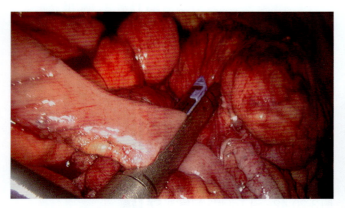

图 3-20-45　切断闭合回肠

Figure 3-20-45　Closing and dividing the small intestine

2. 标本取出　与肛门相比，阴道具备良好弹性、充足血液供应、愈合能力强及易于操作等特性，经阴道取标本也被认为是取出较大体积结直肠标本的理想选择。阴道冲洗后，助手于体外将膀胱拉钩置于阴道内，用其前端顶起阴道后穹隆。在其指示下，术者用超声刀横行切开阴道后穹隆约3cm，然后纵行牵拉切口，使切口扩大为5～6cm（图 3-20-46），助手用卵圆钳经阴道置入保护套入腹腔，助手用卵圆钳夹住保护套远端，经阴道将其取出（图 3-20-47）。同时，术者与助手将全结肠标本逐次置入保护套（图 3-20-48），助手于体外将标本缓缓拉出（图 3-20-49）。

3. 消化道重建　助手经阴道将吻合器抵钉座送入腹腔，判定末端回肠至直肠残端距离，选择回肠吻合点。术者在回肠断端沿着缝合钉剪开2cm小口（图 3-20-50），将抵钉座置入回肠肠腔内（图 3-20-51），调整好位置，用直线切割闭合器闭合回肠断端（图 3-20-52），切下的残端组织可经阴道取出。在回肠预吻合点，打开一小孔，取出抵钉座连接杆（图 3-20-53）。助手经肛门置入环形吻合器，并在直肠残端的一角旋出吻合器穿刺针（图 3-20-54），完成抵钉座与吻合器对接（图 3-20-55），完成回肠 - 直肠侧端吻合，并对吻合口进行加固缝合（图 3-20-56）。检查吻合口上下切缘是否完整。经肛门行注水注气试验，再次检查吻合口是否完整，有无出血（图 3-20-57）。检查无误后，左右下腹部各放置一根引流管于盆腔（图 3-20-58、图 3-20-59），停止气腹，排净腹腔气体，缝合戳卡孔。

4. 阴道切口的缝合　用两把 Allis 钳夹持住阴道切口的前后壁，充分显露切口，用可吸收线间断缝

合（图 3-20-60），检查阴道切口，确认无渗漏和出血后，用一碘附纱团置于阴道后穹隆，48 小时后取出，术毕。

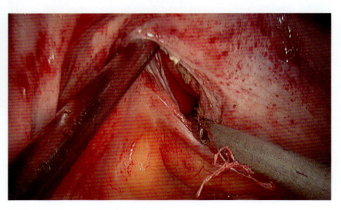

图 3-20-46　切开阴道后穹隆

Figure 3-20-46　Incising the posterior vaginal fornix

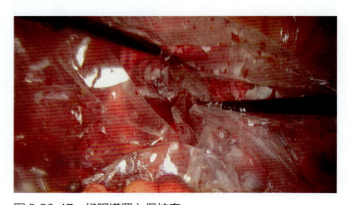

图 3-20-47　经阴道置入保护套

Figure 3-20-47　Inserting a plastic protective sleeve through the vagina

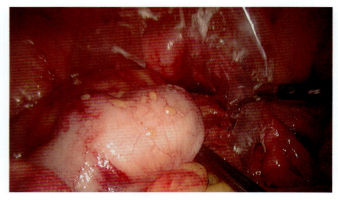

图 3-20-48　将标本置入保护套

Figure 3-20-48　Placing the specimen into the protective sleeve

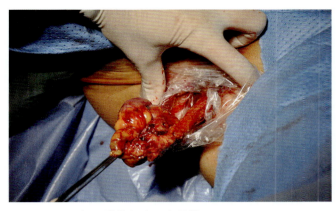

图 3-20-49　经阴道将标本取出体外

Figure 3-20-49　Extracting the specimen through the vagina

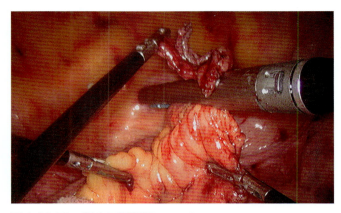

图 3-20-52　闭合回肠断端

Figure 3-20-52　Closing the ileum

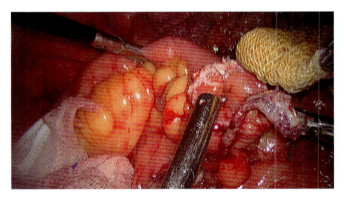

图 3-20-50　切开回肠断端

Figure 3-20-50　Incising the ileal stump

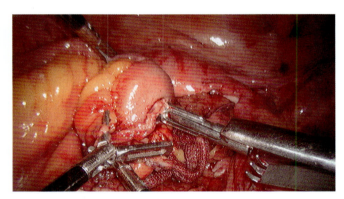

图 3-20-53　取出抵钉座连接杆

Figure 3-20-53　Removing the anvil connector rod

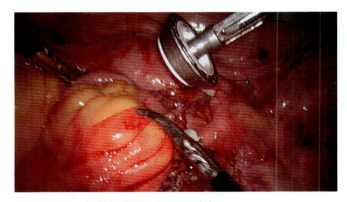

图 3-20-51　将抵钉座置入回肠肠腔内

Figure 3-20-51　Placing the anvil into the ileum cavity

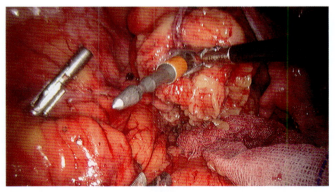

图 3-20-54　经肛门置入环形吻合器

Figure 3-20-54　Inserting the circular stapler through the anus

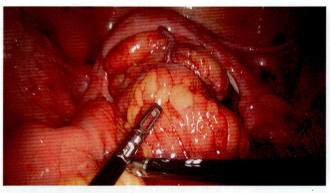

图 3-20-55　行回肠 - 直肠侧端吻合

Figure 3-20-55　Performing side-to-end anastomosis between the ileum and the rectum

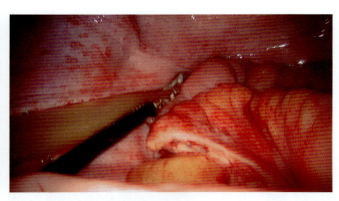

图 3-20-58　置入左侧腹腔引流管

Figure 3-20-58　Inserting left abdominal drainage tube

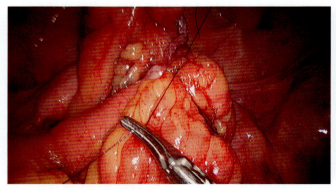

图 3-20-56　吻合口加固缝合

Figure 3-20-56　Reinforcing the anastomosis with sutures

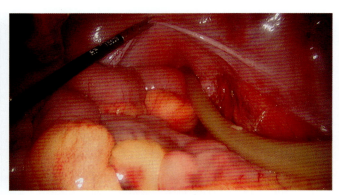

图 3-20-59　置入右侧腹腔引流管

Figure 3-20-59　Inserting right abdominal drainage tube

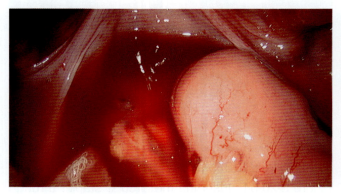

图 3-20-57　注水注气试验

Figure 3-20-57　Air and water injection test

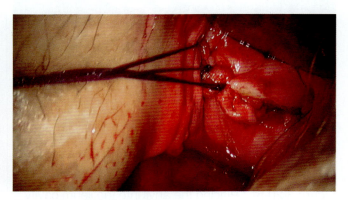

图 3-20-60　间断缝合阴道切口

Figure 3-20-60　Intermittent suturing of the vaginal incision

## 第二十一节　腹部无辅助切口经阴道拖出标本的腹腔镜下横结肠癌根治术

### 【简介】

对于女性横结肠癌患者，可选择经阴道取标本的腹腔镜下横结肠癌根治术。该术式对阴道的术前准备有更严格的要求。由于阴道具有很强的延展性，经阴道取标本的适应证更广泛，但仅限于女性患者。该术式的难点主要体现在 NOSES 特有的腹腔镜下消化道重建，即腹腔镜下使用直线切割闭合器进行重叠式三角吻合。

## 一、适应证与禁忌证

### 【适应证】

1. 女性横结肠癌或良性肿瘤。
2. 肿瘤环周直径为 3～5cm。
3. 肿瘤不侵出浆膜为宜。

### 【禁忌证】

1. 肿瘤体积过大，取出有困难者。
2. 肿瘤侵犯周围组织器官。
3. 过于肥胖者（ BMI>35kg/m$^2$ ）。

## 二、手术操作步骤、技巧与要点

### 【戳卡位置】

1. 腹腔镜镜头戳卡孔（10mm 戳卡）　脐至脐下方

5cm 的范围内均可。

2. 术者主戳卡孔（12mm 戳卡）　左上腹中部，腹直肌外缘。
3. 术者辅助戳卡孔（5mm 戳卡）　左下腹，与腹腔镜镜头戳卡孔不在同一水平线。
4. 助手主戳卡孔（5mm 戳卡）　麦氏点。
5. 助手辅助戳卡孔（5mm 戳卡）　右上腹，右锁骨中线与横结肠投影区交叉处（图 3-21-1 ）。

### 【探查】

1. 常规探查　观察各脏器及腹膜表面有无种植转移等病变。
2. 肿瘤探查　根据肿瘤的位置、大小、侵犯深度，确定手术的可行性。
3. 解剖结构的判定　横结肠毗邻脏器多、血管关系复杂，需判定回结肠动静脉、右结肠动静脉、中结肠动静脉的位置。此外，还需判定升结肠和横结肠游离后可否行腹腔镜下升结肠 - 横结肠重叠式三角吻合。

### 【解剖与分离】

1. 右结肠血管根部的处理　在胰颈下缘横结肠系膜薄弱处行第一刀切割，并向上及向右扩展空间。在右结肠血管根部结扎并切断。
2. 中结肠血管的处理　于胰腺下缘分离出中结肠血管，结扎并切断。

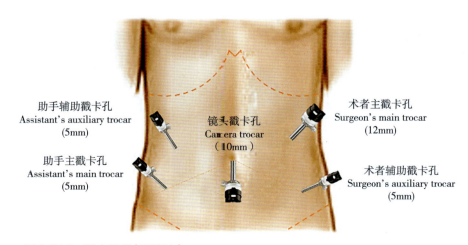

图 3-21-1　戳卡位置（五孔法）

Figure 3-21-1　Trocar placement（five-port method）

3. Henle 干的处理　沿胰前间隙在十二指肠及胰头表面游离,仔细分离后可见副右结肠静脉、胃网膜右静脉、胰十二指肠上前静脉汇成 Henle 干后汇入肠系膜上静脉。在各血管分支根部结扎并切断。

4. 大网膜及第 6 组淋巴结的处理　沿胃网膜右动静脉血管弓外缘向右分离切断胃网膜右动静脉,弓外清扫第 6 组淋巴结。

5. 升结肠系膜的游离及处理　注意保护右侧生殖血管、胰头及十二指肠。于距肿瘤近端约 10cm 处确定升结肠预切除线,裁剪升结肠系膜,并裸化肠管。

6. 横结肠系膜的处理　向横结肠预切除线方向分离裁剪横结肠远端系膜,结扎并切断边缘血管弓,并裸化预切除线部位横结肠肠壁。

### 【标本切除与消化道重建】

1. 标本切除　用直线切割闭合器在横结肠预切除线处闭合切断肠管(图 3-21-2),然后在升结肠近端预切除线,用直线切割闭合器闭合切断升结肠(图 3-21-3)。至此横结肠肿瘤根治切除完成,将标本置于保护套中,置于盆腔(图 3-21-4)。

2. 消化道重建　将横结肠断端向右牵拉摆放,并将升结肠断端拉至上腹部与横结肠重叠摆放(图 3-21-5)。然后将横结肠断端与距升结肠断端 7cm 处肠管缝合固定(图 3-21-6),检查两侧肠管血运良好,估计两侧吻合口无张力后,分别于升结肠断端对系膜侧肠壁与相应位置的横结肠对系膜侧肠壁做 1cm 切口(图 3-21-7、图 3-21-8),酒精或碘附纱条消毒肠壁切口。经术者主戳卡孔置入直线切割闭合器,分别将钉仓两侧置入升结肠及横结肠肠腔,进行必要的调整,确认无误后击发,完成升结肠 - 横结肠侧侧吻合(图 3-21-9、图 3-21-10)。

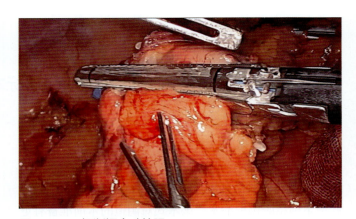

图 3-21-3　切断闭合升结肠

Figure 3-21-3　Closure and transection of the ascending colon

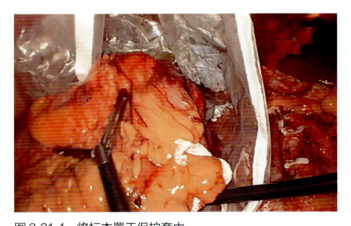

图 3-21-4　将标本置于保护套中

Figure 3-21-4　Placement of specimen into the protective sleeve

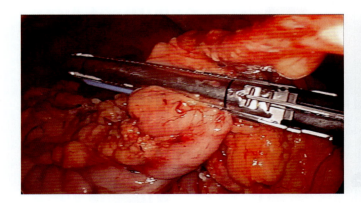

图 3-21-2　切断闭合横结肠

Figure 3-21-2　Closure and transection of the transverse colon

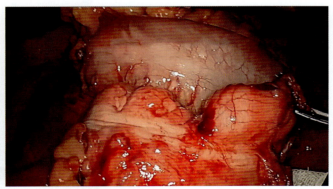

图 3-21-5　升结肠断端与横结肠重叠摆放

Figure 3-21-5　Overlapping of the terminal ascending colon with transverse colon

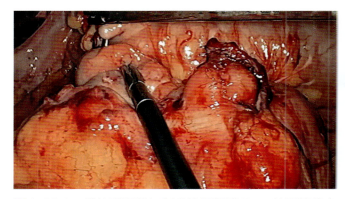

图 3-21-6　横结肠断端与距升结肠断端 7cm 处肠管缝合固定

Figure 3-21-6　Suture of the transverse colon stump with bowel wall 7cm from the terminal ascending colon

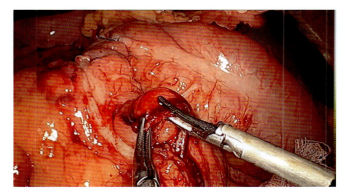

图 3-21-7　升结肠断端对系膜侧肠壁做 1cm 切口

Figure 3-21-7　Making an incision of 1cm long on the antimesenteric border of the terminal ascending colon

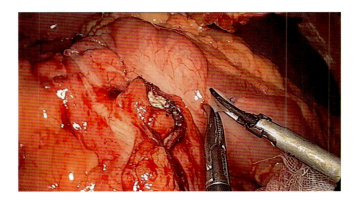

图 3-21-8　相应位置的横结肠对系膜侧肠壁做 1cm 切口

Figure 3-21-8　Making an incision of 1 cm long on the corresponding antimesenteric border of the transverse colon

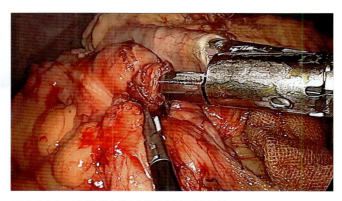

图 3-21-9　直线切割闭合器置入两侧肠管

Figure 3-21-9　Insertion of linear cutting stapler into both sides of the bowel

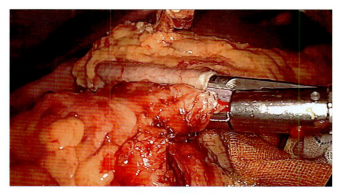

图 3-21-10　完成回肠 - 横结肠侧侧吻合

Figure 3-21-10　Completing the side-to-side anastomosis between the ileum and transverse colon

再次以酒精或碘附纱布消毒升结肠和横结肠,检查肠腔内吻合口有无明显出血,如有出血可以缝合止血(图 3-21-11)。确认无活动性出血后,在两侧肠管共同开口的两端及中间各缝合 1 针用于牵拉固定(图 3-21-12),术者和助手分别牵拉缝线尾端,牵开侧侧吻合口呈 V 形,最后用直线切割闭合器关闭共同开口,完成回肠 - 横结肠重叠式三角吻合(图 3-21-13、图 3-21-14)。

3. 标本取出　消毒阴道后,助手将卵圆钳置于阴道后穹隆并向上下打开起指示作用(图 3-21-15),术者用超声刀横行切开阴道后穹隆 3～5cm(图 3-21-16),助手将卵圆钳经阴道后穹隆切口置入腹腔,夹持住保护套及肠管一端(图 3-21-17、图 3-21-18),缓慢经阴道切口拉出标本及保护套(图 3-21-19)。

腹腔镜下术者应用 V-loc 倒刺线连续缝合阴道后穹隆切口(图 3-21-20、图 3-21-21)。蒸馏水冲洗腹腔,检查器械无误,确认无活动性出血后,经右侧 12mm 戳卡孔留置腹腔引流管一根。停止气腹,排出腹腔气体,关闭戳卡孔。

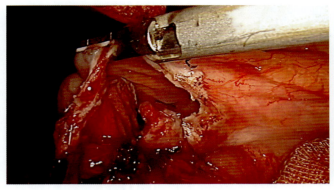

图 3-21-11　查看吻合口情况

Figure 3-21-11　Examination of the condition of anastomosis

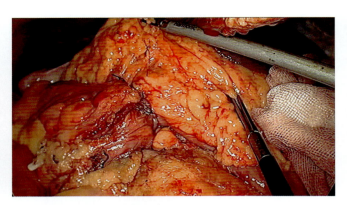

图 3-21-14　重叠式三角吻合

Figure 3-21-14　Overlapped delta-shaped anastomosis

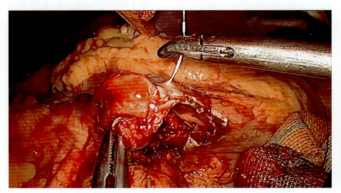

图 3-21-12　两侧肠管共同开口两端及中间各缝合 1 针

Figure 3-21-12　Suture one needle at each of the two ends and the middle of the common opening of the intestinal tubes on both sides

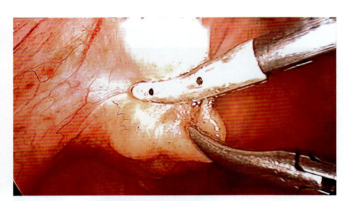

图 3-21-15　用卵圆钳指示切口位置

Figure 3-21-15　Indication of the incision position by the oval forceps

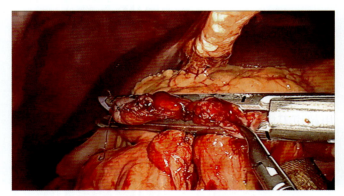

图 3-21-13　用直线切割闭合器闭合两侧肠管共同开口

Figure 3-21-13　Close the enterotomies with a linear cutting stapler

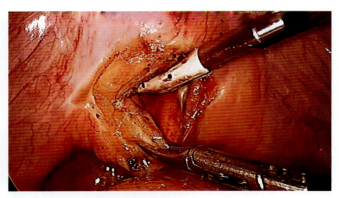

图 3-21-16　切开阴道后穹隆

Figure 3-21-16　Opening the posterior vaginal fornix

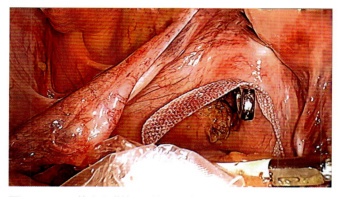

图 3-21-17    将卵圆钳经阴道置入腹腔

Figure 3-21-17    Transvaginal placement of the oval forceps

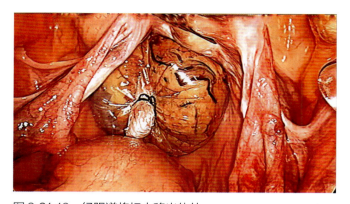

图 3-21-19    经阴道将标本移出体外

Figure 3-21-19    Transvaginal extraction of specimen

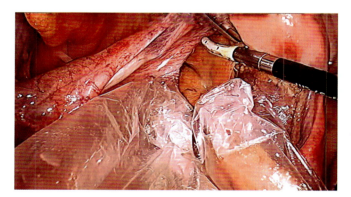

图 3-21-18    卵圆钳夹持住保护套及肠管一端

Figure 3-21-18    Clamp the specimen protective sleeve and one end of the intestinal tube with the oval forceps

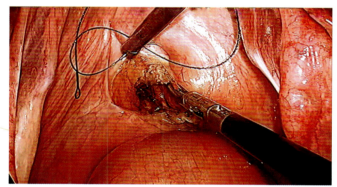

图 3-21-20    腹腔镜下缝合阴道切口

Figure 3-21-20    Closure of the vaginal incision under laparoscopy

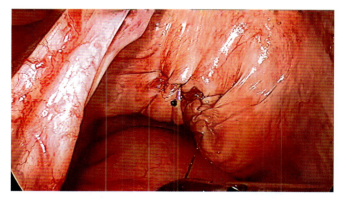

图 3-21-21    完整闭合阴道切口

Figure 3-21-21    Closure of the vaginal incision completely

# 第二十二节　腹部无辅助切口经直肠切口拖出标本的腹腔镜下横结肠癌根治术

## 【简介】

该术式的难点主要体现在 NOSES 特有的腹腔镜下消化道重建，即腹腔镜下使用直线切割闭合器行重叠式三角吻合，重建难度超过其他术式。因此该术式需要更严格地把握适应证，具有清晰的手术思路，以及娴熟的操作技巧。

## 一、适应证与禁忌证

### 【适应证】

1. 横结肠癌或良性肿瘤。
2. 肿瘤环周直径为 3～5cm。
3. 肿瘤不侵出浆膜为宜。

### 【禁忌证】

1. 肿瘤体积过大，取出有困难者。
2. 肿瘤侵犯周围组织器官。
3. 过于肥胖者（BMI>35kg/m²）。

## 二、手术操作步骤、技巧与要点

### 【戳卡位置】

1. 腹腔镜镜头戳卡孔（10mm 戳卡）　脐至脐下方 5cm 的范围内均可。

2. 术者主戳卡孔（12mm 戳卡）　左上腹中部，腹直肌外缘。
3. 术者辅助戳卡孔（5mm 戳卡）　左下腹，与腹腔镜镜头戳卡孔不在同一水平线。
4. 助手主戳卡孔（12mm 戳卡）　麦氏点。
5. 助手辅助戳卡孔（5mm 戳卡）　右上腹，右锁骨中线与横结肠投影区交叉处（图 3-22-1）。

### 【探查】

1. 常规探查　观察各脏器及腹膜表面有无种植转移等病变。
2. 肿瘤探查　根据肿瘤的位置、大小、侵犯深度，确定手术的可行性。
3. 解剖结构的判定　横结肠毗邻脏器多、血管关系复杂，需判定回结肠动静脉、右结肠动静脉、中结肠动静脉的位置。此外，还需判定升结肠和横结肠游离后可否行腹腔镜下升结肠 - 横结肠重叠式三角吻合。

### 【解剖与分离】

1. 右结肠血管根部的处理　在胰颈下缘横结肠系膜薄弱处行第一刀切割，并向上及向右扩展空间。在右结肠血管根部结扎并切断。
2. 中结肠血管的处理　于胰腺下缘分离出中结肠血管，结扎并切断。

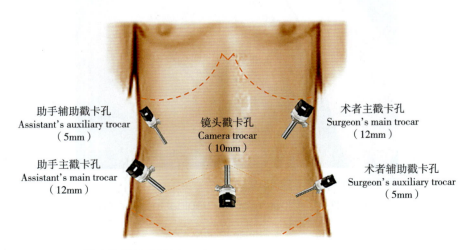

图 3-22-1　戳卡位置（五孔法）
Figure 3-22-1　Trocar placement（five-port method）

3. Henle 干的处理　沿胰前间隙在十二指肠及胰头表面游离,仔细分离后可见副右结肠静脉、胃网膜右静脉、胰十二指肠上前静脉汇成 Henle 干后汇入肠系膜上静脉。在各血管分支根部结扎并切断。

4. 大网膜及第 6 组淋巴结的处理　沿胃网膜右动静脉血管弓外缘向右分离切断胃网膜右动静脉,弓外清扫第 6 组淋巴结。

5. 升结肠系膜的游离及处理　注意保护右侧生殖血管、胰头及十二指肠。于距肿瘤近端约 10cm 处确定升结肠预切除线,裁剪升结肠系膜,并裸化肠管。

6. 横结肠系膜的处理　向横结肠预切除线方向分离裁剪横结肠远端系膜,结扎并切断边缘血管弓,并裸化预切除线部位横结肠肠壁。

【标本切除与消化道重建】

1. 标本切除　用直线切割闭合器在横结肠预切除线处闭合切断肠管(图 3-22-2),然后在横结肠近端预切除线,用直线切割闭合器闭合切断横结肠(图 3-22-3)。至此横结肠肿瘤根治切除完成,将标本置于保护套中,置于盆腔(图 3-22-4)。

2. 消化道重建　将横结肠两侧断端重叠摆放(图 3-22-5)。然后将横结肠远断端与近断端 7cm 处肠管缝合固定(图 3-22-6),检查两侧肠管血运良好,估计两侧吻合口无张力后,分别于横结肠近断端对系膜侧肠壁与相应位置的远端横结肠对系膜侧肠壁做 1cm 切口(图 3-22-7、图 3-22-8),酒精或碘附纱条消毒肠壁切口。经术者主戳卡孔置入直线切割闭合器,分别将钉仓两侧置入横结肠近断端及横结肠远断端肠腔,进行必要的调整,确认无误后击发,完成横结肠侧侧吻合(图 3-22-9 ~ 图 3-22-11)。

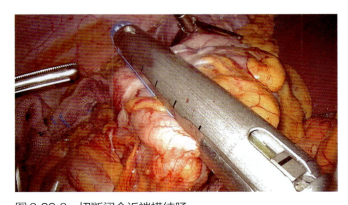

图 3-22-3　切断闭合近端横结肠

Figure 3-22-3　Closure and transection of the proximal transverse colon

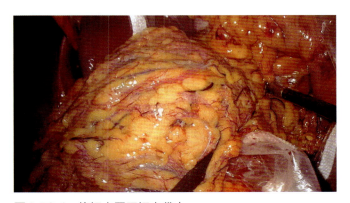

图 3-22-4　将标本置于标本袋中

Figure 3-22-4　Placement of specimen into the sterile specimen bag

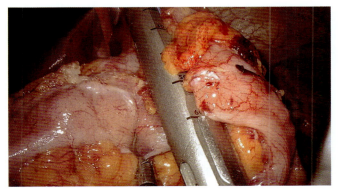

图 3-22-2　切断闭合远端横结肠

Figure 3-22-2　Closure and transection of the distal transverse colon

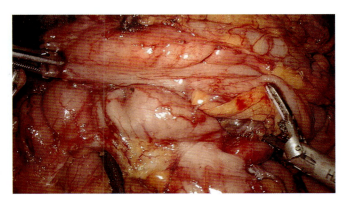

图 3-22-5　横结肠两侧断端重叠摆放

Figure 3-22-5　Overlap of the proximal and distal transverse colon stumps

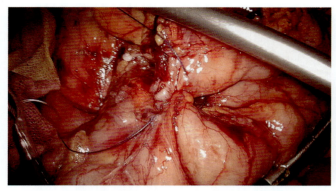

图 3-22-6 横结肠远断端与近断端 7cm 处肠管缝合固定

Figure 3-22-6 Securing the proximal and distal transverse colon stumps with a suture at an overlap of 7cm

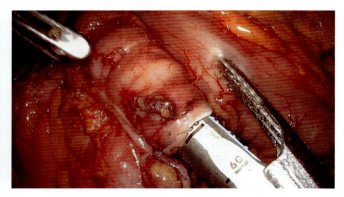

图 3-22-9 直线切割闭合器置入两侧肠管

Figure 3-22-9 Placement of the linear cutting stapler into the lumens of the two bowel stumps

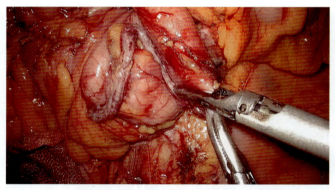

图 3-22-7 横结肠近断端对系膜侧肠壁做 1cm 切口

Figure 3-22-7 A 1cm incision is made on the antimesenteric border of the proximal transverse colon stump

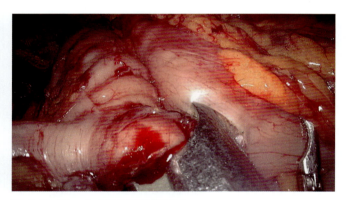

图 3-22-10 完成横结肠侧侧吻合

Figure 3-22-10 Completed side-to-side anastomosis of the transverse colon

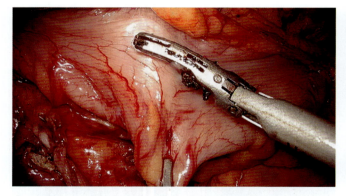

图 3-22-8 在相应位置的远端横结肠对系膜侧肠壁做 1cm 切口

Figure 3-22-8 A 1cm incision is made at the corresponding position on the antimesenteric border of the distal transverse colon

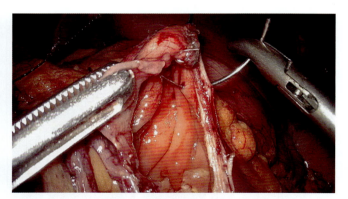

图 3-22-11 两侧肠管断端缺口连续缝合及浆肌层缝合

Figure 3-22-11 Continuous suture of the common opening of the two bowel stumps and suture of the seromuscular layer

再次以酒精或碘附纱布消毒两断端横结肠的共同开口，检查肠腔内侧侧吻合口有无明显出血，如有出血可以缝合止血。确认无活动性出血后，腹腔镜下应用 V-loc 倒刺线连续缝合两侧肠管共同开口。

3. 标本取出　消毒肛门直肠后，助手用卵圆钳夹取碘附纱布置于直肠并向左右打开起指示作用（图 3-22-12），术者用超声刀纵行切开直肠前壁 3～5cm（图 3-22-13），助手将卵圆钳经直肠前壁切口置入腹腔并夹持住保护套及肠管一端（图 3-22-14、图 3-22-15），缓慢经直肠切口拉出标本及保护套，将标本移出体外（图 3-22-16）。

腹腔镜下应用 V-loc 倒刺线连续缝合直肠前壁切口（图 3-22-17、图 3-22-18）。蒸馏水冲洗腹腔，检查器械无误，确认无活动性出血后，经右 12mm Trocar 孔留置腹腔引流管一根。停止气腹，排出腹腔气体，关闭戳卡孔。

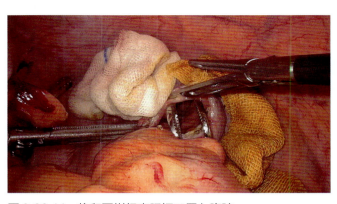

图 3-22-14　将卵圆钳经直肠切口置入腹腔
Figure 3-22-14　Insertion of oval forceps into the abdominal cavity via the rectal incision

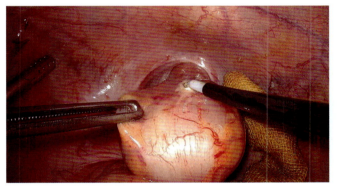

图 3-22-12　用卵圆钳指示直肠前壁切口位置
Figure 3-22-12　Position of anterior rectal wall incision as indicated using oval forceps

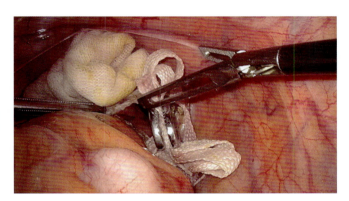

图 3-22-15　卵圆钳夹持住保护套及肠管一端
Figure 3-22-15　Clamping of the specimen protective sleeve and one end of the intestinal tube using oval forceps

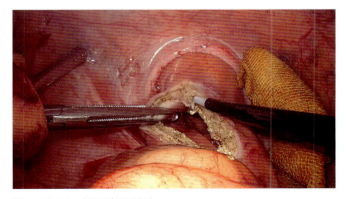

图 3-22-13　切开直肠前壁
Figure 3-22-13　Incision of the anterior rectal wall

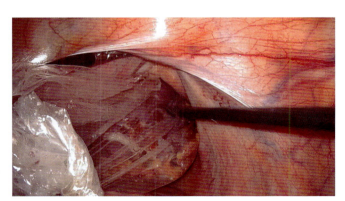

图 3-22-16　标本移出体外
Figure 3-22-16　Specimen extraction

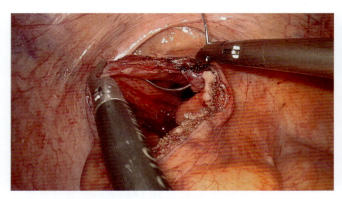

图 3-22-17　腹腔镜下缝合直肠前壁切口

Figure 3-22-17　Laparoscopic suturing of the incision on the anterior rectal wall

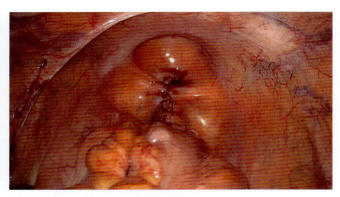

图 3-22-18　完整闭合直肠前壁切口

Figure 3-22-18　Completed closure of the incision on the anterior rectal wall

# 第四章

# 腹腔镜下胃NOSES的标准化流程

## 第一节 腹部无辅助切口经直肠取标本的腹腔镜下远端胃切除术

### （GC-NOSES I式，毕 I 式吻合）

### 【简介】

GC-NOSES I式主要适用于肿瘤位于胃中下 1/3 部位，分期在 $T_3$ 以内，且肿瘤最大径 <5cm，多适用于男性患者。该术式的操作特点：在完成胃周淋巴结清扫后，将标本装入保护套内，可以经直肠将标本取出体外，该术式不需要额外增加腹部的辅助切口，就可以将标本取出体外，腹部仅留有微小的穿刺孔，是真正意义上的腹腔镜下胃癌根治术。

## 一、适应证与禁忌证

### 【适应证】

1. 病变位于胃远端的 $cT_{1\sim3}N_{0\sim1}M_0$ 期胃癌。
2. 肿瘤最大径 ≤5cm。
3. BMI ≤30kg/m²。

### 【禁忌证】

1. 肿瘤体积过大，无法经直肠取出者。
2. 怀疑肿瘤浸透浆膜或累及邻近脏器者。

3. 合并急性胃肠道梗阻或者肿瘤穿孔，需急症手术者。
4. 过于肥胖者（BMI>30kg/m²），尤其是内脏脂肪含量高的患者。
5. 盆腔手术史或存在直肠、肛门畸形等。

## 二、手术操作步骤、技巧与要点

### 【戳卡位置】

1. 腹腔镜镜头戳卡孔（10mm 戳卡） 经脐孔或者根据患者腹型沿脐上下移动 1cm 处。
2. 术者主戳卡孔（12mm 戳卡） 左侧腋前线肋缘下 1~2cm 处。
3. 术者辅助戳卡孔（5mm 戳卡） 左侧锁骨中线平脐处。
4. 助手辅助戳卡孔（5mm 戳卡） 右侧腋前线肋缘下 1~2cm 处。
5. 助手主戳卡孔（10mm 戳卡） 右侧锁骨中线平脐处（图 4-1-1）。

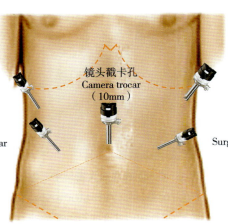

助手辅助戳卡孔
Assistant's auxiliary trocar
（5mm）

助手主戳卡孔
Assistant's main trocar
（10mm）

镜头戳卡孔
Camera trocar
（10mm）

术者主戳卡孔
Surgeon's main trocar
（12mm）

术者辅助戳卡孔
Surgeon's auxiliary trocar
（5mm）

图 4-1-1 戳卡位置（五孔法）
Figure 4-1-1 Trocar placement
（five-port method）

## 【探查】

1. 常规探查　观察各脏器及腹膜表面有无种植转移等病变。

2. 肿瘤探查　根据肿瘤的位置、大小、侵犯深度，确定手术的可行性。

3. 解剖结构的判定　根据肿瘤位置及解剖结构决定手术方案，并估计标本能否经直肠取出。

## 【解剖与分离】

1. 大网膜游离及幽门下区域淋巴结清扫　游离清扫过程中，在保证远端切缘阴性的前提下，保留足够长的十二指肠用于胃十二指肠毕 I 式吻合。

2. 胰腺上区域淋巴结清扫　将胃移向右上腹，充分显露胰腺上平面，依次完成相应区域淋巴结清扫。

3. 小弯侧淋巴结清扫　采取后侧入路，将胃向腹壁及头侧挑起，完成第 1 组和第 3 组淋巴结清扫。

4. 第 4sb 组淋巴结清扫　自脾下极及胰尾前方的胰腺前筋膜面开始，逐步向头侧及脾门区域解剖，于根部结扎并切断胃网膜左血管，从而完成该组淋巴结的清扫。

5. 离断远端胃　距离原发癌灶上极大弯侧 8cm、小弯侧 5～6cm 处，用 60mm 直线切割闭合器两根，离断胃体。

## 【标本切除与消化道重建】

1. 标本切除　距离原发癌灶上极大弯侧 8cm、小弯侧 5～6cm 处，用 60mm 直线切割闭合器两根，离断胃体。

2. 标本取出　患者取头低脚高位，于盆底腹膜反折上方 5～6cm 处，沿直肠系膜对系膜侧肠壁的纵轴，纵行切开直肠前壁 3～5cm（图 4-1-2）。助手将肠钳自肛门引入，从直肠前壁切口处伸出并进入腹腔，术者将标本袋一头递给助手肠钳，左手提起直肠切口处的肠壁轻轻向头侧对抗牵引，此刻，助手缓慢将标本袋自肛门拽出体外，完成经肛门取标本（图 4-1-3）。取出标本后，反复冲洗盆腔后，用 3-0 V-loc 倒刺线连续缝合直肠前壁切口，并间断包埋数针。

3. 消化道重建　在近端残胃大弯侧距离胃断端 5cm 处开孔，同时十二指肠残断端开孔，将 60mm 直线切割闭合器插入上述开孔内，行近端残胃大弯与十二指肠前壁的毕 I 式吻合（图 4-1-4）。击发吻合器后，取出直线切割闭合器，并观察吻合口有无活动性出血（图 4-1-5）。用 3-0 V-loc 倒刺线连续缝

合关闭共同开口（图 4-1-6）。将残胃向腹侧挑起，观察有无吻合口张力，完成胃十二指肠毕 I 式吻合（图 4-1-7）。

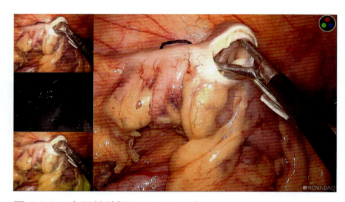

图 4-1-2　直肠前壁切开 3～5cm 小口

Figure 4-1-2　Making an incision about 3-5cm in the anterior rectal wall

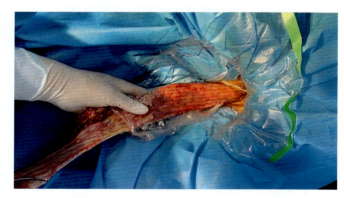

图 4-1-3　经肛门取出标本

Figure 4-1-3　Transanal specimen extraction

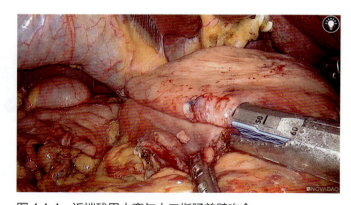

图 4-1-4　近端残胃大弯与十二指肠前壁吻合

Figure 4-1-4　Anastomosis of the proximal remnant stomach and the anterior wall of duodenum

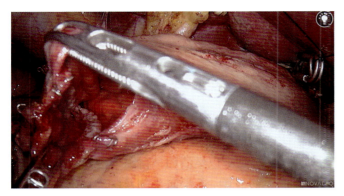

图 4-1-5　经共同开口观察吻合口有无活动性出血

Figure 4-1-5　Observing the anastomosis for active bleeding through the common opening

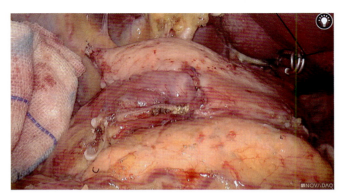

图 4-1-6　用 3-0 V-loc 倒刺线连续缝合关闭共同开口

Figure 4-1-6　Closure of the common opening with 3-0 V-loc barbed suture in a continuous manner

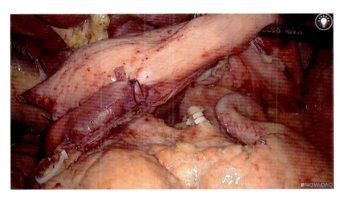

图 4-1-7　胃十二指肠毕 I 式吻合完成

Figure 4-1-7　Completion of Billroth I gastroduodenal anastomosis

# 第二节　腹部无辅助切口经阴道取标本的腹腔镜下远端胃切除术

## （GC-NOSES II 式，毕 I 式吻合）

### 【简介】

GC-NOSES II 式主要适用于肿瘤位于胃中下 1/3 部位，分期在 $T_3$ 以内，且肿瘤最大径 <5cm 的女性患者，多适用于对腹部有一定美容需求者。该术式的操作特点：在完成胃周淋巴结清扫后，将大网膜及远端胃装入标本袋内，可以经阴道将标本取出体外，该术式不需要额外增加腹部的辅助切口，就可以将标本取出体外，腹部仅留有微小的穿刺孔，是真正意义上的腹腔镜下胃癌根治术。

## 一、适应证与禁忌证

### 【适应证】

1. 病变位于胃远端的 $cT_{1\sim3}N_{0\sim1}M_0$ 期胃癌。
2. 肿瘤最大径≤5cm。
3. BMI≤30kg/m²。
4. 女性患者。

### 【禁忌证】

1. 肿瘤体积过大，无法经阴道取出。
2. 怀疑肿瘤浸透浆膜或累及邻近脏器。

3. 合并急性胃肠道梗阻或者肿瘤穿孔，需急症手术者。

4. 过于肥胖者（BMI>30kg/m²），尤其是内脏脂肪含量高的患者。

5. 盆腔或妇科手术史，以及存在阴道畸形等。

## 二、手术操作步骤、技巧与要点

### 【戳卡位置】

1. 腹腔镜镜头戳卡孔（10mm 戳卡）　经脐孔或者根据患者腹形沿脐上下移动 1cm 处。

2. 术者主戳卡孔（12mm 戳卡）　在左侧腋前线肋缘下 1~2cm 处。

3. 术者辅助戳卡孔（5mm 戳卡）　左侧锁骨中线平脐处。

4. 助手辅助戳卡孔（5mm 戳卡）　右侧腋前线肋缘下 1~2cm 处。

5. 助手主戳卡孔（10mm 戳卡）　右侧锁骨中线平脐处（图 4-2-1）。

### 【探查】

1. 常规探查　观察各脏器及腹膜表面有无种植转移等病变。

2. 肿瘤探查　根据肿瘤的位置、大小、侵犯深度，确定手术的可行性。

3. 解剖结构的判定　根据肿瘤位置及解剖结构决定手术方案，并估计标本能否经阴道取出。

### 【解剖与分离】

1. 大网膜游离及幽门下区域淋巴结清扫　游离清扫过程中，在保证远端切缘阴性的前提下，

保留足够长的十二指肠用于胃十二指肠毕 I 式吻合。

2. 胰腺上区域淋巴结清扫　将胃移向右上腹，充分显露胰腺上平面，依次完成相应区域淋巴结清扫。

3. 小弯侧淋巴结清扫　采取后侧入路，将胃向腹壁及头侧挑起，完成第 1 组和第 3 组淋巴结清扫。

4. 第 4sb 组淋巴结清扫　自脾下极及胰尾前方的胰腺前筋膜面开始，逐步向头侧及脾门区域解剖，于根部结扎并切断胃网膜左血管，从而完成该组淋巴结的清扫。

### 【标本切除与消化道重建】

1. 标本切除　距离原发癌灶上极大弯侧 8cm、小弯侧 5~6cm 处，用 60mm 直线切割闭合器两根，离断胃体。

2. 标本取出　助手仔细冲洗阴道确保干净后，调整患者取头低脚高位，将小肠移向上腹部，盆腔无任何阻挡的情况下，用荷包线穿过两侧子宫阔韧带，将子宫向腹侧悬吊起来，这样可以充分显露子宫后方。在盆底腹膜反折处，助手用举宫器将宫颈向腹侧抬起，术者用电钩沿着阴道后穹隆切开长 4~5cm 的切口（图 4-2-2），通过阴道后穹隆切口经腹导入标本袋（图 4-2-3）。将标本袋一端送入阴道后穹隆，助手用抓钳将标本袋经阴道缓缓拖出体外，整个过程轻柔，不宜暴力牵拉，以免造成阴道后穹隆出血（图 4-2-4）。取出标本后，用 3-0 可吸收线连续缝合阴道后穹隆切口，间断缝合加固数针，或者用 V-loc 倒刺线连续加固缝合（图 4-2-5、图 4-2-6）。缝合结束，再次冲洗盆腔干净后，恢复患者头高脚低位，以便进行消化道重建。

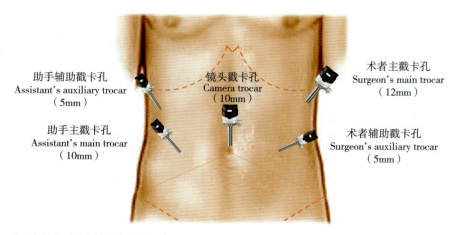

图 4-2-1　戳卡位置（五孔法）

Figure 4-2-1　Trocar placement（five-port method）

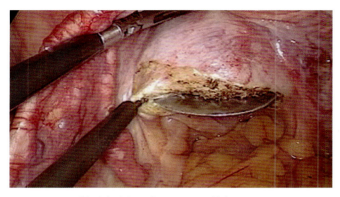

图 4-2-2　阴道后穹隆切开长 4～5cm 的切口

Figure 4-2-2　Making a 4-5cm incision in the posterior vaginal fornix

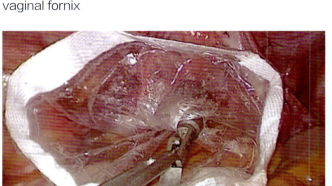

图 4-2-3　通过阴道后穹隆切口经腹导入标本袋

Figure 4-2-3　Transabdominal introduction of specimen bag through the incision in the posterior vaginal fornix

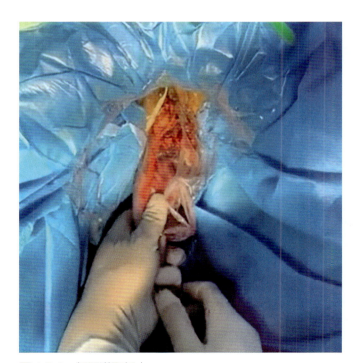

图 4-2-4　经阴道取标本

Figure 4-2-4　Transvaginal specimen extraction

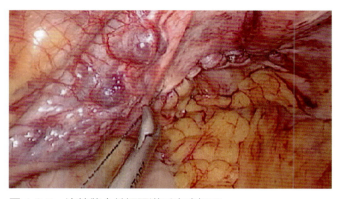

图 4-2-5　连续缝合关闭阴道后穹隆切口

Figure 4-2-5　Closure of incision in the posterior vaginal fornix by continuous suture

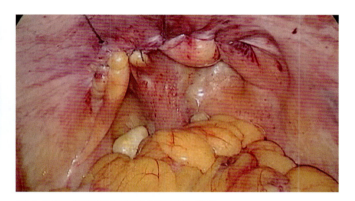

图 4-2-6　阴道后穹隆缝合完毕的术野

Figure 4-2-6　Surgical field after the suture of posterior vaginal fornix

3. 消化道重建　在近端残胃大弯侧距离胃断端 5cm 处开孔，同时十二指肠断端开孔，将 60mm 直线切割闭合器插入上述开孔内，行近端残胃大弯与十二指肠前壁的毕 Ⅰ 式吻合（图 4-2-7）。击发吻合器后，取出直线切割闭合器，并观察吻合口有无活动性出血（图 4-2-8）。用 3-0 V-loc 倒刺线连续缝合关闭共同开口（图 4-2-9）。将残胃向腹侧挑起，观察有无吻合口张力，完成胃十二指肠毕 Ⅰ 式吻合（图 4-2-10）。

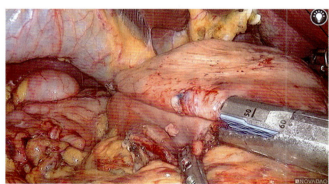

图 4-2-7　近端残胃大弯与十二指肠前壁吻合

Figure 4-2-7　Anastomosis of proximal remnant stomach and the anterior wall of duodenum

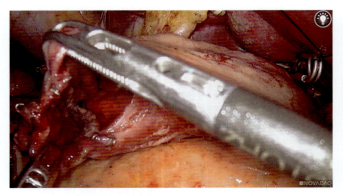

图 4-2-8　经共同开口观察吻合口有无活动性出血

Figure 4-2-8　Observing the anastomosis for active bleeding through the common opening

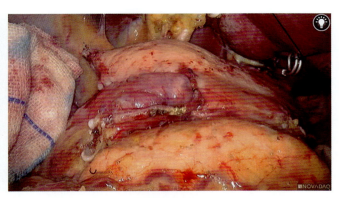

图 4-2-9　用 3-0 V-loc 倒刺线连续缝合关闭共同开口

Figure 4-2-9　Closure of the common opening with 3-0 V-loc barbed suture in a continuous manner

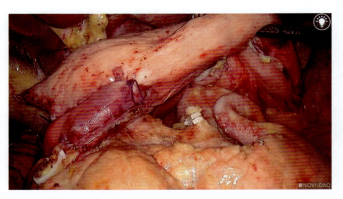

图 4-2-10　胃十二指肠毕 I 式吻合完成

Figure 4-2-10　Completion of Billroth Ⅰ gastroduodenal anastomosis

## 第三节　腹部无辅助切口经直肠取标本的腹腔镜下远端胃切除术

（GC-NOSES Ⅲ式，毕Ⅱ式吻合）

### 【简介】

GC-NOSES Ⅲ式主要适用于肿瘤未浸透浆膜的 $T_3$ 期以内、标本体积较小的男性胃癌患者和部分女性胃癌患者。除了取标本途径与常规腹腔镜手术有所区别，胃肠切除范围、淋巴结清扫范围、手术的游离层次等与常规腹腔镜手术一致。该术式的操作特点：腹腔镜下完成胃癌根治性切除及消化道重建，于直肠上段切开，经直肠将标本取出。这一术式需要术者严格掌握适应证，并评估医生与患者对手术风险的接受程度。

### 一、适应证与禁忌证

#### 【适应证】

1. 病变位于胃远端的 $cT_{1\sim3}N_{1\sim2}M_0$ 期胃癌。
2. 肿瘤最大直径≤4cm 为宜。

#### 【禁忌证】

1. 肿瘤体积过大，无法经肛门取出。
2. 肿瘤浸透浆膜或累及邻近脏器。
3. 合并急性胃肠道梗阻或者肿瘤穿孔，需急症手术者。

4. 过于肥胖者（BMI>30kg/m²）。

5. 盆腔手术史或存在直肠、肛门畸形等。

## 二、手术操作步骤、技巧与要点

### 【戳卡位置】

该术式戳卡位置要同时满足胃癌根治术与经直肠取标本操作的需要。

1. 腹腔镜镜头戳卡孔（10mm 戳卡）　脐下1cm 处。

2. 术者主戳卡孔（12mm 戳卡）　左侧腋前线肋缘下 2cm 处。

3. 术者辅助戳卡孔（5mm 戳卡）　左侧锁骨中线平脐处。

4. 助手辅助戳卡孔（5mm 戳卡）　右侧腋前线肋缘下。

5. 助手主戳卡孔（12mm 戳卡）　右侧锁骨中线平脐处（图 4-3-1）。

### 【探查】

1. 常规探查　观察各脏器及腹膜表面有无种植转移等病变。

2. 肿瘤探查　根据肿瘤的位置、大小、侵犯深度，确定手术的可行性。

3. 解剖结构的判定　根据肿瘤及直肠的情况估计标本能否经直肠取出。

### 【解剖与分离】

1. 分离大网膜　将大网膜向头侧翻起，从横结肠偏左部离断大网膜，进入小网膜囊，向右至结肠肝曲并在结肠系膜前叶后方分离，切除结肠系膜前叶。

2. 胃周淋巴结清扫

（1）清扫第 6 组淋巴结：以中结肠动静脉为标志，进入胃十二指肠和横结肠系膜之间的融合筋膜间隙。显露 Henle 干，于根部离断胃网膜右静脉；继续沿胰头表面解剖，打开胃胰韧带，显露胃十二指肠动脉，裸化胃网膜右动脉，于根部离断，彻底清扫第 6 组淋巴结。

（2）清扫第 4sb 组淋巴结：显露胰尾，定位脾血管，松解结肠脾曲，分离大网膜与脾中下极的粘连，保护胰尾，显露根部，待分出进入脾下极分支后，离断胃网膜左动静脉，清扫第 4sb 组淋巴结。

（3）清扫第 11p、7、8、9 组淋巴结：脾动脉起始段位置相对固定，解剖变异少，因此可将此处作为切入点。助手抓持胃胰皱襞，将胃翻向上方，以利于显露胰腺上缘及脾动脉周围区域。

（4）清扫第 5、12a 组淋巴结：显露肝总动脉，将胰腺向左下方牵拉，沿胃十二指肠动脉及肝总动脉充分显露胃右动脉及肝固有动脉，继续向上分离肝固有动脉前方及外侧，清扫第 12a 组淋巴结。于根部离断胃右血管，并清扫第 5 组淋巴结。于幽门远端用直线切割闭合器离断十二指肠，清扫其周围第 5 组淋巴结。

（5）清扫第 1、3 组淋巴结：紧贴胃壁小弯侧，采用超声刀解剖胃小弯及清扫贲门右侧淋巴结（第 1、3 组淋巴结）。

### 【标本切除与消化道重建】

1. 标本切除　距肿瘤近端 5cm 用腔内直线切割闭合器离断胃，根据胃壁厚度选择合适钉仓（图 4-3-2），

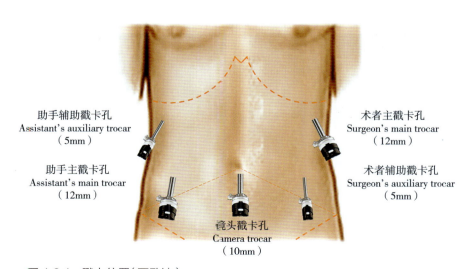

助手辅助戳卡孔
Assistant's auxiliary trocar
（5mm）

助手主戳卡孔
Assistant's main trocar
（12mm）

术者主戳卡孔
Surgeon's main trocar
（12mm）

术者辅助戳卡孔
Surgeon's auxiliary trocar
（5mm）

镜头戳卡孔
Camera trocar
（10mm）

图 4-3-1　戳卡位置（五孔法）

Figure 4-3-1　Trocar placement（ five-port method ）

术者将保护套经主戳卡孔置入腹腔,将切除的标本置入标本袋中(图 4-3-3)。

2. 消化道重建

(1)毕Ⅱ式吻合:在距离屈氏韧带 15～20cm 处的空肠对系膜侧肠壁开孔,在残胃断端与胃大弯交界处开孔,用 60mm 直线切割闭合器行近端胃 - 空肠侧侧吻合。用 4-0 可吸收线间断缝合关闭胃空肠共同开口(图 4-3-4～图 4-3-8)。

(2)远端胃空肠 uncut Roux-en-Y 吻合:胃 - 空肠侧侧吻合及关闭胃空肠共同开口同毕Ⅱ式吻合。使用 60mm 直线切割闭合器对近端空肠与远端空肠行侧侧吻合,输入袢吻合位置距屈氏韧带 7～10cm,输出袢吻合位置距胃空肠吻合口 40～45cm。输入袢阻断位置距胃空肠吻合口约 3cm(图 4-3-9～图 4-3-11)。

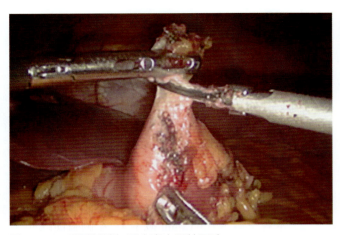

图 4-3-4 残胃断端与胃大弯交界处开孔

Figure 4-3-4 Opening a window at the point of gastric stump and greater curvature

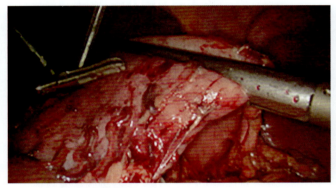

图 4-3-2 距肿瘤近端 5cm 离断胃

Figure 4-3-2 Amputation of the stomach at 5cm from the proximal end of tumor

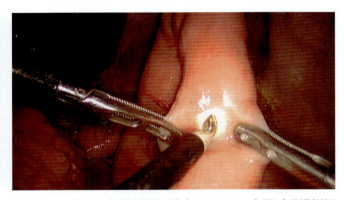

图 4-3-5 自屈氏韧带测量近端空肠 20cm,空肠对系膜侧肠壁开孔

Figure 4-3-5 Measuring a 20cm length of proximal jejunum from the Treitz ligament, a window opening in the antimesenteric intestinal wall

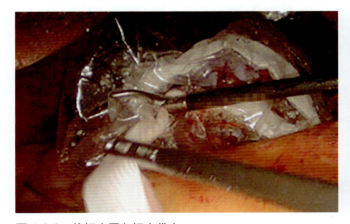

图 4-3-3 将标本置入标本袋中

Figure 4-3-3 Placing the specimen in the specimen bag

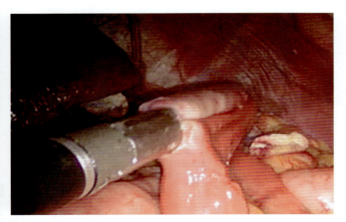

图 4-3-6 结肠前行胃 - 空肠侧侧吻合

Figure 4-3-6 Antecolic side-to-side gastric jejunal anastomosis

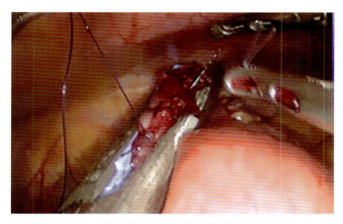

图 4-3-7　用腔内直线切割闭合器关闭胃空肠共同开口

Figure 4-3-7　Closing up the common opening of the stomach and jejunum with a linear cutting stapler

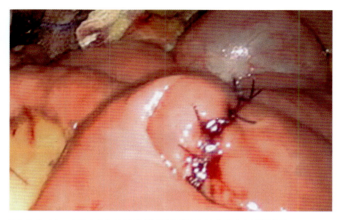

图 4-3-10　用 4-0 可吸收线间断缝合关闭胃空肠共同开口

Figure 4-3-10　Intermittent sutures with 4-0 absorbable suture to close the common opening of the stomach and jejunum

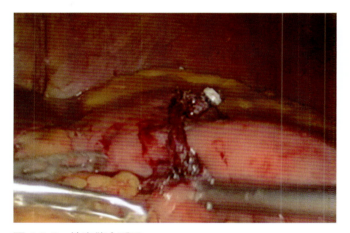

图 4-3-8　检查缝合质量

Figure 4-3-8　Quality check of sutures

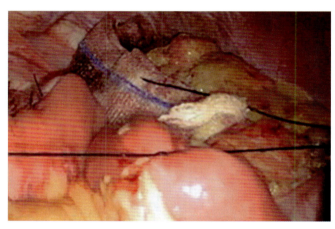

图 4-3-11　距胃空肠吻合口约 3cm 处结扎阻断输入袢

Figure 4-3-11　Blocking the afferent loop at about 3cm from the gastrojejunal anastomosis

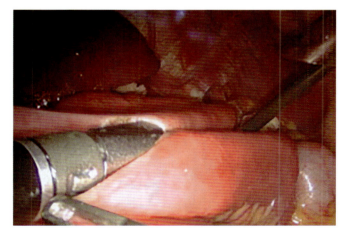

图 4-3-9　近端空肠与远端空肠侧侧吻合

Figure 4-3-9　Side-to-side anastomosis of proximal and distal jejunum

3. 标本取出　完成胃癌根治性切除及消化道重建后，更换为功能截石位，稀碘附溶液消毒会阴区及直肠肠腔。调整腹腔镜监视器至患者足侧，取头低足高右倾位，助手牵拉乙状结肠充分显露直肠上段，使其与身体纵轴平行，术者于直肠上段前壁切开 5～6cm（图 4-3-12）。用稀碘附溶液反复消毒、生理盐水反复冲洗盆腔后置入切口保护套（图 4-3-13、图 4-3-14），自切口保护器将标本自肛门取出（图 4-3-15、图 4-3-16）。连续或间断原位缝合直肠切口并冲洗盆腔（图 4-3-17、图 4-3-18）。

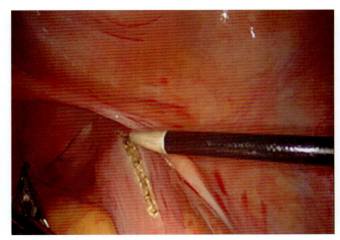

图 4-3-12　反复消毒肠腔后切开直肠上段前壁
Figure 4-3-12　Cutting open the anterior wall of the upper rectum after repetitive disinfection of the bowel cavity

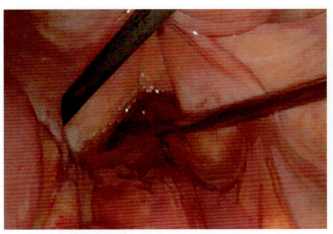

图 4-3-13　稀碘附溶液、生理盐水反复冲洗盆腔
Figure 4-3-13　Irrigation of pelvic cavity with diluted povidone-iodine solution and normal saline

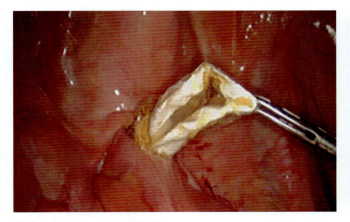

图 4-3-14　置入切口保护器
Figure 4-3-14　Insertion of a protective sleeve

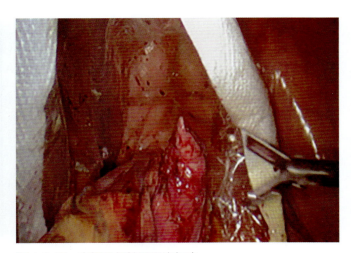

图 4-3-15　自切口保护器取出标本
Figure 4-3-15　Removing the specimen from the protective sleeve

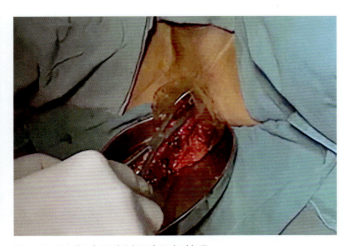

图 4-3-16　标本取出过程中肛门外观
Figure 4-3-16　Anal appearance during specimen removal

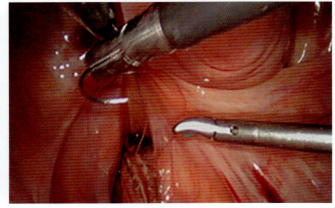

图 4-3-17　3-0 倒刺线连续缝合直肠切开处
Figure 4-3-17　Continuous sutures with barbed suture for rectum incision

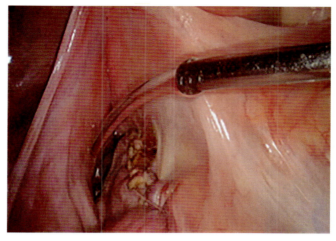

图 4-3-18　检查缝合质量，反复冲洗盆腔

Figure 4-3-18　Quality check of sutures, repetitive irrigation of the pelvic cavity

## 第四节　腹部无辅助切口经阴道取标本的腹腔镜下远端胃切除术

（GC-NOSES Ⅳ式，毕Ⅱ式吻合）

### 【简介】

GC-NOSES Ⅳ式主要适用于肿瘤位于胃中下区的女性患者。在严格遵守常规腹腔镜下胃癌根治术、消化道重建原则的基础上，通过腹腔镜下操作，切开阴道后穹隆，经阴道取出标本。按照《结直肠肿瘤经自然腔道取标本手术专家共识（2017 版）》，该术式属于切除拖出式。

### 一、适应证与禁忌证

#### 【适应证】

1. 女性患者。
2. 病变位于胃远端的 $cT_{1\sim3}N_{0\sim1}M_0$ 期胃癌。
3. 肿瘤最大直径≤4cm 为宜。

#### 【禁忌证】

1. 未育或有再生育计划者。
2. 局部晚期胃癌（$cT_4N_{2\sim3}M_1$）。
3. 肿瘤体积大，无法经阴道后穹隆拖出。
4. 过于肥胖者（BMI>30kg/m²）。
5. 盆腔手术史或存在阴道畸形等。

### 二、手术操作步骤、技巧与要点

#### 【戳卡位置】

1. 腹腔镜镜头戳卡孔（10mm 戳卡）　脐下 1cm 处。
2. 术者主戳卡孔（12mm 戳卡）　左侧腋前线肋缘下。
3. 术者辅助戳卡孔（5mm 戳卡）　左侧锁骨中线平脐处。
4. 助手辅助戳卡孔（5mm 戳卡）　右侧腋前线肋缘下。
5. 助手主戳卡孔（12mm 戳卡）　右侧锁骨中线平脐处（图 4-4-1）。

#### 【探查】

1. 常规探查　观察各脏器及腹膜表面有无种植转移等病变。
2. 肿瘤探查　肿瘤位于胃窦前壁，未浸透浆膜层。
3. 解剖结构的判定　根据肿瘤及阴道的情况估计标本能否经阴道取出。

143

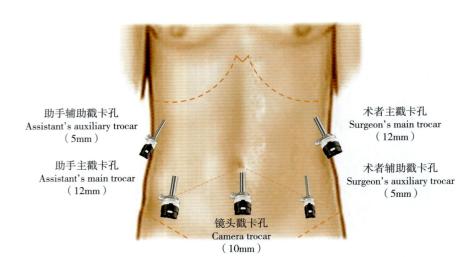

助手辅助戳卡孔
Assistant's auxiliary trocar
（5mm）

助手主戳卡孔
Assistant's main trocar
（12mm）

镜头戳卡孔
Camera trocar
（10mm）

术者主戳卡孔
Surgeon's main trocar
（12mm）

术者辅助戳卡孔
Surgeon's auxiliary trocar
（5mm）

图 4-4-1　戳卡位置（五孔法）
Figure 4-4-1　Trocar placement
（five-port method）

## 【解剖与分离】

1. 分离大网膜　将大网膜向头侧翻起，从横结肠偏左部离断大网膜，进入小网膜囊，向右至结肠肝曲，并在横结肠系膜前叶后方分离，切除结肠系膜前叶。

2. 清扫第 4sb 组淋巴结　显露胰尾，定位脾血管，松解结肠脾曲，分离大网膜与脾中下极的粘连，保护胰尾，显露根部，待分出进入脾下极分支后，离断胃网膜左动静脉，清扫第 4sb 组淋巴结。

3. 清扫第 6 组淋巴结　以中结肠动静脉为标志，进入胃十二指肠和横结肠系膜之间的融合筋膜间隙，离断胃网膜右静脉。继续沿胰头表面解剖，显露胃十二指肠动脉，裸化胃网膜右动脉，离断根部，清扫第 6 组淋巴结。

4. 离断十二指肠　先通过 Kocher 法游离十二指肠，即切开其外侧腹膜并钝性分离，将其向内翻转；然后裸化十二指肠，清理其周围组织，特别是幽门附近并清扫第 6 组淋巴结；最后使用闭合器或缝扎线在预定位置闭合并切断十二指肠，确保断端牢固闭合。

5. 清扫第 8a、12a 组淋巴结　沿胰腺上缘分离，显露肝总动脉，将胰腺压向左下方，沿肝总动脉前方及上缘，清扫第 8a 组淋巴结。助手将肝总动脉向右下牵拉，术者清扫肝固有动脉内侧及门静脉内侧淋巴结、脂肪组织，即第 12a 组淋巴结。于胃右动静脉根部夹闭后离断。

6. 清扫第 11p、7、9 组淋巴结　切开胰腺被膜，紧贴胰腺上缘分离，显露脾动脉近端，清扫第 11p 组淋巴结。由左向右清扫，显露腹腔动脉干，分离胃左动静脉，在根部夹闭后离断，清扫第 7、9 组淋巴结。

7. 清扫胃小弯及贲门右侧淋巴结　紧贴胃壁小弯侧，采用超声刀分层切开腹膜，清扫胃小弯及贲门右侧淋巴结（第 1、3 组淋巴结）。

## 【标本切除与消化道重建】

1. 标本切除　距肿瘤近端 5cm 离断胃（图 4-4-2），根据胃壁厚度选择合适钉仓，将保护套经主戳卡孔置入腹腔，将切除的标本置入标本袋中（图 4-4-3）。

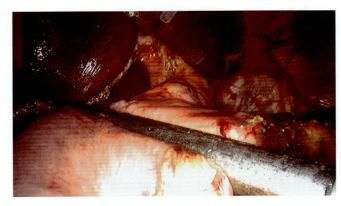

图 4-4-2　距离肿瘤近端 5cm 离断胃
Figure 4-4-2　Transection of the stomach at 5cm from the proximal end of tumor

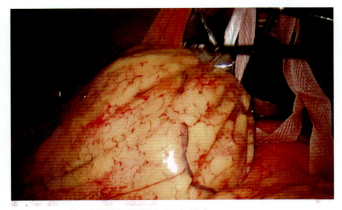

图 4-4-3　将切除的标本置入标本袋中
Figure 4-4-3　Placing the resected specimen in the specimen bag

2. 消化道重建

（1）毕Ⅱ式吻合：在距离屈氏韧带 15～20cm 处的空肠对系膜侧肠壁开孔（图 4-4-4），残胃断端大弯侧开孔（图 4-4-5），用 60mm 直线切割闭合器行近端胃-空肠侧侧吻合（图 4-4-6）。用 4-0 可吸收线间断缝合或用 3-0 倒刺线连续缝合关闭共同开口（图 4-4-7）。

（2）远端胃空肠 uncut Roux-en-Y 吻合：胃-空肠侧侧吻合及关闭胃空肠共同开口同毕Ⅱ式吻合。再用 60mm 直线切割闭合器对近端空肠与远端空肠行侧侧吻合，输入袢吻合位置距屈氏韧带 7～10cm，输出袢吻合位置距胃空肠吻合口 40～45cm（图 4-4-8、图 4-4-9）。输入袢阻断位置距胃空肠吻合口约 3cm（图 4-4-10）。

3. 标本取出　悬吊子宫（图 4-4-11），反复消毒阴道后，用压肠板顶起阴道后穹隆（图 4-4-12），在助手指引下切开阴道后穹隆，不超过两侧子宫骶韧带（图 4-4-13），经阴道置入切口保护套（图 4-4-14），用卵圆钳夹持胃断端沿胃长轴取出（图 4-4-15～图 4-4-17），蒸馏水、希碘附溶液及盐水反复冲洗盆腔（图 4-4-18），用 3-0 倒刺线连续缝合关闭阴道后穹隆切口（图 4-4-19）。

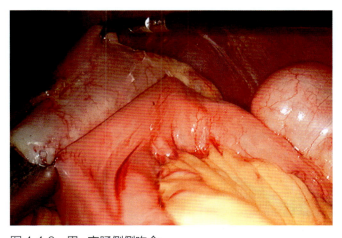

图 4-4-6　胃-空肠侧侧吻合

Figure 4-4-6　Side-to-side gastric jejunal anastomosis

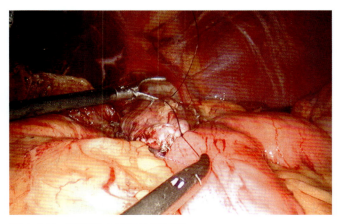

图 4-4-7　间断缝合关闭共同开口

Figure 4-4-7　Closure of the common opening with intermittent suture

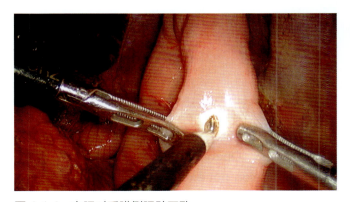

图 4-4-4　空肠对系膜侧肠壁开孔

Figure 4-4-4　Opening a window in the antimesenteric border of the jejunum

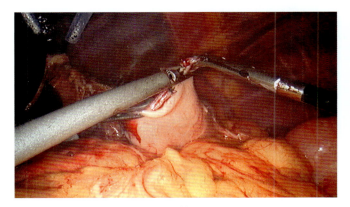

图 4-4-5　残胃断端与大弯交界处开孔

Figure 4-4-5　Opening the window at the point of gastric stump and greater curvature

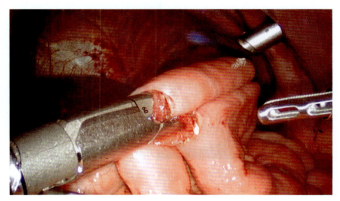

图 4-4-8　近端空肠与远端空肠侧侧吻合

Figure 4-4-8　Side-to-side anastomosis of proximal and distal jejunum

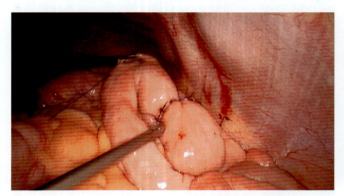

图 4-4-9　用 4-0 可吸收线间断缝合关闭胃空肠共同开口

Figure 4-4-9　Intermittent suture with 4-0 absorbable suture to close the common opening of the stomach and jejunum

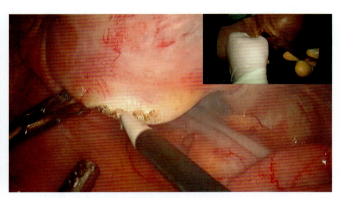

图 4-4-12　反复消毒阴道后用压肠板顶起阴道后穹隆

Figure 4-4-12　Posterior vaginal fornix is withstood with the abdominal spatula after repeated disinfection of vagina

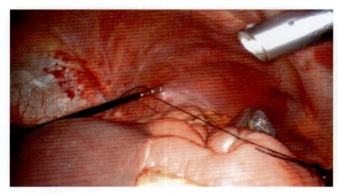

图 4-4-10　距胃空肠吻合口约 3cm 处结扎阻断输入袢

Figure 4-4-10　4-0 Ligation for blocking the afferent loop at about 3cm from the anastomosis position of gastric jejunum

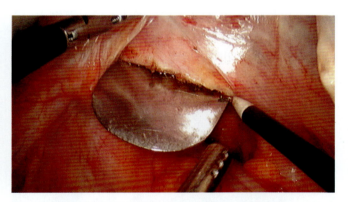

图 4-4-13　切开阴道后穹隆，不超过两侧子宫骶韧带

Figure 4-4-13　Opening the posterior vaginal fornix with the incision not exceeding the bilateral sacral ligaments

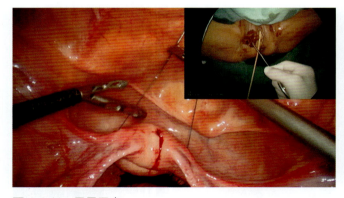

图 4-4-11　悬吊子宫

Figure 4-4-11　Suspension of uterus

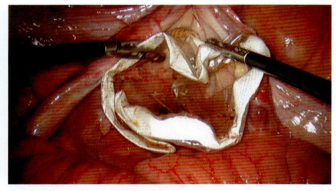

图 4-4-14　经阴道置入切口保护套

Figure 4-4-14　Placement of protective sleeve transvaginally

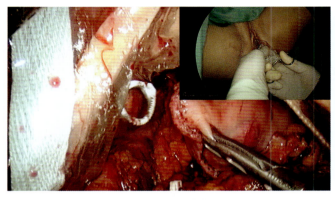

图 4-4-15　卵圆钳夹持胃断端沿胃长轴取出

Figure 4-4-15　The gastric stump is held by the oval forceps and extracted along the long axis of stomach

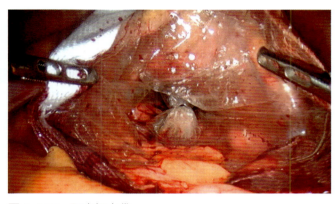

图 4-4-17　取出标本袋

Figure 4-4-17　Extraction of specimen bag

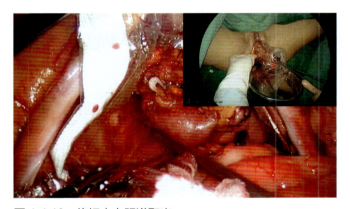

图 4-4-16　将标本自阴道取出

Figure 4-4-16　Transvaginal extraction of specimen

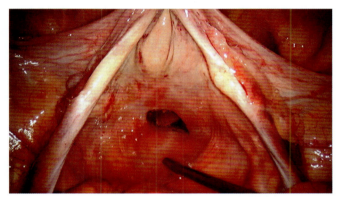

图 4-4-18　蒸馏水、稀碘附溶液及盐水反复冲洗盆腔

Figure 4-4-18　Repeated pelvic irrigation with distilled water, diluted povidone-iodine solution, and saline solution

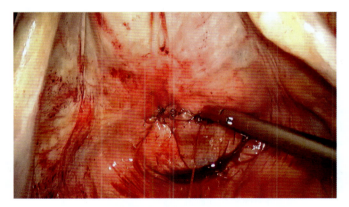

图 4-4-19　用 3-0 倒刺线连续缝合关闭阴道后穹隆切口

Figure 4-4-19　Incision of the posterior vaginal fornix closed by continuous suture with 3-0 barbed suture

## 第五节　腹部无辅助切口经肛门取标本的腹腔镜下近端胃切除术

### （GC-NOSES Ⅴ式）

【简介】

　　近端胃切除术是适用于胃上部（贲门、胃底及部分胃体）早期胃癌或者良性病变的一种标准手术方式，GC-NOSES Ⅴ式主要适用于早期胃上部病变的男性患者和部分女性患者。在严格遵守常规腹腔镜胃癌根治术、消化道重建原则的基础上，切开直肠，经肛门取出标本，体现了微创手术与功能保留手术的结合。该术式属于切除拖出式，其操作特点如下：①全部操作在腹腔镜下完成，包括胃癌根治性切除、淋巴结清扫及消化道重建，与常规腹腔镜手术相比，未明显增加手术难度；②腹壁无辅助切口，最大限度地保留了腹壁功能，减轻术后疼痛。

### 一、适应证与禁忌证

【适应证】

1. $cT_{1\sim2}N_0M_0$ 期胃上部癌。
2. 肿瘤环周直径≤4cm 为宜。

【禁忌证】

1. 局部晚期胃癌（$cT_{3\sim4}N_{1\sim3}M_{0\sim1}$）。
2. 肿瘤体积大无法经肛门拖出者。
3. 合并急性胃肠道梗阻或者肿瘤穿孔者。
4. 过于肥胖者（$BMI>30kg/m^2$）。
5. 盆腔手术史或存在直肠、肛门畸形等。

### 二、体位、戳卡位置与手术团队站位

【患者体位】

　　患者取水平仰卧分腿位（图 4-5-1），切开直肠取标本时，更换为功能截石位（图 4-5-2）。

【戳卡位置】

1. 腹腔镜镜头戳卡孔（10mm 戳卡）　脐下 1cm 处。
2. 术者主戳卡孔（12mm 戳卡）　左侧腋前线肋缘下 2cm 处。

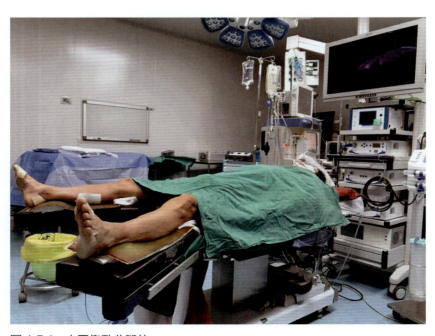

图 4-5-1　水平仰卧分腿位

Figure 4-5-1　Horizontal supine position with legs abduction

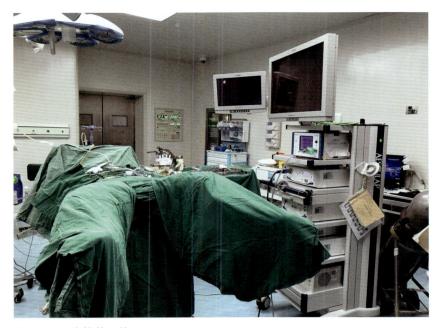

图 4-5-2　功能截石位

Figure 4-5-2　Functional lithotomy position

3. 术者辅助戳卡孔（5mm 戳卡）　左侧锁骨中线平脐处。

4. 助手辅助戳卡孔（5mm 戳卡）　右侧腋前线肋缘下。

5. 助手主戳卡孔（12mm 戳卡）　右侧锁骨中线平脐处（图 4-5-3）。

## 【手术团队站位】

1. 腹腔探查、解剖分离及淋巴结清扫阶段　术者站位于患者左侧，助手站位于患者右侧，扶镜手站立于患者两腿之间（图 4-5-4）。

2. 消化道重建阶段　术者站位于患者右侧，助手站位于患者左侧，扶镜手站立于患者两腿之间（图 4-5-5）。

3. 经肛门拖出标本阶段　术者站位于患者右侧，助手站位于患者左侧，扶镜手站立于助手同侧（图 4-5-6）。此时显示器变换摆放位置，摆放于患者足侧。

## 【特殊手术器械】

超声刀、60mm 腔内直线切割闭合器、3-0 倒刺线、4-0 可吸收线、保护套。

## 三、手术操作步骤、技巧与要点

### 【探查】

在详细术前检查的基础上，进镜观察肝脏、胆囊、胃、脾脏、大网膜、结肠、小肠及系膜表面和盆腔脏器有无种植转移及其他异常。

### 【解剖与分离】

1. 分离大网膜　将大网膜向头侧翻起，从横结肠偏左部离断大网膜，进入小网膜囊，向右至结肠肝曲，并在横结肠系膜前叶后方分离，清除横结肠系膜前叶，注意保留胃网膜右血管。胃网膜右血管是残胃的唯一血供，一旦损伤，需行全胃切除，保护胃网膜右血管至关重要。

2. 游离胃近端与离断血管　从横结肠中部向结肠脾曲方向分离大网膜，于根部离断胃网膜左血管，同时清扫第 4sb 组淋巴结。贴近脾门采用超声刀逐支离断胃短动脉，清扫第 4sa 组淋巴结。

3. 清扫第 7、8a、9、11p、11d 组淋巴结　裸化分离胃左血管，并于根部切断。清扫第 7、9、11p 组淋巴结，沿脾动脉清扫第 11d 组淋巴结，沿肝总动脉、肝固有动脉清扫第 8a 组淋巴结。

4. 清扫第 1、2 组淋巴结及游离裸化食管　继续分离至贲门左侧，离断迷走神经前、后干，裸化食管下段。在肿瘤近端的食管置牵引线，将食管向下牵引，继续向上充分游离食管至保证足够切缘且满足吻合需要。

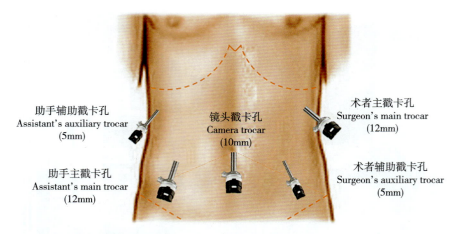

图 4-5-3　戳卡位置（五孔法）

Figure 4-5-3　Trocar placement（five-port method）

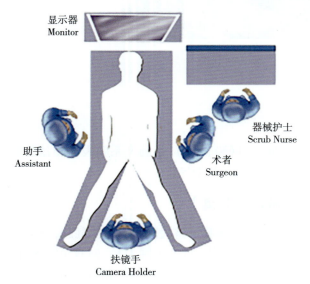

图 4-5-4　手术团队站位 1

Figure 4-5-4　Surgical team position 1

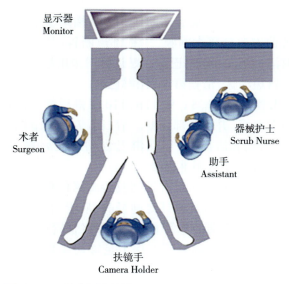

图 4-5-5　手术团队站位 2

Figure 4-5-5　Surgical team position 2

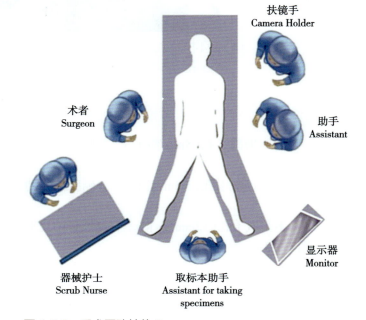

图 4-5-6　手术团队站位 3

Figure 4-5-6　Surgical team position 3

## 【标本切除与消化道重建】

1. 标本切除　于食管胃结合部上 2cm 处用腔内直线切割闭合器离断食管，距肿瘤远端 5cm 处用腔内直线切割闭合器离断胃。将切除的标本置入标本袋中（图 4-5-7 ~ 图 4-5-9）。

2. 消化道重建（Overlap 法）　用 3-0 薇乔线在食管断端左右两侧分别缝合一针，用超声刀自食管断端中央部位切开，在胃管引导下，将腔内直线切割闭合器两臂分别置入食管腔和胃腔内，对食管后壁和残胃前壁进行吻合，用 3-0 倒刺线连续缝合关闭共同开口（图 4-5-10 ~ 图 4-5-13）。

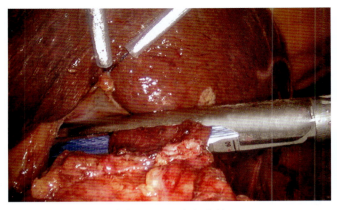

图 4-5-7　食管胃结合部上 2cm 离断食管

Figure 4-5-7　Transection of esophagus at 2cm above the esophagogastric junction

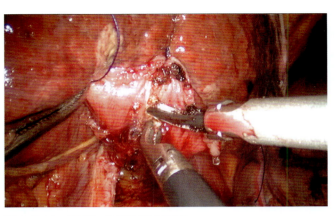

图 4-5-10　胃壁与食管壁缝合固定

Figure 4-5-10　Suture of the gastric wall with the esophageal wall

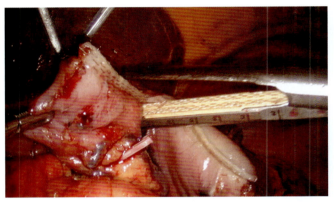

图 4-5-8　距肿瘤远端 5cm 处离断胃

Figure 4-5-8　Transection of the stomach at 5cm from the distal end of tumor

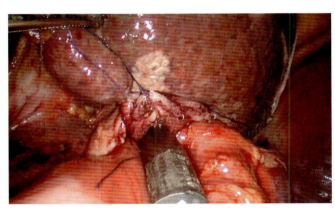

图 4-5-11　食管后壁与残胃前壁吻合（Overlap 法）

Figure 4-5-11　Anastomosis between the posterior wall of the esophagus and the anterior wall of the remnant stomach（Overlap method）

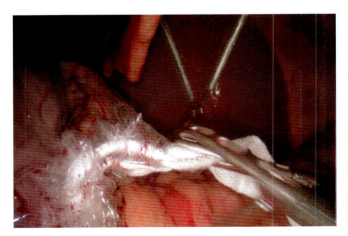

图 4-5-9　将标本置入标本袋中

Figure 4-5-9　Placing the specimen in the specimen bag

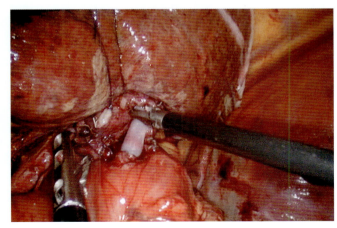

图 4-5-12　放置胃管

Figure 4-5-12　Placement of gastric tube

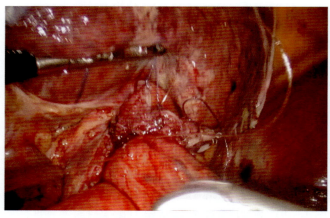

图 4-5-13　用 3-0 倒刺线连续缝合关闭共同开口

Figure 4-5-13　Common opening of gastroesophageal anastomosis closed by continuous suture with 3-0 barbed suture

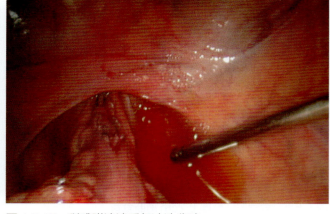

图 4-5-15　稀碘附溶液反复冲洗盆腔

Figure 4-5-15　Repeated irrigation of pelvic cavity with diluted povidone-iodine solution and normal saline

3. 标本取出　完成胃癌根治性切除及消化道重建后，将患者体位更换为功能截石位，碘附消毒会阴区及直肠肠腔。调整腹腔镜监视器至患者足侧，取头低足高右倾位，助手牵拉乙状结肠充分显露直肠上段，术者于直肠上段前壁纵行切开 5～6cm（图 4-5-14）。用稀碘附溶液反复消毒后置入切口保护套（图 4-5-15、图 4-5-16），自保护套将标本经肛门取出（图 4-5-17、图 4-5-18）。3-0 倒刺线连续缝合肠壁并反复冲洗盆腔（图 4-5-19、图 4-5-20）。

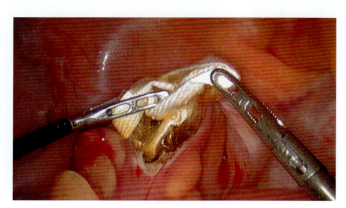

图 4-5-16　经术者主戳卡孔置入保护套

Figure 4-5-16　Insert the protective sleeve through the surgeon's main trocar port

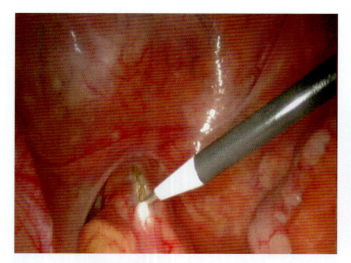

图 4-5-14　反复消毒肠腔后切开直肠上段前壁

Figure 4-5-14　Cutting open the anterior wall of the upper rectum after repeated disinfection of the bowel cavity

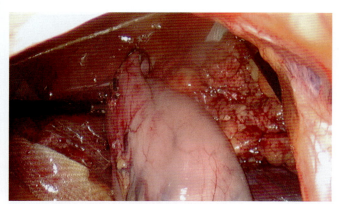

图 4-5-17　经肛门取标本（自腹腔内照片）

Figure 4-5-17　Transanal specimen extraction （intraperitoneal picture）

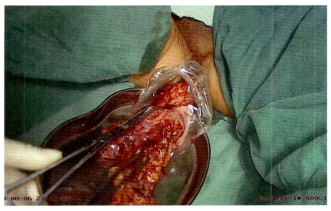

图 4-5-18　经肛门取标本（外景照片）

Figure 4-5-18　Transanal specimen extraction（extracorporeal picture）

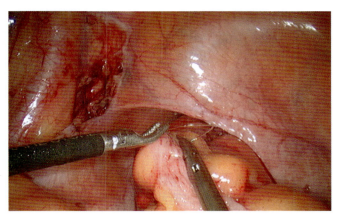

图 4-5-19　3-0 倒刺线连续缝合肠壁切口

Figure 4-5-19　Continuous suture of rectal incision with 3-0 barbed suture

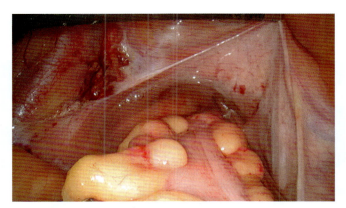

图 4-5-20　检查缝合质量，反复冲洗盆腔

Figure 4-5-20　Inspection of the quality of the rectal suture and repeated irrigation of pelvic cavity

## 第六节　腹部无辅助切口经阴道取标本的腹腔镜下近端胃切除术
### （GC-NOSES Ⅵ式）

### 【简介】

GC-NOSES Ⅵ式是一种保留胃功能的手术，主要适用于较早期胃上部癌、胃食管结合部癌的女性患者。在保证淋巴结充分清扫的前提下，严格遵守常规腹腔镜胃癌根治、消化道重建原则，通过切开阴道后穹隆经阴道取出标本，对腹腔镜手术操作及贯彻无菌、无瘤原则提出了更高的要求。该术式属于切除拖出式。

### 一、适应证与禁忌证

#### 【适应证】

1. 女性患者。
2. $cT_{1\sim2}N_{0\sim1}M_0$ 期胃上部癌或胃食管结合部癌。
3. 肿瘤环周直径≤4cm 为宜。

#### 【禁忌证】

1. 未婚或已婚但有再生育计划的女性。

2. 局部晚期胃癌（$cT_{3\sim4}N_{1\sim3}M_{0\sim1}$），肿瘤体积大。

3. 合并急性胃肠道梗阻或者肿瘤穿孔者。

4. 过于肥胖者（BMI>30kg/m$^2$）。

5. 盆腔严重粘连或存在阴道畸形等。

## 二、体位、戳卡位置与手术团队站位

### 【患者体位】

患者先取水平仰卧分腿位（图 4-6-1），切开阴道后穹隆取标本时，更换为功能截石位（图 4-6-2）。

### 【戳卡位置】（图 4-6-3）

1. 腹腔镜镜头戳卡孔（10mm 戳卡） 脐下 1cm 处。

2. 术者主戳卡孔（12mm 戳卡） 左侧腋前线肋缘下。

3. 术者辅助戳卡孔（5mm 戳卡） 左侧锁骨中线平脐处。

4. 助手辅助戳卡孔（5mm 戳卡） 右侧腋前线肋缘下。

5. 助手主戳卡孔（12mm 戳卡） 右侧锁骨中线平脐处。

### 【手术团队站位】

1. 腹腔探查、解剖分离及淋巴结清扫阶段 术者站位于患者左侧，助手站位于患者右侧，扶镜手站位于患者两腿之间（图 4-6-4）。

2. 消化道重建阶段 术者站位于患者右侧，助手站位于患者左侧，扶镜手站位于患者两腿之间（图 4-6-5）。

3. 经阴道取标本阶段 术者站位于患者右侧，助手站位于患者左侧，扶镜手站位于助手同侧（图 4-6-6）。此时显示器变换摆放位置，摆放于患者足侧。各戳卡孔功能做相应变动（图 4-6-7）。

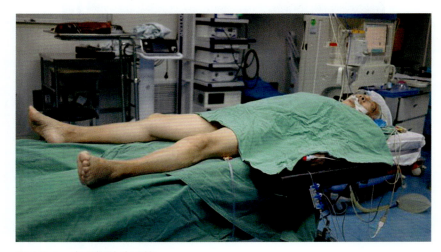

图 4-6-1 水平仰卧分腿位

Figure 4-6-1 Horizontal supine position with legs abduction

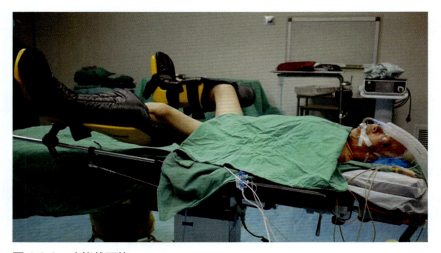

图 4-6-2 功能截石位

Figure 4-6-2 Functional lithotomy position

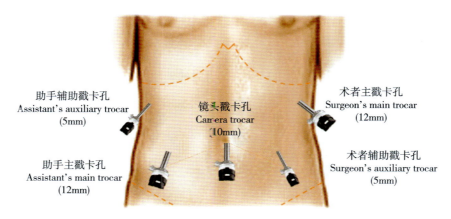

图 4-6-3　戳卡位置（五孔法）

Figure 4-6-3　Trocar sites（five-port method）

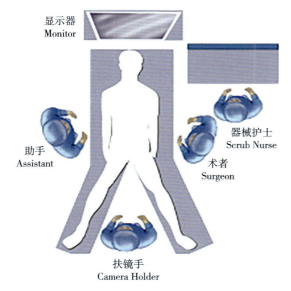

图 4-6-4　手术团队站位 1

Figure 4-6-4　Surgical team position 1

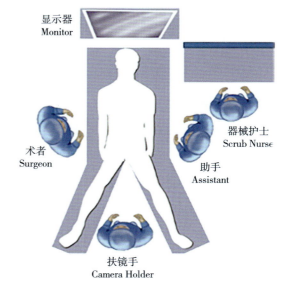

图 4-6-5　手术团队站位 2

Figure 4-6-5　Surgical team position 2

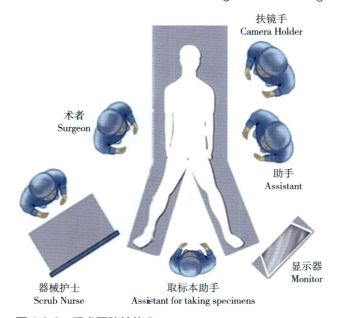

图 4-6-6　手术团队站位 3

Figure 4-6-6　Surgical team position 3

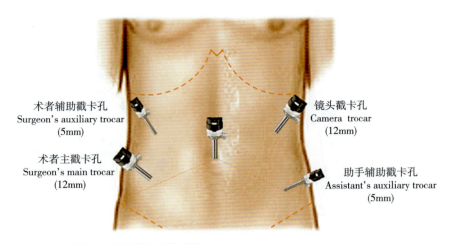

术者辅助戳卡孔
Surgeon's auxiliary trocar
(5mm)

术者主戳卡孔
Surgeon's main trocar
(12mm)

镜头戳卡孔
Camera trocar
(12mm)

助手辅助戳卡孔
Assistant's auxiliary trocar
(5mm)

图 4-6-7　取标本阶段戳孔功能变动

Figure 4-6-7　Changes in trocar function during specimen extraction

【特殊手术器械】

超声刀、60mm 腔内直线切割闭合器、3-0 倒刺线、4-0 可吸收线、保护套。

## 三、手术操作步骤、技巧与要点

【探查】

在详细术前检查的基础上，进镜观察肝脏、胆囊、胃、脾脏、大网膜、结肠、小肠及系膜表面和盆腔脏器有无种植转移及其他异常。

【解剖与分离】

1. 肝脏悬吊及胃食管 - 膈肌脚分离　打开肝胃韧带，于肝胃韧带肝侧缘置牵引线，悬吊肝左叶以充分暴露术野；在胃食管结合部与右侧膈肌脚之间锐性分离，进入 Gerota 间隙。

2. 分离大网膜及胃脾韧带　将大网膜向头侧翻起，从横结肠偏左部离断大网膜，向右至结肠肝曲，并在横结肠系膜前叶后方分离，切除横结肠系膜前叶，注意保留胃网膜右血管。患者取左高右低位，显露胃脾韧带，从结肠中部向结肠脾曲离断大网膜，于根部离断胃网膜左血管，清扫第 4sb 组淋巴结。贴近脾门采用超声刀离断胃短动脉，清扫第 4sa 组淋巴结。

3. 清扫第 7、8a、9、11p、11d 组淋巴结　紧贴胰腺上缘分离，显露脾动脉近端，清扫第 11p 组淋巴结。显露腹腔动脉干，分离胃左血管，在根部夹闭后离断，清扫第 7、9 组淋巴结。继续沿肝总动脉分离清扫第

8a 组淋巴结。进一步沿脾动脉清扫第 11d 组淋巴结，根据肿瘤位置及脾门淋巴结是否肿大决定是否清扫第 10 组淋巴结。

4. 清扫第 1、2 组淋巴结及裸化食管　离断胃前、后迷走神经，游离食管达足够长度。当食管游离长度不足时，于食管膈肌裂孔穹隆部向正前方打开膈肌 4～5cm，在膈肌脚中下部充分离断两侧膈肌脚，将胸膜继续向两侧推开。在肿瘤上方食管置牵引线，尽量将食管向下牵引，继续在后纵隔向上充分游离食管至保证足够切缘。

【标本切除与消化道重建】

1. 标本切除　于食管胃结合部上 2cm 处用腔内直线切割闭合器离断食管，距肿瘤远端 5cm 处用腔内直线切割闭合器离断胃。将切除的标本置入标本袋中（图 4-6-8）。

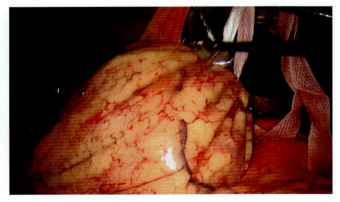

图 4-6-8　标本置入标本袋中暂置于左下腹

Figure 4-6-8　Placing the specimen in the specimen bag and temporarily placing it in the left lower abdomen

2. 消化道重建

（1）器械吻合法（Overlap 法）：于食管后壁及残胃前壁开口，分别置入直线切割缝合器两臂，击发后完成食管后壁 - 残胃前壁侧侧吻合。然后用 3-0 倒刺线缝合关闭共同开口。

（2）手工缝合法：使用 3-0 薇乔线缝合 3 针固定残胃前壁与食管后壁，切开残胃前壁与食管后壁行手工吻合。胃前壁与食管后壁吻合采用 3-0 薇乔线间断全层缝合，共同开口吻合采用 3-0 倒刺线连续缝合。

3. 标本取出　更换为功能截石位，调整腹腔镜监视器至患者足侧，碘附消毒会阴区及阴道；取头低足高右倾位，悬吊子宫显露阴道后穹隆（图 4-6-9）压肠板顶起阴道后穹隆，横行切开约 5cm，置入切口保护套（图 4-6-10～图 4-6-12），自切口保护套将标本取出（图 4-6-13～图 4-6-15）。3-0 倒刺线连续缝合

关闭阴道后穹隆切口并反复冲洗盆腔（图 4-6-16～图 4-6-19）。

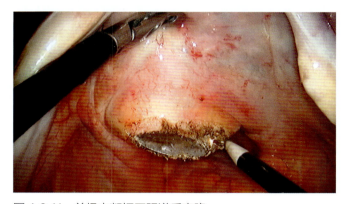

图 4-6-11　单极电凝切开阴道后穹隆

Figure 4-6-11　Open the posterior vaginal fornix with monopolar electrocoagulation

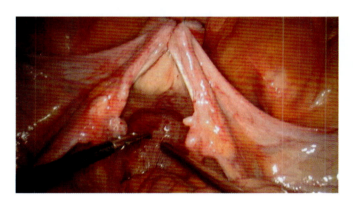

图 4-6-9　悬吊子宫

Figure 4-6-9　Suspension of uterus

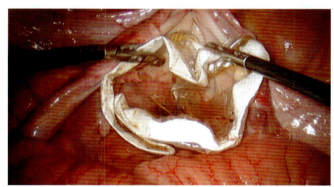

图 4-6-12　经术者主戳卡孔置入保护套

Figure 4-6-12　Insertion of protective sleeve through the surgeon's main trocar port

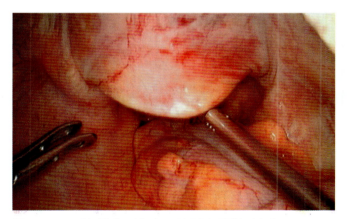

图 4-6-10　反复消毒阴道后压肠板顶起阴道后穹隆

Figure 4-6-10　Posterior vaginal fornix is withstood with the abdominal spatula after repeated disinfection of vagina

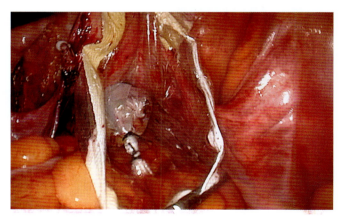

图 4-6-13　取出标本及标本袋

Figure 4-6-13　Extraction of specimen and specimen bag

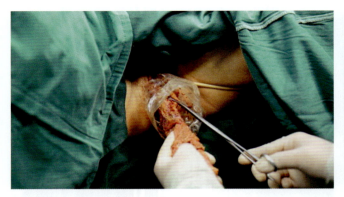

图 4-6-14　将标本自阴道取出

Figure 4-6-14　Transvaginal extraction of specimen

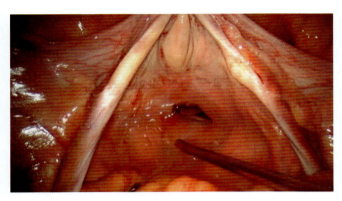

图 4-6-17　生理盐水反复冲洗

Figure 4-6-17　Repeated irrigation with normal saline

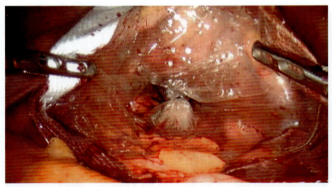

图 4-6-15　取出保护套

Figure 4-6-15　Extraction of protective sleeve

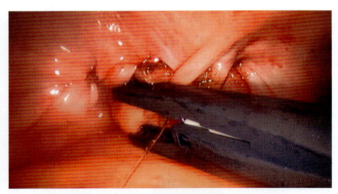

图 4-6-18　用 3-0 倒刺线连续缝合关闭阴道后穹隆切口

Figure 4-6-18　Incision of the posterior vaginal fornix closed by continuous suture with 3-0 barbed suture

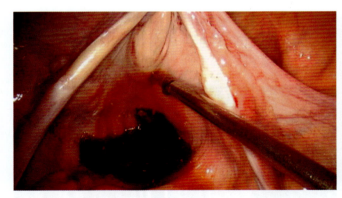

图 4-6-16　稀碘附溶液反复冲洗

Figure 4-6-16　Repeated irrigation with diluted povidone-iodine solution

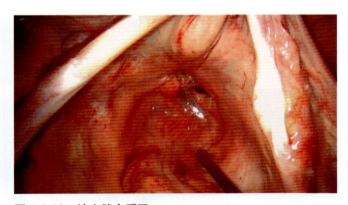

图 4-6-19　检查缝合质量

Figure 4-6-19　Quality check of sutures

## 第七节　腹部无辅助切口经肛门取标本的腹腔镜下全胃切除术

### （GC-NOSES Ⅶ式）

### 【简介】

GC-NOSES Ⅶ式属于切除拖出式。其操作特点：腹腔镜下完成胃癌根治性切除及消化道重建，于直肠上段切开，经肛门将标本取出。该术式符合微创手术理念，在满足手术基本原则的前提下，通过优化手术入路，改进手术操作并保留腹壁的结构与功能，有助于减少创伤、提高患者的生活质量。

## 一、适应证与禁忌证

### 【适应证】

1. 病灶累及胃体、胃中上部或胃食管结合部的 $cT_{1\sim3}N_{1\sim2}M_0$ 期胃癌。

2. 肿瘤环周直径≤4cm 为宜。

3. 男性患者和部分不适宜经阴道取标本的女性患者。

### 【禁忌证】

1. 肿瘤体积过大，无法经肛门拖出。

2. 肿瘤浸透浆膜或累及邻近脏器。

3. 合并急性胃肠道梗阻或者肿瘤穿孔者。

4. 过于肥胖者（BMI>30kg/m²）。

5. 盆腔手术史或存在直肠、肛门畸形等。

## 二、手术操作步骤、技巧与要点

### 【戳卡位置】

1. 腹腔镜镜头戳卡孔（10mm 戳卡）　脐下1cm 处。

2. 术者主戳卡孔（12mm 戳卡）　左侧腋前线肋缘下 2cm 处。

3. 术者辅助戳卡孔（5mm 戳卡）　左侧锁骨中线平脐处。

4. 助手辅助戳卡孔（5mm 戳卡）　右侧腋前线肋缘下。

5. 助手主戳卡孔（12mm 戳卡）　右侧锁骨中线平脐处（图 4-7-1）。

### 【探查】

1. 常规探查　观察各脏器及腹膜表面有无种植转移等病变。

2. 肿瘤探查　根据肿瘤的位置、大小、侵犯深度，确定手术的可行性。

3. 解剖结构的判定　根据肿瘤位置及解剖结构决定手术方案，并估计标本能否经肛门取出。

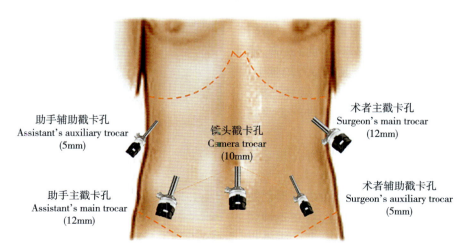

图 4-7-1　戳卡位置（五孔法）

Figure 4-7-1　Trocar placement（five-port method）

## 【解剖与分离】

1. 分离胃结肠韧带，剥离横结肠系膜前叶　将大网膜向头侧翻起，打开胃结肠韧带，从横结肠偏左部离断大网膜，进入小网膜囊，向右至结肠肝曲，并在横结肠系膜前叶后方分离，清除系膜前叶。

2. 清扫第 6 组淋巴结　显露 Henle 干，于根部离断胃网膜右静脉；继续沿胰头表面解剖，打开胃胰韧带，显露胃十二指肠动脉，裸化胃网膜右动脉，于根部离断，彻底清扫第 6 组淋巴结。

3. 清扫第 4sb、10 组淋巴结　进入网膜囊，显露胰尾和脾血管，松解结肠脾曲，分离大网膜与脾中下极的粘连，保护胰尾，显露胃网膜左血管，于根部进行离断，清扫第 4sb 组淋巴结，并进一步清扫第 10 组淋巴结。

4. 清扫第 4sa 组淋巴结　将胃及大网膜向左侧牵拉，继续向上方分离，离断胃短血管，并清扫第 4sa 组淋巴结。

5. 清扫第 8a、12a、5 组淋巴结　显露肝总动脉，将胰腺向左下方牵拉，沿肝总动脉前方及上缘分离，清扫第 8a 组淋巴结。沿胃十二指肠动脉及肝总动脉充分显露胃右动脉及肝固有动脉，继续向上分离肝固有动脉前方及外侧，清扫第 12a 组淋巴结。于根部离断胃右血管，并清扫第 5 组淋巴结。于幽门远端用直线切割闭合器离断十二指肠，清扫其周围第 5 组淋巴结。于肝总动脉、胃十二指肠动脉及胰腺上缘夹角处打开门静脉前方筋膜，显露门静脉，将肝总动脉向腹前壁挑起，沿门静脉前方分离，清扫门静脉与肝固有动脉间淋巴结。沿门静脉内缘向上分离至肝门部，将肝总动脉向右下方牵拉，清扫肝固有动脉内侧及门静脉内侧淋巴结、脂肪组织。

6. 清扫第 11 p、7、9 组淋巴结　将大网膜置于肝脏下方，助手抓持胃胰皱襞，将胃翻向上方。清扫胰腺前被膜，紧贴胰腺上缘分离，显露脾动脉近端，清扫第 11p 组淋巴结。由左向右清扫，显露腹腔动脉干，分离胃左血管，于根部离断，清扫第 7、9 组淋巴结。沿脾动脉向远端分离，切断胃后血管，并进一步清扫第 11p 组淋巴结。

7. 清扫胃小弯淋巴结　紧贴胃壁小弯侧，用超声刀分层切开，清扫胃小弯淋巴结。

8. 游离食管下段，并清扫贲门右侧及左侧淋巴结　紧贴食管用超声刀分层切开，显露胃前、后迷走神经并离断，清扫贲门右侧及左侧淋巴结（第 1、2 组淋巴结）。当食管游离长度不足时，可在后纵隔分离，或在食管膈肌裂孔穹隆部向正前方打开膈肌 4~5cm，分离

过程中注意将胸膜继续向两侧推开，避免损伤胸膜。将食管向下牵引，充分游离食管，保证上切缘安全。

## 【标本切除与消化道重建】

1. 标本切除　距离肿瘤上缘 3cm 切断食管，将标本置入标本袋中，暂置于左下腹，待经肛门取标本（图 4-7-2~图 4-7-4）。

2. 消化道重建（腹腔镜下食管空肠 Roux-en-Y 吻合、Overlap 法）　以 3-0 薇乔线在食管断端左右两侧各缝合一针，用超声刀自食管断端中央部位切开（图 4-7-5），距屈氏韧带 20cm 处离断空肠（图 4-7-6、图 4-7-7），对远端空肠与食管行 Overlap 法吻合（图 4-7-8）。以 3-0 倒刺线连续缝合关闭共同开口（图 4-7-9~图 4-7-11）。食管与空肠吻合后，在距离食管空肠吻合口 40cm 处空肠对系膜侧肠壁开孔，使用直线切割闭合器行近端空肠 - 远端空肠侧侧吻合，使用 3-0 薇乔线间断缝合关闭空肠共同开口（图 4-7-12、图 4-7-13）。

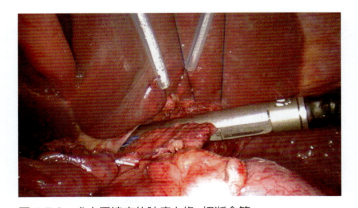

图 4-7-2　术中胃镜定位肿瘤上缘，切断食管

Figure 4-7-2　Intraoperative gastroscopy for the localization of the proximal edge of tumor, and transection of the esophagus

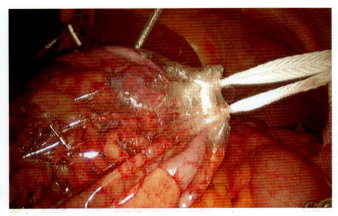

图 4-7-3　将标本置入标本袋中，并暂置左下腹

Figure 4-7-3　Placing the specimen in the specimen bag and temporarily placing it in the left lower abdomen

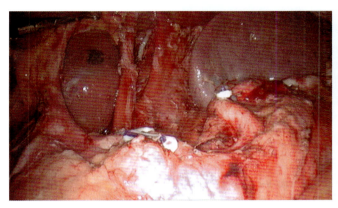

图 4-7-4 第 10、11 组淋巴结清扫后状态

Figure 4-7-4 Status after the dissection of group 10 and 11 lymph nodes

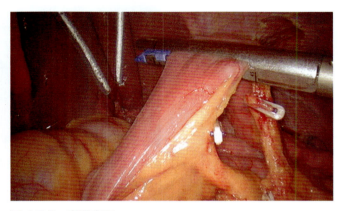

图 4-7-7 离断空肠

Figure 4-7-7 Transection of jejunum

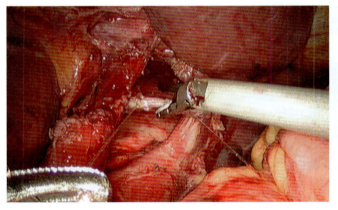

图 4-7-5 自食管断端中央部位切开

Figure 4-7-5 Open the middle of the esophageal stump

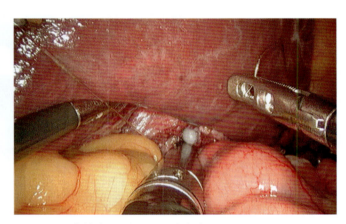

图 4-7-8 食管空肠 Overlap 法吻合

Figure 4-7-8 Overlap anastomosis of esophagus and jejunum

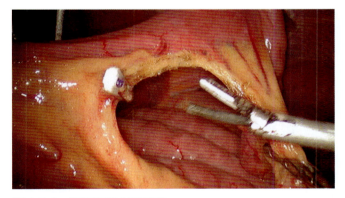

图 4-7-6 切断近端空肠系膜

Figure 4-7-6 Transection of proximal mesojejunum

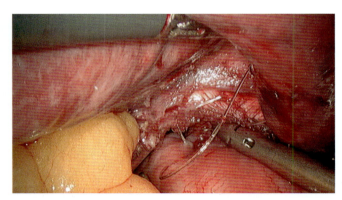

图 4-7-9 3-0 倒刺线连续缝合关闭共同开口

Figure 4-7-9 Common opening is closed by suture in a continuous pattern with 3-0 barbed suture

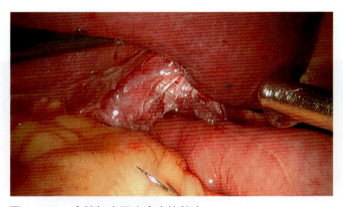

图 4-7-10　食管与空肠吻合完毕状态

Figure 4-7-10　Status after esophagojejunal anastomosis

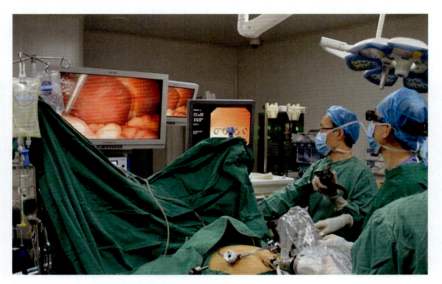

图 4-7-11　术中胃镜检查吻合口缝合质量

Figure 4-7-11　Intraoperative gastroscopy to check the quality of anastomosis

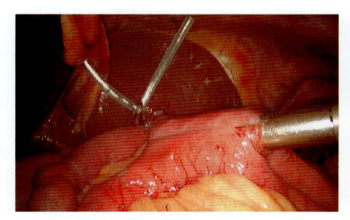

图 4-7-12　空肠侧侧吻合

Figure 4-7-12　Side-to-side jejunal anastomosis

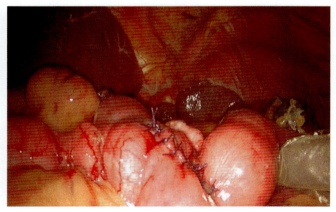

图 4-7-13　3-0 薇乔线间断缝合关闭空肠共同开口

Figure 4-7-13　Common opening of jejunum closed in an intermittent pattern with 3-0 Polyglactin 910 suture

3. 标本取出 完成胃癌根治性切除及消化道重建后，将患者体位更换为功能截石位，碘附消毒会阴区及直肠肠腔；调整腹腔镜监视器至患者足侧，取头低足高位，助手牵拉乙状结肠，充分显露直肠上段，术者于直肠上段前壁切开 5～6cm（图 4-7-14）。用碘附纱布反复消毒后置入保护套（图 4-7-15、图 4-7-16），经保护套将标本自肛门取出（图 4-7-17、图 4-7-18）。3-0 倒刺线连续缝合肠壁并冲洗盆腔（图 4-7-19～图 4-7-21）。

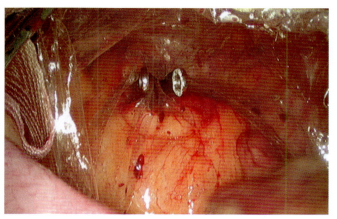

图 4-7-16 经术者主戳卡孔置入保护套

Figure 4-7-16 Insert the protective sleeve through the surgeon's main trocar port

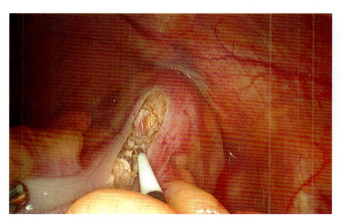

图 4-7-14 反复消毒肠腔后切开直肠上段前壁

Figure 4-7-14 Cutting open the anterior wall of the upper rectum after repeated disinfection of the bowel cavity

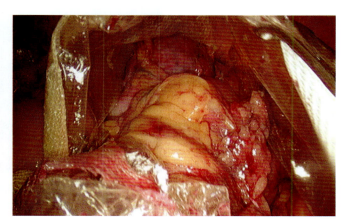

图 4-7-17 自切口保护套取出标本

Figure 4-7-17 Specimen extraction from the protective sleeve

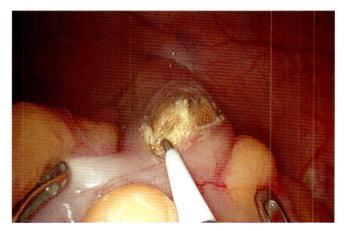

图 4-7-15 碘附纱布反复消毒肠腔

Figure 4-7-15 Repeated disinfection of the bowel lumen with the iodoform gauze

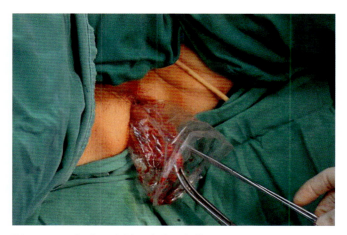

图 4-7-18 标本取出过程中会阴部外观

Figure 4-7-18 Perineal appearance during specimen extraction

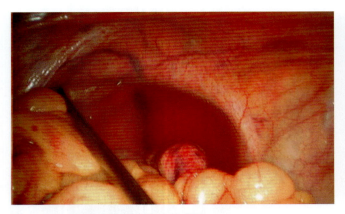

图 4-7-19　稀碘附溶液反复冲洗盆腔

Figure 4-7-19　Repeated irrigation of pelvic cavity with diluted povidone-iodine solution

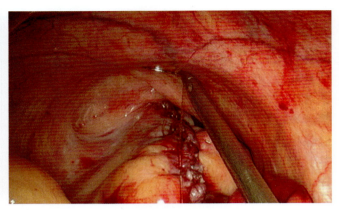

图 4-7-20　3-0 倒刺线双重连续缝合直肠切开处

Figure 4-7-20　Continuous double sutures with 3-0 barbed suture for rectum incision

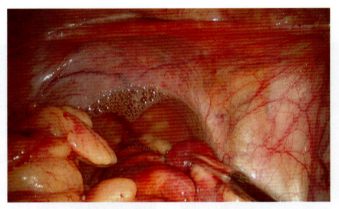

图 4-7-21　稀碘附溶液再次冲洗盆腔，并行直肠注水注气试验

Figure 4-7-21　Irrigate the pelvic cavity again with diluted povidone-iodine solution, followed by a rectal air and water injection test

# 第八节　腹部无辅助切口经阴道取标本的腹腔镜下全胃切除术

## （GC-NOSES Ⅷ式）

### 【简介】

GC-NOSES Ⅷ式主要适用于胃中上部癌及胃食管结合部癌的女性患者。与常规腹腔镜胃癌根治术一样，需严格遵循肿瘤根治、消化道重建的原则，除了取标本途径与常规腹腔镜手术不同外，胃肠道切除、淋巴结清扫范围、手术游离层次等方面均与常规腹腔镜手术一致，本术式为切除拖出式。其操作特点：腹腔镜下完成胃癌根治性切除及消化道重建，切开阴道后穹隆，经阴道将标本取出。在腹腔镜下重建时更容易判断肠管远近端方向，可有效避免小切口辅助下吻合后肠管扭转、吻合口张力过大等情况。经阴道取标本，避免了腹壁的辅助切口，最大限度地保留了腹壁功能，减轻术后疼痛，便于患者早期离床活动，同时能够加快康复，减少手术所带来的心理创伤。

## 一、适应证与禁忌证

### 【适应证】

1. 病变位于胃中上部及胃食管结合部的 $cT_{1\sim3}N_{1\sim2}M_0$

期胃癌。

2. 肿瘤环周直径≤4cm 为宜。

【禁忌证】

1. 肿瘤体积过大，无法经阴道取出。
2. 肿瘤浸透浆膜或累及邻近脏器。
3. 过于肥胖者（BMI>30kg/m²）。
4. 有严重心、肺、肝、肾疾病等不能耐受手术者。

## 二、手术操作步骤、技巧与要点

【戳卡位置】（图 4-8-1）

1. 腹腔镜镜头戳卡孔（10mm 戳卡） 脐下 1cm 处。
2. 术者主戳卡孔（12mm 戳卡） 左侧腋前线肋缘下。
3. 术者辅助戳卡孔（5mm 戳卡） 左侧锁骨中线平脐处。
4. 助手辅助戳卡孔（5mm 戳卡） 右侧腋前线肋缘下。
5. 助手主戳卡孔（12mm 戳卡） 右侧锁骨中线平脐处。

【探查】

1. 常规探查 观察各脏器及腹膜表面有无种植转移等病变。
2. 肿瘤探查 根据肿瘤的位置、大小、侵犯深度，确定手术的可行性。
3. 解剖结构的判定 根据肿瘤位置及解剖结构决定手术方案，并估计标本能否经阴道取出。

【解剖与分离】

1. 打开横结肠附着处大网膜，剥离横结肠系膜前叶 将大网膜向头侧翻起，从横结肠偏左部离断大网膜，进入小网膜囊，向右至结肠肝曲，并在横结扬系膜前叶后方分离，清除结肠系膜前叶。

2. 清扫第 6 组淋巴结 以中结肠血管为标志，进入胃十二指肠和横结肠系膜之间的融合筋膜间隙，显露胰十二指肠上前静脉，在其与胃网膜右静脉汇合处上方离断胃网膜右静脉。继续沿胰头表面解剖，显露胃十二指肠动脉，裸化胃网膜右动脉根部后离断，彻底清扫第 6 组淋巴结。

3. 清扫第 4sb 组淋巴结 显露胰尾，显露胃网膜左血管，于根部离断，并进一步原位清扫脾门淋巴结，即沿脾血管向远侧分离，直至显露出脾门各分支血管，清扫第 4sb 组淋巴结。

4. 清扫第 11p、11d、7、9 组淋巴结 紧贴胰腺上缘分离，显露脾动脉近端，清扫第 11p 组淋巴结，进一步沿脾动脉清扫第 11d 组淋巴结，根据肿瘤位置及脾门淋巴结是否肿大决定是否清扫第 10 组淋巴结。显露腹腔动脉干，分离胃左血管，在根部夹闭后离断，清扫第 7、9 组淋巴结。

5. 清扫第 12a 组淋巴结 采用直线切割闭合器于幽门远端 2cm 处离断十二指肠，打开肝十二指肠韧带被膜，裸化肝固有动脉前侧及左侧，于胃右血管根部夹闭后离断。助手将肝总动脉向右下方牵拉，清扫肝固有动脉内侧及门静脉内侧第 12a 组淋巴结。

6. 裸化食管 用超声刀紧贴食管分层切开黏膜下层，显露胃前、后迷走神经并离断，游离食管至足够长度，清扫第 110 组淋巴结。当食管游离长度不足时，可在后纵隔分离，或在食管膈肌裂孔穿隆部向正前方打开膈肌 4～5cm，分离过程中注意将胸膜继续向两侧推开，避免损伤胸膜。将食管向下牵引，充分游离食管，保证上切缘安全。

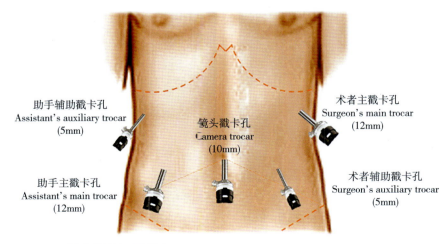

图 4-8-1 戳卡位置（五孔法）
Figure 4-8-1 Trocar placement（five-port method）

**【标本切除与消化道重建】**

1. 标本切除　食管游离完毕后，距离肿瘤上缘 3cm 采用直线切割闭合器横断食管（图 4-8-2），将标本置入标本袋中，暂置于左下腹，待经阴道取标本。

2. 消化道重建

（1）器械吻合法（Overlap 法）：距屈氏韧带 25cm 处离断空肠（图 4-8-3），于食管后壁及远端空肠对系膜侧肠壁各戳一小孔，分别置入直线切割闭合器两臂，击发后完成食管 - 空肠侧侧吻合（图 4-8-4 ～图 4-8-6）。然后采用 3-0 倒刺线连续缝合关闭共同开口（图 4-8-7）。

（2）手工缝合法（Roux-en-Y 吻合）：采用先吻合后离断方式完成食管与空肠吻合，即先将屈氏韧带 25cm 肠管上提至食管裂孔处，再与食管后壁缝合 3 针进行

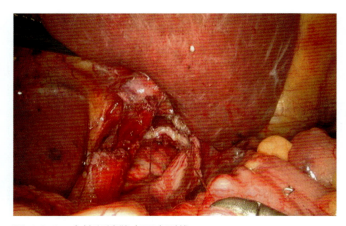

图 4-8-4　食管断端缝合两牵引线

Figure 4-8-4　The esophageal stump is sutured with two traction stitches

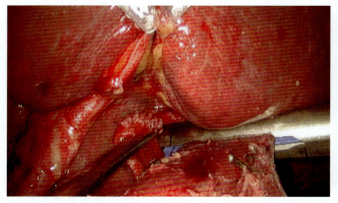

图 4-8-2　肿瘤近端 3cm 横断食管

Figure 4-8-2　Transection of the esophagus at 3cm from the proximal end of tumor

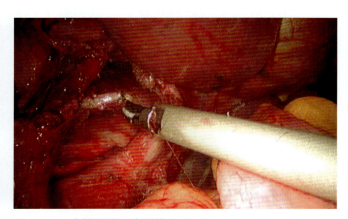

图 4-8-5　食管断端两牵引线之间开口

Figure 4-8-5　Opening of the esophageal stump between the two traction stitches

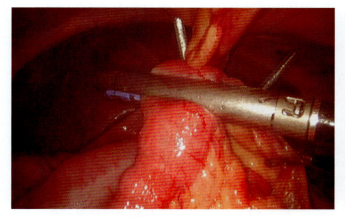

图 4-8-3　距屈氏韧带 25cm 处离断空肠

Figure 4-8-3　Transection of the jejunum at 25cm from the Treitz's ligament

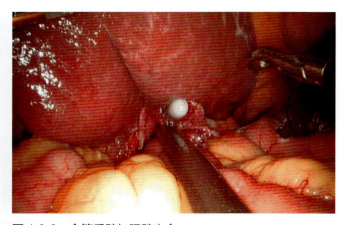

图 4-8-6　食管后壁与肠壁吻合

Figure 4-8-6　Anastomosis between the posterior wall of the esophagus and bowel wall

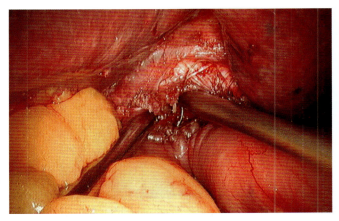

图 4-8-7 3-0 倒刺线连续缝合关闭共同开口

Figure 4-8-7 Common opening is closed in a continuous pattern with 3-0 barbed suture

固定，切开空肠侧壁及食管后壁行手工吻合（图 4-8-8、图 4-8-9）。食管后壁和空肠侧壁吻合采用可吸收线间断全层缝合（图 4-8-10）。共同开口采用倒刺线连续缝合（图 4-8-11）。完成食管与空肠吻合后，距吻合口 3cm 离断近端空肠，距离食管空肠吻合口 40cm 空肠对系膜侧肠壁开孔，使用直线切割闭合器将近端空肠与远端空肠行侧侧吻合，采用 3-0 可吸收线间断或 3-0 倒刺线连续缝合关闭空肠共同开口（图 4-8-12～图 4-8-14）。

3. 标本取出 完成胃癌根治性切除及消化道重建后，变换患者体位为功能截石位，碘附消毒会阴区及阴道；调整腹腔镜监视器至患者足侧，取头低足高位，悬吊子宫显露阴道后穹隆，于阴道后穹隆横向切开 5～6cm（图 4-8-15）。用稀碘附溶液反复消毒后经术者主戳卡孔置入切口保护套（图 4-8-16），经切口保护套将标本自阴道取出（图 4-8-17、图 4-8-18）。稀碘附溶液及生理盐水反复冲洗盆腔（图 4-8-19、图 4-8-20）。3-0 倒刺线连续缝合关闭阴道后穹隆切口（图 4-8-21）。

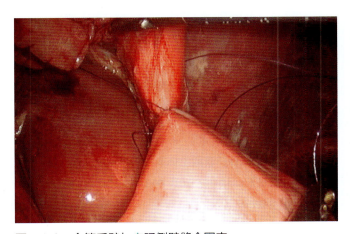

图 4-8-8 食管后壁与空肠侧壁缝合固定

Figure 4-8-8 Suturing of the posterior wall of the esophagus and the lateral wall of the jejunum

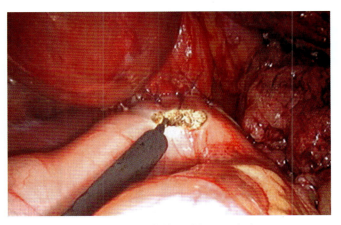

图 4-8-9 切开空肠侧壁及食管后壁行手工吻合

Figure 4-8-9 Perform a hand-sewn anastomosis by incising the lateral wall of the jejunum and the posterior wall of the esophagus

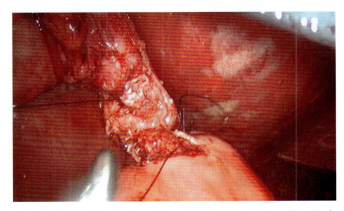

图 4-8-10 空肠侧壁及食管后壁吻合采用 3-0 薇乔线间断全层缝合

Figure 4-8-10 An anastomosis between the lateral wall of the jejunum and the posterior wall of the esophagus is performed using interrupted full-thickness sutures with 3-0 Polyglactin 910 suture

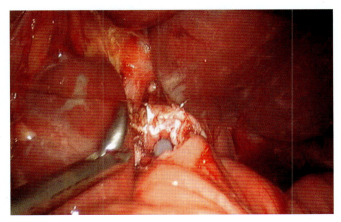

图 4-8-11 共同开口采用 3-0 倒刺线连续缝合

Figure 4-8-11 The common opening is closed with continuous suturing using 3-0 barbed sutures

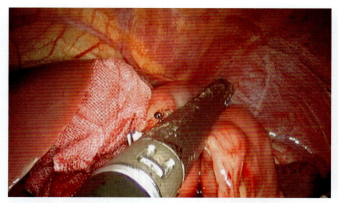

图 4-8-12　食管与空肠吻合后离断近端空肠

Figure 4-8-12　Esophagojejunal anastomosis followed by transection of the proximal jejunum

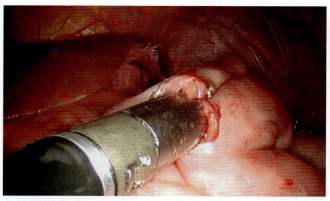

图 4-8-13　空肠侧侧吻合

Figure 4-8-13　Side-to-side jejunal anastomosis

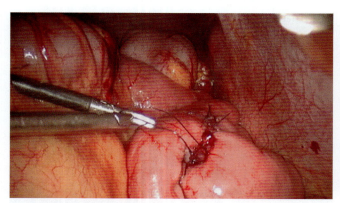

图 4-8-14　缝合关闭共同开口

Figure 4-8-14　Closure of the common opening

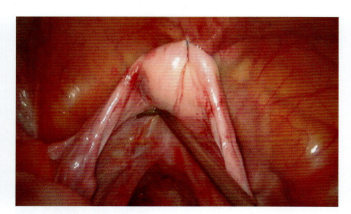

图 4-8-15　悬吊子宫

Figure 4-8-15　Suspension of uterus

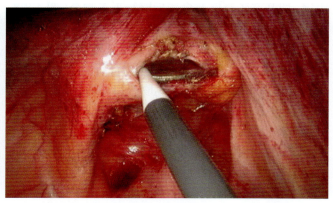

图 4-8-16　用电钩切开阴道后穹隆

Figure 4-8-16　Opening the posterior vaginal fornix with a cautery hook

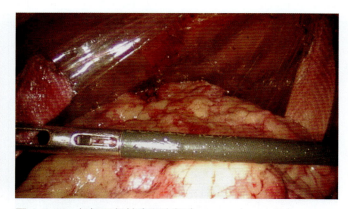

图 4-8-17　经切口保护套取出标本

Figure 4-8-17　Specimen extraction through the protective sleeve

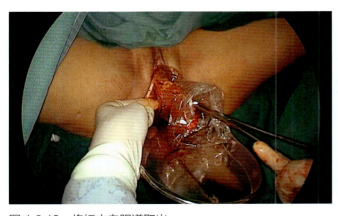

图 4-8-18　将标本自阴道取出

Figure 4-8-18　Transvaginal extraction of specimen

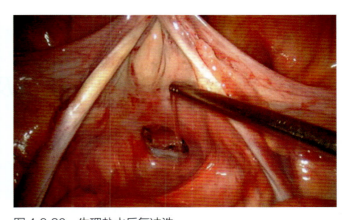

图 4-8-20　生理盐水反复冲洗

Figure 4-8-20　Repeated irrigation with normal saline

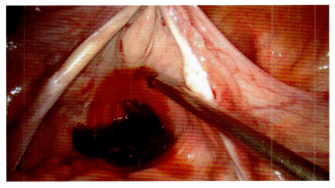

图 4-8-19　稀碘附溶液反复冲洗

Figure 4-8-19　Repeated irrigation with diluted povidone-iodine solution

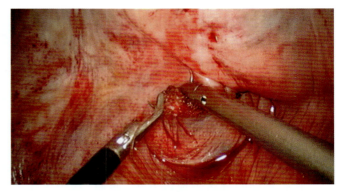

图 4-8-21　采用 3-0 倒刺线连续缝合关闭阴道后穹隆切口

Figure 4-8-21　Incision of the posterior vaginal fornix closed by continuous suture with 3-0 barbed suture

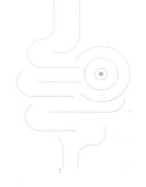

# 第五章
# 消化道 NOSES 常见并发症及处理

NOSES 在标本取出方式及消化道重建方式上具有特殊性,但在手术并发症方面与开腹手术、常规腹腔镜手术类似。本章列举了胃肠 NOSES 相关并发症的原因、临床表现及处理原则。

## 一、腹腔感染

胃肠手术相关腹腔感染的致病菌多来自胃肠道,以大肠埃希菌为主的革兰氏阴性杆菌占主导地位。NOSES 发生腹腔感染的原因主要包括以下几点:术前肠道准备不充分,术中无菌操作不规范,术后吻合口漏,腹腔引流不充分,患者状态差,伴发糖尿病、高龄、营养不良等因素。因此,预防腹腔感染的关键在于加强上述各环节的管理,控制相关危险因素,以降低腹腔感染的概率。

腹腔感染的临床表现以发热、腹痛、腹膜炎体征为主,常伴有恶心、呕吐、腹胀、低血压、脉速、气促、白细胞增多等中毒现象。晚期可导致全身衰竭,出现重度失水、代谢性酸中毒或感染性休克。

腹腔感染的诊断除依据病史、临床表现外,还需根据引流液的性状及辅助检查综合分析。如患者出现发热、腹痛等症状,需密切观察引流液的性状。如引流液呈黄色,多为脓性,考虑腹腔感染可能。如为吻合口漏导致的腹腔感染,引流液中还可见粪便沉渣,且多伴臭味。辅助检查包括实验室检查(如白细胞计数及中性粒细胞比例、生化检查等)、影像学检查(如 X 线、彩超或 CT)、腹水分析、细菌培养等。对于无引流管或引流管已脱落的患者,可通过腹部穿刺抽取积液,以明确积液的性质。

治疗原则包括一般治疗、全身支持治疗、抗感染治疗、腹腔引流治疗和手术治疗。

一般治疗:①卧床休息。宜取 30°~45° 半卧位,有利于腹腔内渗出液积聚在盆腔而便于引流,并能使腹肌松弛,膈肌免受压迫,有利于呼吸、循环的改善。②禁食及胃肠减压。可减轻肠胀气,改善肠壁血液循环,减少肠穿孔时肠内容物的渗出,以及促进肠蠕动的恢复。

全身支持治疗:若全身症状明显,必要时可输血、给予补液,以纠正电解质酸碱平衡紊乱。给予肠外、肠内营养,以改善患者的全身状态,增强免疫力。

抗感染治疗:主要针对革兰氏阴性肠道杆菌,可选用 β- 内酰胺类、氨基糖苷类药物,并根据细菌培养及药敏试验结果进行调整。

存在吻合口漏时,腹腔引流极为关键。开放式引流容易引起逆行性或外源性感染,可用庆大霉素及生理盐水定期冲洗引流管,也可通过负压作用将蓄积的液体吸出,以使包裹区域迅速缩小。如腹腔感染症状较重或有腹腔脓肿形成,经保守治疗无效或症状持续无好转时,需行手术治疗。

目前,我国 79 家中心共同开展的 NOSES 回顾性研究结果表明,仅有 0.8% 的患者术后出现了腹腔感染。这一结果也能证明,只要做好充分准备,熟练掌握手术技巧,NOSES 完全可以做到无菌操作。

## 二、吻合口出血

吻合口出血是术后早期并发症之一,腹腔镜手术一般采用机械吻合,造成吻合口出血最主要原因是吻合口所在肠系膜裸化不全而存在血管,吻合钉未能有效闭合血管导致出血。吻合口出血通常在术后 48 小时内出现,盆腔血肿经吻合口后壁破入出血通常在术后 7 天后出现。我国 79 家中心共同开展的 NOSES 回顾性研究结果表明,0.9% 的 NOSES 术后出现了吻合口出血。

吻合口出血关键在于预防,术中吻合消化道时,需仔细检查吻合口有无出血,可行注水注气试验检查吻合确切与否。有条件的医院可于术中用腹腔镜检查吻合口情况,必要时可对吻合口,尤其是吻合部位的"危险三角区"进行加固缝合。

多数患者术后早期表现为无明显诱因的持续性便血,颜色鲜红或暗红,便血的颜色取决于吻合口与肛门的距离及出血量。查体可发现引流液呈淡粉色或红色。部分患者可伴局部压痛。如吻合口出血较重或继发感染,引起吻合口漏的发生,患者可出现寒战、高热、腹痛、腹膜刺激征等表现。

绝大多数吻合口出血能自行停止,少部分患者需要采取干预措施。干预措施主要包括药物治疗、内镜治疗和手术治疗。药物治疗包括口服或肌内注射止血药，当出血量较大时，可在内镜下找到出血点并用止血夹钳夹止血。若内镜治疗不成功，可行手术治疗，结扎出血点及加固缝合吻合口。此外，对于低位、超低位保肛吻合口出血，可采用经肛加固缝合进行止血。

## 三、腹腔出血

NOSES 术后腹腔出血原因包括：手术时止血或血管结扎不牢固；患者有血液系统或其他系统疾病造成凝血功能障碍，未采取有效措施；各种原因造成的组织坏死或血管结扎部位脱落发生自发性大出血。

腹腔出血的预防关键在于术中仔细认真操作，切勿追求手术速度而忽略质量，确保血管结扎确切可靠。对于高龄或动脉硬化者，切忌过度裸化血管。对于高血压患者，注意避免术中、术后血压波动过大。术中出血，尤其大血管损伤造成的出血，必须进行确切止血。如直肠癌根治术中，肠系膜下动脉的出血处理需要一定的经验和技巧，须根据不同情况采取不同的处理方式。

腹腔出血的临床表现取决于出血部位、出血量及出血时间。患者可有腹部不适、轻度腹胀的表现。出血部位有局限性隆起，可伴轻度压痛，局部浊音区扩大。出血量较大时，叩诊移动性浊音阳性，伴有生命体征不稳定、脉搏细速、呼吸频率加快、血压下降。腹腔出血后引流液多呈鲜红色，引流量持续不减少或增加。一般情况下，引流管内的血性引流液往往提示存在活动性出血的可能。根据腹腔出血的临床表现，不难诊断。

术后出现少量出血时，可口服或肌内注射止血药，并密切观察患者病情变化。若出现大量出血，应密切监测血压、脉搏等生命体征，并做好随时手术探查的准备。一旦发现腹腔内活动性出血且出血量较大，应及时行二次手术探查并止血。在手术过程中，应尽快清除腹腔内的积血及血块，在原手术部位探查，寻找出血点并予以钳夹或缝扎止血，再次检查原手术部位。因术后出血而二次手术的患者中60%~70%找不到明确出血点，应彻底清除积血，冲洗观察后关腹。

## 四、吻合口漏

吻合口漏的发生包括全身因素、局部因素及技术因素。全身因素包括营养状态不良、长期应用糖皮质激素类药物、术前放化疗、伴发糖尿病等慢性疾病；局

部因素包括吻合口血运障碍、吻合口张力大、吻合口周围感染、吻合口区域肠管水肿等；技术因素包括缝合不严密、机械挤压强度较大、吻合器械本身(钉针高度)问题等。另外，预防吻合口漏需做好上述几点，还需通过注水注气试验来检查吻合口通畅，有无出血和渗漏。在条件允许的医院，术中进行结肠镜检查，会使手术过程更为安全可靠。

多数吻合口漏患者以发热或腹痛为首发症状，可伴有腹膜刺激征，腹腔感染较重者可出现中毒性休克及多器官衰竭。发热症状可出现在吻合口漏的任一阶段，有时表现为术后体温持续居高不下，或呈逐步升高态势。腹痛早期可表现为下腹坠胀不适，也可为突发剧烈腹痛，并伴有压痛、反跳痛等急性腹膜炎的症状和体征。如腹腔炎症局限，可呈局限性腹膜炎或可触及肿大包块。若留置了引流管，一旦发生吻合口漏，肠内容物便会从引流管流出。此时，引流液会突然增多，且变得混浊，伴有粪样物质及腐臭气味。引流口周围皮肤会出现红肿现象，有时还可看到有气泡冒出。

吻合口漏一旦确诊，应尽早治疗。局部通畅引流、控制感染是早期治疗的关键。大多数吻合口漏通过引流冲洗能达到自行愈合。如较长时间不能自愈，应考虑手术治疗，可行粪便转流或再次行肠切除吻合术，合理的治疗可使其转化为可控性漏或者局限性漏，直至痊愈。

目前，我国 79 家中心共同开展的 NOSES 回顾性研究结果显示，NOSES 术后吻合口漏的发生率为3.5%。虽然 NOSES 不增加吻合口漏的发生，但术者需要做好预防，关键是要保证吻合口无张力、无感染、良好血运，还需注意肠蠕动时产生的"蠕动张力"。笔者并不提倡对所有直肠癌患者均给予预防性造口，因其并不降低术后吻合口漏的发生率，还会带来一系列问题。但对于以下情况，不反对进行预防性造口：术前肠道准备不佳，合并不完全性肠梗阻；高龄体弱，合并糖尿病等相关基础疾病；合并重度贫血，营养不良；术前施行新辅助放化疗；骨盆狭小致手术不易操作或肥胖等特殊高危体质；肿瘤位置低，行超低位吻合保肛手术。

## 五、直肠阴道瘘

经阴道取标本的手术方式在腹腔镜手术中早已有之，在早期的研究中，腹部尚需要做辅助切口。笔者团队经过多年的实践和随访，已经验证了经阴道取标本的可行性和安全性。

术中切断肠管时，部分肠内容物极有可能流出，而取出标本过程中肠管受挤压也会致使肠腔内液体流入腹腔，上述两种情况均会增加腹腔内感染风险。如

在此基础上出现吻合口漏,加之存在阴道切口,便会增加直肠阴道瘘的风险。

直肠阴道瘘的原因可分为患者自身因素和医源性因素。患者的基础疾病、营养不良、免疫低下和年龄等,均可能增加瘘管发生的风险。而医源性因素,尤其是手术操作,与直肠阴道瘘的发生有重要的关系。直肠癌病变位置一般较低,手术牵拉及视野不清可导致阴道后壁被闭合在吻合口内或挤压性损伤。因此,良好的术野显露和在吻合器击发前确认阴道后壁与直肠关系,对于预防直肠阴道瘘的发生尤为关键。此外,加固缝合时也要注意勿将阴道后壁与吻合口一同缝合。

直肠阴道瘘是一种复杂的并发症,虽然发生率不高,但不可小视,对于术后直肠阴道瘘,特别是医源性直肠阴道瘘,应慎重选择手术时机,切勿因患者迫切要求而立即手术。在急性期,可采取保守治疗,期待其能自然愈合。具体措施为通过阴道冲洗、坐浴的方式保持局部清洁。如果瘘孔较小,自然愈合的概率相对较大。形成陈旧瘘后,建议等待局部及全身炎症消退、瘢痕软化(一般 3 个月)后进行修补术。瘘口位置较低时,可经阴道修补。

## 六、肠梗阻

肠梗阻是腹部手术后的常见并发症,术后的粘连、内疝、扭曲及感染等因素均可导致肠梗阻的发生。术后早期肠梗阻多为麻痹性肠梗阻,与全身状态不良、腹腔内感染、水电解质酸碱平衡紊乱等有关。术后晚期肠梗阻常由肠粘连或粘连带所致,多为机械性肠梗阻。少数患者也可由于肠扭转、肠套叠导致机械性肠梗阻。目前,我国 79 家中心共同开展的 NOSES 回顾性研究结果显示,NOSES 术后肠梗阻的发生率为 0.6%。主要表现为腹痛、腹胀、呕吐、停止排气排便等症状。由于肠梗阻的病因、类型、部位和程度各不相同,临床表现各有特点。如为绞窄性肠梗阻,病情进展迅速,可出现休克症状,因此,早期监测患者症状及体征可为治疗提供重要依据。

关于术后肠梗阻的预防,在技术层面上应尽量避免肠内容物外溢,若术中出现污染,应彻底清洗腹腔。关腹时仔细检查腹腔有无异物残留,将小肠按照正常的生理顺序和位置进行排序,并用大网膜覆盖。应鼓励患者早期下床活动,减少术后肠粘连的发生。此外,有研究报道戳孔疝导致肠梗阻的病例,因此,关闭缝合戳卡孔也至关重要。

肠梗阻作为常见结直肠癌术后并发症,其临床诊治并不难。治疗原则是解除梗阻的同时纠正内环境紊乱,根据肠梗阻的原因、性质、部位,以及全身情况和病情严重程度确定治疗方法。

## 七、肠扭转

肠扭转既可发生在术后早期,也可发生于术后晚期,通常是一段肠管甚至全部小肠及其系膜沿系膜轴扭转 360°～720°。因此,既有梗阻表现,又有肠系膜血液循环受阻表现,该并发症发病凶险、进展迅速,是最严重的术后并发症之一。

术后肠管粘连,肠内容物较多,均是形成肠扭转的潜在因素,在强烈肠蠕动或体位改变的刺激下,肠袢产生不同步的运动,进而引起肠袢的扭转。肠扭转的预防应重视术后宣教,叮嘱患者注意术后相关事项,避免因腹压突然增大而导致肠扭转。

肠扭转可在短期内发生肠绞窄、肠坏死,及时手术治疗将扭转的肠袢复位可降低死亡率,更可减少小肠大量切除后短肠综合征的发生。对于腹膜炎体征不明显、无结肠坏死,且纤维结肠镜示无肠壁坏死的患者,可在肠镜引导下,让软导管缓慢穿过梗阻部位,进入扭转的肠袢,进而排出大量气体和粪便,使肠扭转自行恢复。如肠壁已部分坏死,则需手术治疗。如腹膜炎体征明显,考虑结肠坏死者,也应果断给予手术治疗。手术方式为肠粘连松解,切除坏死结肠及部分冗长结肠,以此恢复结肠的正常解剖位置。

## 八、腹内疝

内疝是指腹腔内的脏器通过腹腔先天性或继发性孔隙(如肠系膜裂孔、网膜孔等)进入另一个腹腔间隙,但未突出到体表,多缺乏典型临床表现,故极易造成误诊。内疝通常以腹胀、腹痛、腹部不适为主要表现,部分患者伴有慢性肠梗阻症状。故术前选择合适的影像技术进行科学诊断是提高确诊率、为医生提供手术依据的关键。可考虑在术中关闭系膜裂孔来预防腹内疝的发生。

X 线检查仅显示液气平面、肠管扩张等肠梗阻征象。CT 检查可协助判断内疝的部位、范围、大小,即使内疝的部位较为隐蔽,也能为诊断提供准确的参考依据。一旦诊断明确,往往需要及时手术治疗,避免肠缺血、肠坏死。腹内疝的预防在于精细操作,尽可能关闭系膜裂孔,注意不能过于自信,操作完成后要仔细检查,以排除危险因素,一旦发现问题及早处理。

## 九、戳卡孔和阴道切口肿瘤种植

NOSES 无腹部辅助切口,戳卡孔和阴道切口是可能造成肿瘤种植的位置,一般认为 $CO_2$ 气腹可造成肿瘤细胞雾化状态,促进肿瘤种植。预防措施包括在术中注意无瘤操作，取标本过程中应用保护套隔离肿瘤，术中排烟时，应从戳卡阀门外接的排气管缓慢排烟。手术结束时，待腹腔内气体排尽后再将戳卡拔出，避免通过戳卡孔直接排气而造成烟囱效应。避免在腹壁上来回移动戳卡，应尽量使用带有螺纹的防脱戳卡，术中如发现戳卡密封圈损坏出现漏气现象，应及时更换，以确保整个气腹的密闭性。此外，为了减少腹腔种植，对于 $T_4$ 期肿瘤患者不建议采用 NOSES 手术方式。笔者在术中通常采用碘附溶液和蒸馏水冲洗腹腔和阴道，蒸馏水为低渗性，冲洗腹腔可使肿瘤细胞肿胀破裂而失活，同时，肿瘤组织受热后，癌细胞微小血管内会形成栓塞，致使癌细胞出现缺氧、酸中毒及代谢障碍，最终裂解。与之不同的是，正常组织细胞能够通过血管扩张、散热等机制维持自身正常状态。严格实施无瘤操作是 NOSES 的基本要求，也是改善患者预后的关键点之一。

## 十、十二指肠残端漏

十二指肠残端漏是胃癌患者在接受 NOSES 行毕 Ⅱ 式吻合或全胃切除术后可能出现的严重并发症。十二指肠残端漏是影响患者术后恢复甚至导致死亡的主要因素之一。其发生的可能原因除贫血、营养不良等全身因素外，还包括胃癌 NOSES 中残端缝合钉的脱落、超声刀对十二指肠的热损伤、输入袢不全梗阻，以及张力过大等。术中正确处理十二指肠残端，是预防十二指肠残端漏的关键因素之一，技术熟练的医生在腹腔镜下采用倒刺线进行十二指肠残端大荷包包埋是简单、有效的方法。十二指肠残端漏多发生在术后 3～8 天，患者表现为突发上腹部剧烈疼痛或胀痛，伴有体温升高、心率增快，以及右上腹压痛和肌紧张，白细胞升高。留有腹腔引流管的患者可引流出含胆汁的肠液，或者超声检查可见腹腔积液，腹腔穿刺抽出黄色胆汁、脓液。在治疗方面，大部分患者可通过充分腹腔引流、肠外营养支持等保守治疗手段即可实现治愈。如为输入袢梗阻导致的十二指肠残端漏，需再次手术行 Roux-en-Y 吻合。

## 十一、输入袢梗阻

胃癌术后输入袢梗阻较罕见，是胃癌术后特有的高位肠梗阻，主要由胆汁、胰液、肠液淤积在吻合口以上的肠腔内所致，是一种闭袢机械性肠梗阻，易发生肠绞窄，需要手术才能解除梗阻。典型症状是上腹部突然发生剧烈疼痛，频繁出现恶心、呕吐，吐出少量不含胆汁的胃内容物，右上腹压痛，有时可扪及包块。消化道造影检查可见造影剂能顺利通过吻合口进入输出袢空肠，而不能进入输入袢空肠，或者仅有少量造影剂缓慢进入输入袢，且输入袢空肠呈现明显扩张改变。超声检查可发现十二指肠扩张，呈液性暗区。对于未发生肠绞窄者，手术原则是去除病因，解除梗阻并建立符合生理的通道；对于已发生肠绞窄者，需手术去除病灶、解除梗阻、加强引流，若十二指肠第二、三段坏死，则须行胰十二指肠切除术。

## 十二、输出袢梗阻

胃癌术后输出袢梗阻不多见，其发生原因可能是腹腔粘连造成输出袢成角或者粘连带压迫肠管，输出袢逆行性套叠，输出袢肠段和吻合口成角，输出袢内疝等。主要表现为高位小肠梗阻的征象，上腹部饱胀，伴恶心、呕吐，呕吐物为食物及胆汁，诊断主要依靠上消化道造影，CT 有助于显示扩张的肠管。在治疗方面，可先行保守治疗，经保守治疗无好转或者不能排除机械性肠梗阻者，可考虑手术探查，手术原则是去除肠梗阻原因，可切除坏死肠段，恢复肠道通畅。

## 十三、术后胰腺炎及胰瘘

随着胃癌腹腔镜 $D_2$ 根治术在国内的广泛开展及推广，高频电刀和超声刀在胃癌 NOSES 的应用，术后胰腺炎及胰瘘的发生率似乎呈上升趋势，文献报道腹腔镜胃癌术后胰瘘的发生率为 0.9%。胰液具有腐蚀性，可导致脏器穿孔、出血及严重感染等并发症。胃癌术后胰腺炎的诊断存在一定难度，若未能及时发现并给予有效治疗，患者病情极有可能迅速恶化，甚至会危及生命。胃癌手术区域特殊的解剖特点及手术过程中的机械性损伤均可能导致术后胰腺炎及胰瘘的发生。术后胰腺炎及胰瘘多发生于术后第 3～10 天，临床症状缺乏特异性，主要表现为上腹痛，且疼痛位置不明确，常伴有腰背部放射性疼痛，同时还会出现难以用其他原因解释的恶心、呕吐、腹胀等症状。患者胃肠功能恢复迟缓，与疾病正常恢复进度不匹配；此外，还会出现持续性发热或白细胞计数增高的情况，病情严重者甚至会进展至败血症，或出现多器官功能衰竭。胰瘘主要依据腹腔引流液淀粉酶、血尿淀粉酶水平，结合临床症状来确诊。腹腔引流液淀粉酶升高指术后 3 天及 3 天后，腹腔引流液淀粉酶高于正常血清淀粉酶测定值上限 3 倍。动态增强 CT 是临床诊断胃癌术后胰腺炎有无坏死及判断坏死程度的金标准。一旦出现胰瘘，应立即采取措施保持腹腔引流通畅，同时让患者禁食，给予胃肠减压，并及时使用抑制胰腺分泌的药物，必要时实施外科手术引流和灌洗。

## 十四、术后淋巴漏

胃癌手术后，淋巴管主要分支破损引起的乳糜液溢出，称为淋巴漏，亦称乳糜漏。由于胃癌 NOSES 采用超声刀进行切割、分离，理论上较传统手术发生淋巴漏的概率更低。淋巴漏的发生与术中对淋巴管的处理方式密切相关，因此，术中预防是避免发生术后淋巴漏的关键。患者术后进食，若腹腔乳白色引流物增多，同时无发热、疼痛等症状，且引流液乳糜试验阳性，即可确诊。术后淋巴漏以保守治疗为主，包括全肠外营养、内环境维持和补充白蛋白，以及尝试性夹管观察。绝大多数淋巴漏经保守治疗在 2 周内愈合，很少需要手术治疗。

## 十五、术后胃轻瘫

术后胃轻瘫是胃肠手术后以胃排空障碍为主的综合征，主要见于胃部手术后，也见于肠道、胰腺和其他腹部及妇科手术后。由于手术方式及手术切除范围等的不同，术后胃排空延迟的发生率不尽相同，国外文献报道发生率为 0.6%～7.4%，国内文献报道发生率为 5.0%～10.0%。术后胃排空延迟的发病机制尚未完全明确，可能与手术改变正常神经激素和肌源性因素对胃排空的调控有关。通常发生在术后 2～3 天，饮食由禁食改为流质或流质改半流质时。患者出现恶心、呕吐，呕吐物多为残胃内容物。术后胃轻瘫的诊断标准尚未统一，但核心条件是排除残胃流出道的机械性梗阻。治疗上多采用禁食、持续胃肠减压、促进胃肠蠕动、加强肠外营养等措施，并做好与患者的沟通，树立信心，经保守治疗多可治愈。近年来，中医药在术后胃排空延迟治疗方面取得了一定的成功，针灸、艾灸、中药敷贴可加快术后胃瘫的康复。

# Basics and Training of
# Natural Orifice Specimen Extraction Surgery —
Gastrointestinal Surgery

Chief     Editors  |  Xishan Wang   Kefeng Ding   Petr V.Tsarkov

Associate editors  |  Jim Khan   Cüneyt Kayaalp   Sergey Efetov   Guiyu Wang

                    Haitao Zhou   Junhong Hu   Danbo Wang   Wei Zhang

                    Fanghai Han   Zheng Liu   Xu Guan   Jiaxing Meng

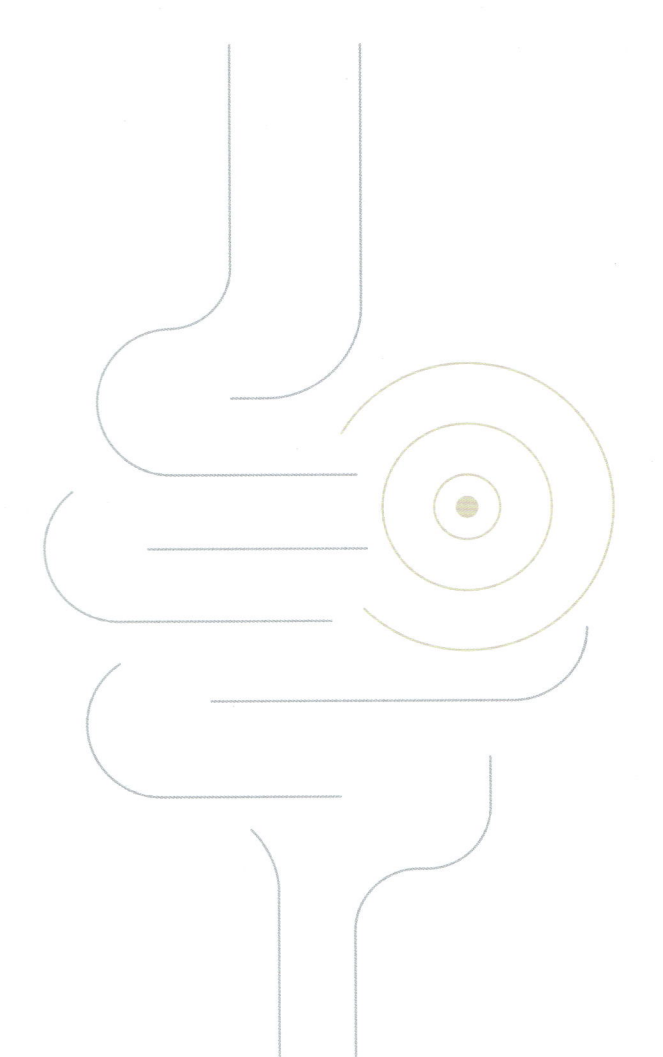

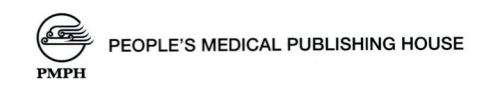
PEOPLE'S MEDICAL PUBLISHING HOUSE

# Editorial Board

| | |
|---|---|
| Jiaxing Meng | Matilda International Hospital |
| Xianwei Mo | Guangxi Medical University Cancer Hospital |
| Jian Peng | Xiangya Hospital of Central South University |
| Tianyu Qiao | The Second Affiliated Hospital of Harbin Medical University |
| Jichuan Quan | Cancer Hospital Chinese Academy of Medical Sciences |
| Peng Sun | Cancer Hospital Chinese Academy of Medical Sciences,Shenzhen Center |
| Jianqiang Tang | Cancer Hospital Chinese Academy of Medical Sciences |
| Qingchao Tang | The Second Affiliated Hospital of Harbin Medical University |
| Yantao Tian | Cancer Hospital Chinese Academy of Medical Sciences |
| Song Wang | Zibo Municipal Hospital |
| Danbo Wang | Cancer Hospital China Medical University |
| Guiyu Wang | The Second Affiliated Hospital of Harbin Medical University |
| Xishan Wang | Cancer Hospital Chinese Academy of Medical Sciences |
| Xiaoming Wang | Zibo Municipal Hospital |
| Zejun Wang | The Affiliated Cancer Hospital of Guizhou Medical University |
| Ye Wei | Huadong Hospital Affiliated to Fudan University |
| Dehai Xiong | Chongqing University Three Gorges Hospital |
| Zhiguo Xiong | Hubei Cancer Hospital |
| Su Yan | Qinghai University Affiliated Hospital |
| Yefeng Yin | Cancer Hospital Chinese Academy of Medical Sciences |
| Gang Yu | Zibo Municipal Hospital |
| Guanyu Yu | Changhai Hospital, First Affiliated Hospital of Naval Medical University |
| Shaojun Yu | The Second Affiliated Hospital Zhejiang University School of Medicine |
| Lei Yu | The Second Affiliated Hospital of Harbin Medical University |
| Ziming Yuan | The Second Affiliated Hospital of Harbin Medical University |
| Qian Zhang | Cancer Hospital University of Chinese Academy of Sciences |
| Wei Zhang | Changhai Hospital, First Affiliated Hospital of Naval Medical University |
| Jinzhu Zhang | Cancer Hospital Chinese Academy of Medical Sciences |
| Mingguang Zhang | Cancer Hospital Chinese Academy of Medical Sciences |
| Tiemin Zhang | The Second Affiliated Hospital of Hainan Medical University |
| Xiaoqian Zhang | Cancer Hospital Chinese Academy of Medical Sciences |
| Zhixun Zhao | Cancer Hospital Chinese Academy of Medical Sciences |
| Chaoxu Zheng | Cancer Hospital Chinese Academy of Medical Sciences |
| Haitao Zhou | Cancer Hospital Chinese Academy of Medical Sciences |
| Xiaoming Zhu | Changhai Hospital, First Affiliated Hospital of Naval Medical University |
| Meng Zhuang | Cancer Hospital Chinese Academy of Medical Sciences |

**Writing Secretary**  Jialiang Liu   Zheng Liu   Xiyue Hu

# Preface One

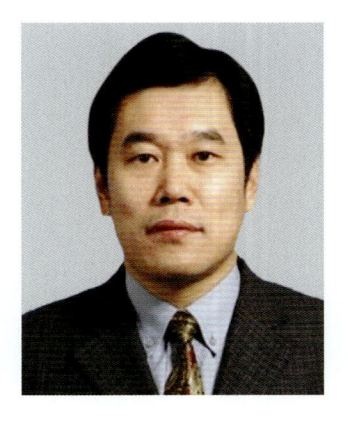

In recent years, with the continuous advancement and progress of surgery, the purpose of tumor surgery has gone beyond curative resection; minimal invasiveness and organ function preservation have become the higher pursuits in surgical treatment. Against this backdrop, Professor Xishan has made outstanding contributions to advancing minimally invasive surgical treatment and enhancing surgical techniques. As a leading figure in the field of colorectal cancer in China, his multiple technological innovations, particularly in the natural orifice specimen extraction surgery (NOSES) , have become an exemplary model driving industry development.

Professor Xishan has undertaken extensive efforts to promote NOSES, leading the development of over ten international and Chinese NOSES guidelines and consensus documents, establishing industry standards for the implementation NOSES worldwide. To enrich the theoretical framework of NOSES, the scope of indications for NOSES has been continuously expanded. It has been expanded from colorectal tumors in the first edition to gastrointestinal tumors in the second edition, then extended to abdominal and pelvic tumors in the third edition. By the fourth edition, surgeries for thoracic tumors, esophageal cancer, etc. have also been systematically included. His works have been translated by renowned international experts into multiple languages, including English, Korean, Russian, Japanese, and French, for global dissemination. This objectively reflects not only the feasibility and significant societal value of NOSES,but also highlights the international reputation and status of Chinese NOSES, underscoring the vast prospects of NOSES application.

To better promote the standardized application of NOSES , a comprehensive training system and standardized training materials are essential. Therefore, Professor Xishan organized the compilation of a bilingual textbook, NOSES International Structured Training and Certification Course: *Basics and Training of Natural Orifice Specimen Extraction Surgery-Gastrointestinal Surgery*. This textbook

covers the core theories and surgical essentials of NOSES, aiming to help physicians worldwide systematically master the essence of NOSES, enabling this minimally invasive technique to be refined in theory and widely practiced globally. Notably, the textbook content is systematic and thorough, covering every critical step from procedure selection to intraoperative operation and postoperative management, making it an invaluable reference for surgeons worldwide.

The publication of this textbook represents not only a milestone for Chinese NOSES but also a solid step toward introducing NOSES globally. I am confident that this textbook will profoundly impact the field of global surgery.

Jie He
December 2024

# Preface Two

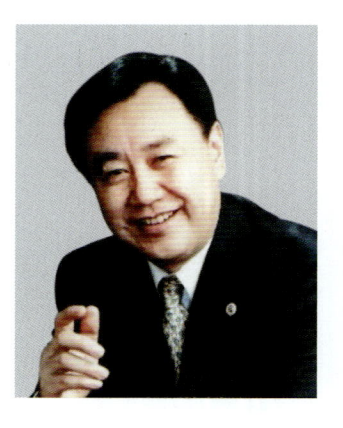

With the advancement of integrated medical concepts, deep integration across disciplines has enabled modern medicine to develop rapidly toward optimizing diagnostic and therapeutic approaches from a holistic perspective. Professor Xishan keenly captured this trend. After more than a decade of continuous exploration and practice, he led his domestic and international colleagues to successfully build a systematic NOSES integrated theory and technology system, opening up a new height for minimally invasive surgery, making it more innovative and clinically valuable.

As a surgical technique, NOSES has not only achieved breakthroughs in minimally invasive treatment,but also achieved comprehensive development in horizontal and vertical integration. Horizontally, NOSES connects multiple disciplines such as gastro intestinal surgery, hepatobiliary-pancreatic-splenic surgery, thoracic surgery, gynecology, and urology, and promotes its deep development of NOSES in multidisciplinary collaboration and integration. Vertically, NOSES systematically integrates knowledge from fundamental theory to surgical operations and patient management, comprehensively covering every aspect of clinical application. This system not only helps surgeons achieve effective treatment without abdominal incisions,but also significantly improves patients' quality of life and treatment experience. NOSES embodies a patient-centered diagnostic and therapeutic approach, reflecting Professor Xishan's profound understanding and practice of integrated medicine.It is not limited to the medical technology itself, but also touches upon the integration of fields such as psychology and sociology, thus creating a brand-new perspective for diagnosis and treatment.

The textbook NOSES International Structured Training and Certification Course: *Basics and Training of Natural Orifice Specimen Extraction Surgery-Gastrointestinal Surgery*, edited by Professor Xishan, is more comprehensive, practical, and accessible, with a strong focus on surgical details and clinical standards, providing invaluable guidance. Presented in both Chinese and English, this textbook facilitates

learning and training for colleagues worldwide, building a bridge for exchange and promoting the standardized global adoption of NOSES. This innovative textbook serves not only as a clinical operations guide but also as a vital vehicle for spreading the NOSES concept, providing practical support for surgeons applying NOSES.

With the guidance of this textbook, NOSES will undoubtedly enable China's minimally invasive surgery to shine at the intersection of medicine and surgery. I hope this book will serve as a valuable reference for colleagues exploring the field of NOSES, supporting NOSES in reaching international frontiers and benefiting more patients.

Daiming Fan
December 2024

# Foreword

    Time waits for no one, and the seasons flow like a river. Looking back, it has been more than ten years since the concept of NOSES was proposed. Over these years, it has passed through its budding stage, initial stage, development stage, and now, its stage of maturity. Colleagues from across the country have collectively contributed to refining both the technical and theoretical frameworks of NOSES, and everyone has devoted their wisdom and effort to this endeavor. As I approach my sixties, I reflect on the many experiences along the journey of NOSES' development-the novelty, inspiration, effort, pay, doubts, criticism, praise, applause, and accolades...These reflections have left me with many insights. NOSES is not just a matter of a technical system and a theoretical system, but more importantly, it involves reflections and deliberations on human nature, the so-called "worldly affairs", and the meaning of life. Moreover, I am deeply aware of the advancement of science and academia, the importance of education and training, and the power of reflection and legacy. Shouldering the mission of benefiting patients, the responsibility of cultivating talents, and the responsibility of discipline development, I wish to gather my thoughts here and share them with everyone.

## 1. Innovation and Reflection

- The knowledge, experience and inertial thinking we currently possess are at times the greatest enemy of innovation, and a justification for the denial of others.
- Innovation in norms, pragmatism in innovation. Seek truth in pragmatism and move forward in truth-seeking.
- You can limit my hands, but can not limit my brain. That is why thinking is one of the essential qualities of a surgeon.
- The perfection of the human body makes up for the shortage of medicine and our self-righteousness.

## 2. Personal Growth and Professional Development

- A surgeon's fall into a pit, a gain in the whole profession's wit.
- When a surgeon dares to deny himself, he really grew up.
- The moment our effort paid off marked our achievements as a thing of the past. Now is the time to set sail for the next destination.
- Power speaks, practice matters.
- Desire stimulates potential and goals are born alive.

- The wise lead the way, the kind shape the future.
- Lead the field with skill, win the future with virtue.

## 3. Medical Ethics and Professional Culture

- See others' achievements with appreciative perspectives, but see our own inadequacy with captious perspectives.
- There is no self-respect to speak of when you have no accomplishments to show for it, for your self-respect is worth nothing compared to the life of a patient!
- Kindness can't touch the meanness, integrity can't melt the shameless, but we shouldn't stop being kind and upright because of that.
- Team Culture

Two ones

One motto: Those who are not as virtuous as Buddha should not practice medicine, and those whose medical skills are not as miraculous as those of immortals should not practice medicine.

One goal: Aim at our own health and the recovery of the patients we treat.

Two twos

Two senses: a doctor should always have a sense of achievement and guilt. Sense of achievement makes our career persistent forward momentum; guilt can be corrected for our career.

Two pursuits: every action of a surgeon should reflect wisdom, and a surgeon should have three-dimensional anatomical thinking.

Two threes

Three principles of medical practice:

Practice medicine in according with the law-Principle.

Practice medicine with a humanistic approach-Flexibility.

Practice medicine scientifically-Scientific.

The three realms of being a doctor:

Craftsman- "hand" to see the disease

Family- "brain" to see the disease

Teacher- "heart" to see the disease

4. Medicine and Social Insights

· The development of medicine depends on the development of other disciplines, such as optics, electricity, engineering, pharmacology, aesthetics, etc. Medicine is a complex of human scientific and technological progress, social progress, and human civilization.

· Greedy favours are not rewarded, and rewards are given without favours.

· To make someone grateful for a lifetime-hard; to make someone hate a lifetime-easy.

· The bystander sees things clearly because their own interests are not involved.

· Civilisation stems from the accumulation and inheritance of culture, inheritance stems from the confidence and mission of the nation, gratitude stems from the piety and reverence of the heart, and development stems from the innovation and faith of the country.

· The "Six Truths" philosophy for physicians: True faith, true capability, true collaboration, true teaching, true effort and true compassion.

· It's hard for a person to succeed, it takes a myriad of factors in his favor, while it's easy to fail, it only takes one factor.

· These are my reflections from different stages of my life, the famous quote that I remembered and a record of my personal journey. I am eager to share these insights with my students and trainees, and if they benefit the readers in any way, I would feel deeply gratified! The purpose of editing the *Basics and Training of Natural Orifice Specimen Extraction Surgery-Gastrointestinal Surgery* (*Chinese-English in one*) is to provide domestic and international trainees with a resource for learning, applying, and promoting NOSES. I hope that all trainees will become caring, compassionate, warm and philosophical international NOSES people who benefit patients and bless society to push surgery forward.

    NOSES belongs to China, and it also belongs to the world!


· Respecting with a devout heart and adhering to the medical ethics serve as the preface!


Xishan Wang

December 2024

# Contents

## Chapter Ⅳ
## Standardized Procedures of Laparoscopic Gastric NOSES　|　065

## Chapter V
## The Common Complications and Management of
## Gastrointestinal NOSES    |    084

# Video Directory

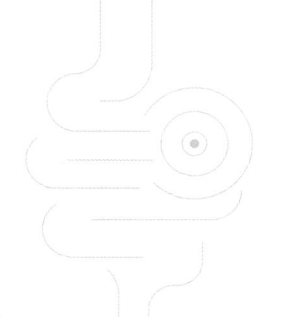

# Chapter I

# General Statement of NOSES

With the rapid development of surgical techniques and the widespread acceptance of minimal invasiveness, minimally invasive surgery has undisputedly become the focal point of new medical technology. Natural orifice transluminal endoscopic surgery (NOTES) has overturned the conventional concept and pushed minimally invasive **surgery** to the extreme of "no incision". Recently, as one of the new techniques in minimally invasive surgery, natural orifice specimen extraction surgery (NOSES) has gradually attracted extensive attention and heated discussion both domestically and overseas.

It is well known that NOSES is a new type of hybrid surgical procedure with the "no incision" idea of NOTES and the surgical techniques of laparoscopic surgery, and demonstrates a perfect minimally invasive effect with satisfying safety and operability. Currently, the application of NOSES is not only limited to the colorectal field, but has also extended gradually to perform gastrointestinal, hepatobiliary, splenopancreatic, urogynecologic and thoracic surgeries, reflecting the vitality and potentiality of NOSES.

## 1 Definition and Classification of NOSES

NOSES is defined as follow: Unassisted incision surgery of the abdominal wall using equipment such as conventional laparoscopic instruments, transanal endoscopic microsurgery (TEM) , or soft endoscopes and robotic surgical platform to complete intra-abdominal surgical operations (resections, reconstructions), with lesion specimens taken through the natural orifice (rectum, vagina, or mouth). The biggest difference between NOSES and conventional laparoscopic surgery is that the lesion specimen is removed through the natural orifice, which avoids the auxiliary incision of the abdominal wall to take the specimen, and only a few small scars remain on the abdominal wall after surgery (Figure 1-1-1).

According to different routes of specimen extraction, NOSES is divided into three categories: transanalspecimen extraction, transvaginal specimen extraction and transoral specimen extraction (Figure 1-1-2). The former two procedures are used more commonly in clinical practice, especially the transanal specimen extraction. The

transanal specimen extraction is mainly applied to the patients with small-sized specimen, easy to be removed via anus. The transvaginal specimen extraction is applied to the female patients with large-sized specimen, which are difficult to be removed transanally. Considering that the esophagus is long and narrow with low elasticity, the indications of transoral specimen extraction procedure should be strict.

According to the different procedures of specimen extraction, NOSES can also be classified into three categories: ①Specimen eversion and extra-corporeal resection (eversion-resection procedure) ; ②Specimen extraction and extra-corporeal resection (extraction-resection procedure); ③Intra-abdominal specimen resection and extra-corporeal extraction (resection-extraction procedure) (Figure 1-1-3). Different surgical procedures carry different operation characteristics and require specific surgical skills, however, the decisive factor in choosing an appropriate surgical procedure is the tumor location. In colorectal NOSES, the eversion-

resection procedure is mainly used for the lower rectal tumors, the extraction-resection procedure is mainly used for the middle rectal tumors, and the resection-extraction procedure is used more widely, including for the tumors in the upper rectum, the sigmoid colon, the left half colon, the right half colon, and the whole colon. Besides colorectal, other organs follow the resection-extraction procedure of NOSES to extract the specimen.

# 2    Concepts and Principles for Conducting NOSES

The relationship between the development of surgical oncology and the birth of NOSES can be viewed as a gradual technological evolution. Surgical oncology has gone through many technological advances from traditional open surgery to laparoscopic and robotic-assisted surgery, which laid the foundation for the birth of NOSES. Surgical oncology has promoted the creation of NOSES through technological advances, deepening of minimally invasive concepts, and changes in patient needs, while the birth of NOSES has further promoted the development of minimally invasive techniques in surgical oncology. NOSES inherits the core concepts of surgical oncology of oncological safety and preservation of organ function, and at the same time, through the innovative way of specimen removal, it advances the minimally invasive surgery to a new height and meets the patient's demand for less trauma and faster recovery. NOSES is a part of radical oncologic surgery and colorectal surgery, therefore, the operation of this technique must meet the three concepts and two principles of radical surgery and colorectal surgery. The three concepts are the function preservation in oncology surgery concept (FPOSC), the surgical risk-benefit balance concept (SRBBC), and concept of aseptic and tumor-free surgical practice (CATFSP); the two principles refer to the need to comply with the total mesorectal excision (TME) and the complete mesocolic excision (CME).

## 2.1    Three Concepts

### 2.1.1    FPOSC

NOSES has become a surgical treatment option for many tumor patients due to its many advantages. The selection of the extent of resection for NOSES for gastrointestinal tumors must follow the FPOSC concept, which is to maximize tumor resection to ensure cure and maximize the preservation of normal tissue and organ function. The concept reflects the surgeon's ability to make trade-offs and should never be done for the sake of surgery. For example, in the same transanal external resection of a tumor, the length of the externalized bowel was 3-4cm in one patient and 10cm or more of the bowel in the other (Figure 1-2-1). Although both underwent NOSES, the former was right and the latter was wrong, the error being that the latter did not conform to the FPOSC concept. Another example is the preservation of the middle colonic artery in right hemicolectomy and the protection of pelvic floor nerve function in rectal NOSES, both of which exemplify FPOSC. The FPOSC followed during surgical oncology is not only the equal importance of tumor eradication and preservation of function, but also focuses on the clinical outcome of the oncology patient, especially the quality of life in the postoperative period. Surgery should not be performed for the sake of surgery.

### 2.1.2    SRBBC

To date, for most solid tumors, surgery is still the means of curing the tumor, and thus the reasonable choice of the surgical procedure is very important. The so-called SRBBC refers to the comparison of the trauma, damage and blow caused by the surgical removal of a tumor with the endurance and benefit to tissues, organs and the body, physical endurance and overall benefit i.e., which patients should be operated on, and what kind of surgery should be performed so that the patients can get the maximum benefit with the minimum damage. If the specimen can be removed both anally and vaginally, choose to take the specimen transanally, which avoids unnecessary damage to the vagina and is more consistent with SRBBC. The SRBBC reflects the surgeon's selection ability. Through accurate assessment, it can ensure that the appropriate

surgical procedure is applied to the suitable patients, and ensure the safety of patients and at the same time safeguards the surgeon's own operational safety. It is imperative that there be successful surgery and failed treatment.

### 2.1.3  CATFSP

To ensure the successful implementation of NOSES, asepsis and tumor-free operation are the basic requirements for its operation. First, the surgeon must have a basic CATFSP, and strictly follow the technique of probing from far to near, no-contact isolation, the principle of whole resection, the principle of prioritizing blood vessels, and try to perform sharp dissection as much as possible. Second, adequate bowel and vaginal preparation must be performed preoperatively. Third, certain surgical operation skills must be mastered, and the overall cooperation of the surgical team must be emphasized, especially the digestive tract reconstruction and specimen removal sessions, which are the core steps to accomplish high-quality NOSES. Fourth, the rational use of antitumor drugs and antibacterial drugs. Intraperitoneal drugs can be administered to colorectal cancer patients with high risk of recurrence, especially those with tumor invasion to the plasma membrane, lymph node metastasis, positive or suspected positive free cancer cells on cytological examination of abdominal lavage fluid, and those whose tumors have been excessively extruded or ruptured intraoperatively. Injecting chemotherapy drugs into the abdominal cavity during the operation directly acts on the implanted and detached cancer cells within the abdominal cavity. maintaining a relatively high effective drug concentration in the abdominal cavity. This is one of the important means for preventing and treating abdominal implantation and metastasis of colorectal cancer. At present, the commonly used clinical intraperitoneal drugs for colorectal cancer include raltitrexed, lobaplatin, tumor necrosis factor, fluorouracil implants and so on.

## 2.2  Two principles

### 2.2.1  TME principle

The TME principle is a principle of standard surgical technique used in the treatment of rectal cancer to ensure complete tumor resection and lymph node dissection through precise resection of the rectum and its mesenteric tissues within the plane of the membranous anatomy outside the mesorectum. TME focuses on integrity of resection extent and autonomic nerve preservation, which ensures the radical tumor resection and reduces postoperative dysfunction, such as loss of sexual or voiding function. It effectively reduces the rate of local recurrence and improves patients' quality of life.

### 2.2.2  CME principle

The CME principle is a standard surgical technique principle based on anatomy and used for the treatment of colon cancer. By completely removing the colon and its mesenteric tissues within the plane of the membranous anatomy, it ensures that all relevant tissues, including the lymph nodes around the tumor, are completely excised. CME emphasizes high ligation of blood vessels and thorough lymph node dissection in order to reduce the risk of local recurrence, while at the same time guaranteeing a tumor-free operation to prevent the dissemination of tumor cells. This improves the disease-free survival rate and overall prognosis of colon cancer patients.

## 3  Indications Selection for NOSES

Since the NOSES is performed based on the laparoscopy platform, the indications of NOSES should meet the basic requirements of laparoscopic surgery. In general, the following conditions need to be met to perform minimally invasive **surgery** such as laparoscopy **surgery**: ①The surgeon has experience in laparoscopic operation; ②Don't indicated for locally advanced cancer; ③Don't indicated for acute intestinal obstruction or perforation of intestine; ④Thorough abdominal exploration is required; ⑤Consider localizing the lesion before the operation. In brief, in the application of NOSES, the basic indications of laparoscopic surgery

should be met.

Besides, since the specimen extraction is performed through natural orifices, there are corresponding requirements for the indication of NOSES. According to new edition of the *Expert Consensus of Natural Orifice Specimen Extraction Surgery in Colorectal Neoplasm*, the specific indications of NOSES for colorectal cancer mainly include:the depth of tumor invasion is preferably $T_2$-$T_3$, the circumferential diameter of the specimen taken through the **anus** is preferably less than 5cm,and the circumferential diameter of the specimen taken through the vagina is preferably 5-7cm. Relative contraindications include a relatively advanced local stage of the tumor, a large-sized specimen and a body mass index (BMI) more than 30kg/m$^2$. As it is still not clear whether the incision of posterior vaginal fornix  affects women's reproductive function or not, the transvaginal specimen extraction

is best to be avoided in unmarried or childbearing women. The specific indications of NOSES are mainly mentioned for the operative link of specimen extraction through the natural orifice ,which mainly involve three considerations, namely, the size of the specimen, the depth of tumor invasion, and the BMI.

For patients with colorectal cancer accompanied by local organ invasion who require combined resection of organs, as well as patients with colorectal cancer accompanied by distant metastasis or lesions in other parts who require simultaneous surgical resection, complex surgical NOSES can also be chosen. The surgical indications for NOSES in the combined resection of organs and multi-organ resection are more stringent, especially, it puts forward more stringent requirements for doctors' operating techniques.

# 4    Normalization of Specimen Extraction through the Natural Orifice

Specimen extraction through the natural orifice is the most characteristic core step in NOSES and is also the most concerned and hotly debated surgical procedure. The operation of specimen extraction through the natural orifice reflects strong individual differences, which is related not only to the anatomical and physiological conditions of the patient's natural orifice, but also to the doctor's cognitive level and operational experience regarding specimen extraction.

## 4.1    Transanal specimen extraction

There are many surgical methods to take specimens through the natural passage of the anus, and the majority of doctors are also proficient. To sum up, there are three ways.

### 4.1.1    Transanal specimen extraction by eversion-resection

Transanal specimen extraction by eversion-resection is applicable to patients with lower rectal tumors, those with relatively small lesions, and those whose circumferential invasion is less than half of the circumference. This method is to make use of the elasticity of the healthy side of

the bowel wall to turn the distal rectum containing tumor outside the anus, and then use iodophor water to rinse it abundantly, especially at the reflexes of the bowel wall. This allows for clear visualization of the subcutaneous margins of the tumor under direct vision and ensures that the tumor is isolated with safe margins.

### 4.1.2    Specimen extraction through the stump of rectum

It is currently the most widely applied and least invasive preferred approach for specimen extraction in colorectal NOSES. In order to consider the safety and feasibility of the specimen extraction, the requirements of operation are as follows: ①It is necessary to perform sufficient anal dilatation before the specimen extraction. ②Rectal stump must be irrigated with a large amount of iodophor water. ③The protective sleeve should be placed before specimen extraction to avoid contact between the specimen and the natural orifice. ④The specimen should be handled gently and slowly during specimen extraction to avoid the damage of specimen integrity by violent pulling. If the resistance during specimen extraction is

hard, the anesthesiologist can be instructed to administer muscular relaxant appropriately to reduce the tension of anal sphincter. Whether specimen extraction through the stump of rectum will damage the anal sphincter and affect defecation function is a focal issue of concern in NOSES. According to the current findings, transanal specimen extraction does not significantly increase the risk of anal injury as long as reasonable indications are met.

### 4.1.3 Specimen extraction through the incision of rectum

It is primarily used for right or left hemicolectomy or transverse colectomy of male. This method needs an extra rectal incision and increases the risk of postoperative rectal leakage. Therefore, the doctors should communicate fully with patients and their family members and the consent must be obtained before the operation. There are two obstacles in specimen extraction through the incision of rectum. Firstly, how to extract the specimen through the anus.The key operative point is the same as the techniques of specimen extraction through the stump of rectum. Secondly, how to choose the site of rectal incision and what are the operative specifications. Intraoperative colonoscopic confirmation may be used in medical units where available.

It is recommended that the rectal incision should be chosen on the anterior wall of the middle rectum above the peritoneal reflection. The length of incision is about 3cm, and the incision direction should be parallel to the direction of rectum. The contralateral rectal wall should not be damaged during incising.It is recommended that continuous suture should be performed from the distal to the proximal. After suturing, air and water injection test should be performed to examine whether the rectal incision is fully sutured. Intraoperative colonoscopy can be used to confirm in medical units where conditions permit.

## 4.2 Transvaginal specimen extraction

The vaginotomy and vaginal suture are the difficulties of transvaginal specimen extraction. It is recommended to prioritize the posterior vaginal fornix as the site for the vaginal incision. The rectouterine pouch has unique anatomical advantages. It is easy to locate and expose under laparoscopy, which can effectively reduce the risk of collateral damage. At the same time, the posterior vaginal fornix has a good healing ability, and there are no important blood vessels and nerves around it. There will be no scar after the mucosa heals, and it has relatively little impact on the patient's sexual life, and the surgeon can choose according to their operation habits. The length of vaginal incision is recommended to be 3-5cm and the direction should be transverse. The depth of incision is the full thickness of the vaginal wall. After the specimen is extracted, the vagina needs to be rinsed intraperitoneally. Suture of vaginal incision includes transvaginal extra-abdominal suture and laparoscopic suture. Most of the suture methods are continuous full-thickness suture with the barbed thread from one end of the vaginal incision to another. After the suture, vaginal or anal examination is required to check whether the incision is properly sutured and whether there is any damage to the rectum.

## 4.3 Transoral specimen extraction

In addition to the transanal specimen extraction and the transvaginal specimen extraction, some scholars have begun to try to carry out NOSES with the transoral specimen extraction, including sleeve gastrectomy, gastric mesenchymal tumor resection, liver biopsy, cholecystectomy, and splenectomy. The stomach is connected to the esophagus and the oral cavity, the transoral specimen extraction can be performed for gastric tumors with small lesions. There is no need to take another way to take the specimen through the mouth, and it does not involve the incision and suture of the natural orifice and the transportation of the specimen, and the main operation point is to take out the specimen through the esophagus and the mouth. In the process of transoral specimen extraction, it is recommended to put the specimen into a protective sleeve for closure and complete the specimen extraction under the guidance of endoscopy. However, due to the long and narrow lumen of the esophagus and the poor elasticity of the wall, the surgeon must strictly grasp the indications for transoral specimen extraction.

## 4.4 Experiences and skills of the natural orifice specimen extraction

### 4.4.1 The method of mesorectal priority is applied to the transanal specimen extraction by eversion-resection.

In the conventional laparoscopic rectum eversion and extraction resection for rectal cancer surgery, if the tumor is small and the mesentery is thin, the direct turn-out method can be used to easily turn out the distal rectum. However, for patients with large tumor or hypertrophied mesentery, this method may easily lead to failure of external rotation and tumor fragmentation. The method of mesorectal priority overcomes the difficulties of large tumors, hypertrophied mesentery, and clusters of tumors stuck at the anal opening. The anterior wall of the rectum is cut (about 3cm), and the cut mesentery is pulled out of the rectal cavity, which reduces the pressure for turning out, and the operation will be much easier when the intestinal tract with the tumor is everted by means of pulling it outwards and pushing it from the inside. There are many skills in the method of mesorectal priority, such as the method of pulling and pushing the specimen externally and internally, and the obese and large tumors can be successfully turned out. However, it is necessary to make an accurate judgment and avoid causing unnecessary damage.

### 4.4.2 Skills of expanding anus in the transanal specimen extraction

It is necessary to give the muscular relaxant before the anal dilatation; The protective sleeve is placed through the 12mm trocar site via abdominal approach; When the assistant extracts the specimen through the anus, the root of mesentery can be dragged out first ; The surgeon should avoid to drag the protective sleeve when extracting the specimen and the protective sleeve can play the roles of isolation and anal dilation; When the largest part of the tumor is dragged into the anal canal, the protective sleeve should be tightened and the specimen can be pulled outward together with the protective sleeve; Under laparoscopy, the surgeon and the assistant should cooperate and tighten the inner opening of the protective sleeve. At this time, the first assistant can aspirate to prevent the liquid inside the specimen into the abdominal cavity.

### 4.4.3 Operational skills in the transvaginal specimen extraction

Selection of incision: According to previous experience, after laparoscopic incision, a cup can be lifted or gauze can be inserted to expose the posterior vaginal fornix, and the surgeon can make a transverse incision of the posterior vaginal fornix with a length of 3-5cm under direct vision under laparoscopic vision. Due to the well ductility of the vagina, we can expand the incision to 5cm by pulling upwards and downwards, to meet the requirements of specimen extraction.

Suture of incision: Vaginal incision can be sutured extracorporeally under direct vision or laparoscopically. Extracorporeal suture is the first choice, especially for surgeons who cannot master the skills of laparoscopic suture since it is relatively easy according to the experience. ①Extracorporeal suture: Due to the deep position of the posterior fornix, it is necessary to fully expose the incision of the posterior fornix when performing extracorporeal suture. In clinical practice, instruments such as vaginal scopes or right-angled retractor are often used to fully expose the vagina, and the two sides of the posterior fornix are important parts of the vagina. Two Alice forceps are used to clamp the upper and lower edges of the vaginal incision respectively, pull the vaginal incision outward properly, and then perform intermittent or continuous sutures for several stitches. When exposure is unsatisfactory, a full open suture of the vaginal incision can be considered, and the gauze can be tamponade vaginally to avoid the residual blood cavity affecting healing, and can be removed after 24-48 hours of compression. ②Laparoscopic suture: This suture technique is relatively difficult, which needs high requirements on the surgeon's ability. Barbed thread (15cm is sufficient, the line is too long and will affect the operation) is needed for laparoscopic suture. Continuous full-thickness sutures are usually applied from one end of the vaginal incision to the other. After suturing, vaginal or rectal digital examination should be performed.In the process of suturing, the upper and lower edges of the vaginal incision should be pulled inwards, and the pulling force should not be too large to cause vaginal bleeding.

# 5 Normalization of Digestive Tract Reconstruction

Total laparoscopic digestive tract reconstruction should be performed in NOSES, which is the important and difficult part in NOSES. Digestive tract reconstruction of NOSES should follow the basic principles of open surgery and conventional laparoscopic surgery as followed: ①On the premise of guaranteeing radical resection of tumor, select a safe and feasible method of digestive tract reconstruction according to the extent of digestive resection. ②The anastomosis should be provided with sufficient blood supply without tension and stenosis. ③FPOSC should be followed, so as to reduce unnecessary tissue damage and take into account the physiological functions of the gastrointestinal tract. ④For low rectal cancer, ultra-low anastomosis anus-preserving surgery, if the risk of anastomosis leakage is high or the patient was treated with neoadjuvant radiochemotherapy, protective ileostomy should be performed.

## 5.1 Selection of digestive tract reconstruction methods (colorectal)

There are three different ways of digestive tract reconstruction, end-to-end anastomosis, functional end-to-end anastomosis and functional side-to-side anastomosis. The anastomotic organs include colon-rectal anastomosis, colon-colonic anastomosis, ileocolonic anastomosis and colon-anal anastomosis. Colon-rectal anastomosis can be used for digestive tract reconstruction of the rectal NOSES and the end-to-end anastomosis is recommended. Functional side-to-side anastomosis is suitable for transverse colon, left hemicolon, and right hemicolon resection surgeries. The ileo-colic anastomosis is suitable for right hemicolectomy surgery. Functional end-to-end anastomosis is mostly used for right hemicolectomy surgery (Figure 1-5-1).

## 5.2 Precautions for digestive tract reconstruction

In the process of digestive tract reconstruction, attention should be paid to the selection of surgical instruments, the inspection of anastomosis quality, and the prevention of high-risk factors. Through scientific and reasonable steps and strict control of details, the success rate of surgery can be effectively improved and the risk of complications can be reduced.

### 5.2.1 Selection of surgical instruments

For the reconstruction of the digestive tract in NOSES, the selection of surgical instruments is crucial for laparoscopic surgical procedures. Appropriate use of devices such as motorized linear cutting stapler with pre-chip technology, motorized circular stapler with 3D anastomosis technology, and curved tip stapler can help complete anastomoses more stably and precisely. These devices are easy to operate and have stable performance, which can significantly improve the anastomotic effect and reduce the possibility of intraoperative and postoperative adverse events.

### 5.2.2 Inspection of anastomosis quality

Before anastomosis, it is necessary to check the blood flow of the intestinal wall, anastomotic tension, and whether the direction of the mesentery is twisted; after anastomosis, it is necessary to check whether there is leakage and bleeding at the anastomotic site, as well as the degree of patency and other conditions. In the quality assessment of anastomosis, the exact degree of anastomosis can be evaluated by checking the integrity of the anastomosis of the upper and lower cutting edges, observing whether the anastomotic staple is exposed or not, and evaluating the anastomosis by finger touch to see whether there is any reversal of the staple. At the same time, the air and water injection test can be used to detect whether there is leakage from the anastomosis. In addition, intraoperative colonoscopy can provide an effective visual field to facilitate the determination of the degree of patency of the anastomosis, the width of the anastomotic staples encircling the tissues and the presence of other hidden dangers.

### 5.2.3　Prevention of high-risk factors

In patients with high-risk factors, additional measures are needed to minimize the risk of anastomotic complications. For example, in cases of incomplete anastomosis or risk of leakage, the anastomosis can be reinforced laparoscopically, often with continuous barbed sutures or interrupted reinforcement using absorbable sutures. The anastomosis can also be reinforced transanally during anus-preserving surgery. For the area known as the "danger triangle", a figure-of-eight reinforcement suture is often used to further improve the stability of the anastomosis. After completion of the digestive tract reconstruction, a drain should be placed adjacent to the anastomosis to maintain drainage and reduce the incidence of anastomotic complications.

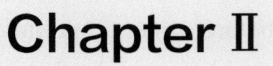
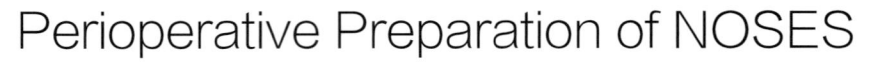

# Chapter II

## Perioperative Preparation of NOSES

Perioperative preparation is a routine procedure before gastrointestinal surgery. With the widespread adoption of enhanced recovery after surgery (ERAS), the content of perioperative preparation is continuously adjusted and improved. Due to the specific nature of NOSES operations,good perioperative preparation is particularly important and involves many aspects such as bowel preparation, vaginal preparation , and **surgical team and instrument preparation**. Only by adequately preparing in all these aspects can the most satisfactory surgical outcomes be achieved.

## 1　Bowel Preparation

There are significant differences between NOSES and conventional laparoscopic surgery in terms of the specimen extraction and the digestive tract reconstruction. Asepsis is involved in many operations of NOSES, so the bowel preparation is strictly required. If preoperative preparation is insufficient and there is a large amount of intestinal content, it can easily lead to spillage of the contents into the abdominal cavity during surgery, resulting in contamination, postoperative infection, and even serious complications such as anastomotic leakage.

Bowel preparation refers to diet control, catharsis, and enema combined with oral antibiotics. The concept of bowel preparation was initially proposed in the 1950s. It is believed that the bowel preparation can decrease or eliminate stool mass and decrease the rate of infection and anastomotic complications. In the traditional concept, the ideal bowel preparation shares the following common features: ①Complete evacuation of colon; ②Safe, convenient, and quick operation; ③ Effective reduction of bacteria in the bowel; ④Reduction of antibiotic usage; ⑤Maintenance of water and electrolyte balance; ⑥Low irritation to patients and well tolerated by patients; ⑦Cost-effective and encouragement of patient compliance; ⑧Minor effect on bowel function and quick bowel function recovery.

Among bowel preparation drugs, electrolyte solution, mannitol, compound polyethylene glycol, magnesium sulfate, sodium phosphates oral solution, and phenolphthalein tablets belong to the drugs with relatively intense effects. The surgeons should be mindful of water and electrolyte disturbances and supplement as needed. However , castor oil, liquid paraffin, and a small dose of senna leaf granules have the characteristics of slow onset and mild action, and can be used in combination with a liquid diet for patients with incomplete intestinal obstruction.

For NOSES, the bowel preparation is indispensable as it serves as a strong safeguard for asepsis during the operation. According to the guidelines on bowel preparation in elective colon and rectal surgery released in 2019 by the American Society of Colon and Rectal Surgeons (ASCRS), for elective colorectal resections, mechanical bowel preparation combined with preoperative oral antibiotics is typically recommended which reduces the rates of surgical site infection, anastomotic leakage, and readmission.

For patients scheduled to undergo NOSES,the following preoperative bowel preparation plan can be referred to: ①Dietary adjustments. Commence a semi-liquid diet three days before the surgery, followed by a

liquid-only diet two days before the surgery. The day before the surgery should involve fasting. Depending on the patient's nutritional status, consider providing at least one day of intravenous nutritional support. ②Mechanical bowel preparation and preoperative oral antibiotics. The current common method for patients without obstructive symptoms is to administer oral compound polyethylene glycol the day before surgery. Additionally, they are prescribed non-absorbable or poorly absorbable antibiotics that cover both Gram negative bacterium and anaerobe, such as neomycin, erythromycin, metronidazole, etc.

## 2    Vaginal Preparation

In transvaginal NOSES, as the vagina serves as the primary route for specimen extraction, strict sterilization and preparation are crucial.

We recommend the following vaginal preparation and related procedures for patients undergoing the transvaginal specimen extraction: ①Rinse the vagina with 3‰ iodophor or 1‰ benzalkonium bromide once a day 3 days before operation; ②Rinse the vagina, disinfect the cervix with 3‰ iodophor, dry the vagina mucosa and cervix with gauze ball, and indwell urinary catheter on the day of operation; ③D uring surgical site disinfection, areas such as the vulva, vagina, and perianal region need to be disinfected two additional times on top of the standard procedure ; ④Strict aseptic and tumor-free principles should be followed during operation; ⑤An iodophor gauze can be indwelled in the vagina after operation, and the gauze should be extracted 48 hours postoperative.

## 3    Surgical Team and Instrument Preparation

The core of establishing your own team is that the team members must cooperate and perform their own duties during the surgical operation. In the early stages of team formation, there may be issues with coordination. In particular, the lead surgeon may unintentionally overstep boundaries and frequently take on the assistant's tasks. This should be avoided. Give the assistant the opportunity to practice as growth takes time.

As is well known, open surgery can often be performed solo, with the lead surgeon assisted by a visiting doctor or intern. However, the laparoscopic surgery is quite different from open surgery, especially for NOSES, which requires a lot of skills in the operation. NOSES requires a high degree of tacit cooperation between the surgeon and the assistant, especially in terms of aseptic operation and tumor-free operation. In this case, the establishment of a fixed surgical team is required, and the goal of tactic understanding and integration of surgeons with laparoscopic tools can only be achieved through long-term run-in and practice.

"One can't make bricks without straw". To complete NOSES with high quality, in addition to close team cooperation, adequate preparation of surgical instruments is also required. The main differences between NOSES and conventional laparoscopic surgery are the digestive tract reconstruction and the method of specimen extraction. To complete these two surgical procedures, we must first understand which surgical instruments need to be prepared.

Different gastrointestinal NOSES procedures require different surgical instruments for digestive tract reconstruction. In right hemicolectomy NOSES, digestive tract reconstruction is most often completed using a laparoscopic linear cutting stapler (e.g., Endo-GIA). In transverse colon NOSES, a "V-shaped **triangular** anastomosis" is often adopted, which is essentially a variant of side-to-side

anastomosis and also requires the use of a laparoscopic linear cutting stapler for the procedure. In NOSES for the left-sided colon, sigmoid colon, and rectum, the methods of digestive tract reconstruction vary according to different tumor locations and different operating habits of doctors. The methods mainly include end-to-end anastomosis and side-to-end anastomosis, both of which must use a tubular anastomosis. The model of the stapler should be selected according to the bowel caliber, e.g., a 3D electric tubular anastomosis will ensure the quality of the anastomosis and thus reduce the risk of anastomotic leakage. The author emphasizes that "end-to-end anastomosis" should be used if the length of the bowel permits. This can avoid the stump on one side of the bowel in "side-to-end anastomosis" and reduce the risk of anastomotic leakage. In addition, based on the design of the stapler, the method of removing the anvil from the bowel also varies. If the anvil shaft is hollow, the "fixed extrusion method" can be used to remove the anvil. If the anvil shaft has a counter-puncture needle, the "stringing method" is recommended for removing the anvil.

In the specimen extracting procedures, as in the transabdominal operation, NOSES also requires an auxiliary device for the specimen extraction to ensure the implementation of aseptic operation and tumor-free operation to the greatest extent. According to the retrieved literature and clinical practice, the instruments used for assisting in specimen extraction include incision protector, protective sleeve for ultrasonic scalpel, sterile specimen bag, self-made plastic cannula, transanal minimally invasive surgery cannula, and transanal endoscope, etc. (Figure 2-3-1). Although there are many types of specimen extraction devices, they can be mainly classified into two types: hard and soft. Both types of devices have their own advantages. Soft devices have good plasticity and elasticity. Not limited by the size of the specimen, they can be removed as long as the condition of the natural orifice permits. Hard devices have strong tenacity and they can play a strong supporting role. If the circumferential diameter of the specimen is smaller than the caliber of the device, the specimen can be easily removed. However, if the circumferential diameter of the specimen is larger than the caliber of the device, it will be difficult for the specimen to be removed. Therefore, when selecting a specimen extraction device, we must understand the features of various devices and make a comprehensive judgment according to the size of the specimen and the specific conditions of the natural orifice. Only in this way, we can perform the specimen extraction correctly and properly.

"If a craftsman wants to do his work well, he must first sharpen his tools." The research and development of NOSES-related instruments must be an important direction for the future development. It is also an important condition for the standardization of NOSES.

# Chapter III

## Standardized Procedures of Laparoscopic Colorectal NOSES

**1** Laparoscopic Radical Surgery for Low Rectal Cancer with Transanal Specimen Extraction by Eversion-Resection and Auxiliary Incision-Free Abdomen

(CRC-NOSES IA, IB, Eversion Method)

### [Introduction]

CRC-NOSES I is predominantly suited for patients with small tumors located at the lower rectum. Compared to conventional laparoscopic radical surgery for rectal cancer, CRC-NOSES I exhibits no differences in terms of the extent of resection and lymph node dissection. The primary distinctions between the conventional laparoscopic surgery and CRC-NOSES I lie in the methods of the digestive tract reconstruction and the specimen extraction. The key operative steps of CRC-NOSES I are to evert the rectum to the outside of the body through the anus, resect the rectal tumor under direct vision outside the body, and then perform end-to-end anastomosis between the sigmoid colon and the rectum under total laparoscopic conditions. Notably, this technique enables direct visual determination of the distance from the tumor's distal edge to the dentate line, potentially avoiding positive distal resection margins and significantly enhancing the feasibility of anus-preserving surgery for ultra-low rectal cancer. Currently, CRC-NOSES I encompasses two main approaches for the digestive tract reconstruction: CRC-NOSES IA (Figure 3-1-1) and CRC-NOSES IB (Figure 3-1-2). While there are minor differences between these two methods, CRC-NOSES IA incorporates a tumor-free operation, which CRC-NOSES IB does not. Consequently, CRC-NOSES IB has a broader range of

indications than CRC-NOSES IA, yet both approaches yield equivalent surgical outcomes. By ensuring radical resection, CRC-NOSES I offers distinct benefits such as reduced trauma, accelerated recovery, and improved cosmetic results. It is indeed a valuable technique that merits mastery and widespread adoption by surgeons.

### 1.1 Indications and contraindications

#### [Indications]

1. Lower rectal tumor or benign tumor.

2. Infiltrative and ulcerated tumor, involving less than 1/2 of the rectal circumference.

3. Protuberant-type tumors with a circumferential diameter less than 3cm.

4. The distance from the distal edge of the tumor to the dentate line should be 2-5cm.

#### [Contraindications]

1. Tumors with an extent of invasion exceeding 1/2 of the rectal circumference.

2. Tumors with a circumferential diameter greater than 3cm.

3. Mucinous adenocarcinoma or signet ring cell carcinoma, where the status of the distal resection margin is uncertain.

4. Severely obese patients (BMI>35kg/m$^2$).

## 1.2 Surgical procedures, techniques, and key points

### [Trocar placement]

1. The camera trocar (10mm trocar) is positioned 1-2cm above the umbilicus.

2. The surgeon's main trocar (12mm trocar) is placed below the McBurney's point.

3. The surgeon's auxiliary trocar (5mm trocar) is located approximately 10cm to the right of the umbilicus.

4. The assistant's auxiliary trocar (5mm trocar) is placed opposite to the McBurney's point.

5. The assistant's main trocar (5mm trocar) is situated on the left at the upper umbilical level, near the lateral edge of the rectus abdominis (Figure 3-1-3).

### [Exploration]

1. General exploration

Explore the liver, gallbladder, stomach, spleen, greater omentum, colon, small intestine, rectum, and pelvic cavity.

2. Tumor exploration

Low rectal tumors are often undetectable under laparoscopy. The surgeon can perform a digital rectal examination with the right hand and coordinate with the forceps operated by the left hand to determine the location and size of the tumor and assess whether the patient is suitable for this procedure.

3. Evaluation of anatomical structures

This includes evaluating the thickness of the sigmoid colon and rectal mesentery, the length of the vascular arch, and determining the range for the proposed resection.

### [Dissection and separation]

1. First incision point

The incision starts 3-5cm below the sacral promontory, often at a thin spot, using an ultrasonic scalpel to open the mesentery and enter the Toldt's space.

2. Mobilization and division of inferior mesenteric vessels

Expanding the Toldt's space, dissection continues headward to the root of the inferior mesenteric artery and laterally to the left gonadal vessels. Lymph nodes around the root of the inferior mesenteric artery are dissected, and the inferior mesenteric vessels are ligated and transected.

3. Mobilization of the posterior rectum

Proceeding dissection distally along the Toldt's space into the presacral space, the rectosacral fascia is incised, entering the superior musculus levator ani. The dissection continues distally to the hiatus of musculus levator ani.

4. Mobilization of the right side of the rectum

Dissection is carried out along the boundary between the mesorectum and the right pelvic wall to the peritoneal reflection, which is then transversely incised on the right side.

5. Mobilization of the sigmoid colon and the left side of the rectum

Open the adhesions between the sigmoid colon and the left abdominal wall, connect with the medial Toldt's space, and proceed cephalad in dissection. If necessary, mobilize the splenic flexure of colon. Continue the dissection caudally along the boundary to the peritoneal reflection, where it meets with the right side.

6. Mobilization of the anterior rectal wall

Incise the peritoneal reflection and proceed dissection distally to the anterior rectal space, ensuring to preserve the integrity of Denonvillier's fascia. Continue to dissect distally to the level of the musculus levator ani. Dissection to this level marks the endpoint of TME, where the rectum typically has no mesentery and does not require isolation of the rectum.

7. Trimming the sigmoid mesocolon

Divide the mesocolon reversely, starting at the horizontal pre-cut line and dissecting the sigmoid mesocolon retrograde from distal to proximal.

### [Specimen resection and digestive tract reconstruction]

CRC-NOSES I, Method A (Video 3-1)

1. Specimen resection

Adhering strictly to aseptic and tumor-free principles, a protective sleeve is inserted through the anus, extending 5cm above the tumor. Using oval forceps to grip the anvil, it is slid through the protective sleeve at the opposite side of the tumor, reaching just above the pre-cut line (Figure 3-1-4, Figure 3-1-5). A linear cutting stapler is used to resect and close the sigmoid colon at

the pre-cut line on the isolated bowel (Figure 3-1-6), leaving the anvil inside the lumen of the sigmoid colon. The stump is disinfected with the iodoform gauze. The oval forceps, inserted through the anus, reach the rectal stump, gripping both the mesentery and the bowel wall to evert the rectum and pull it out of the anus (Figure 3-1-7, Figure 3-1-8). Once the specimen is everted outside the body, the tumor location becomes clearly visible. After irrigation with iodine solution and verification, the rectum is transected 1-2cm below the tumor margin using the stapler (Figure 3-1-9). The specimen is removed, and the rectal stump can return to the abdominal cavity on its own.

2. Digestive tract reconstruction

Fully dilate the anus and instill iodine solution through the anus. Under laparoscopic observation, check for any leakage at the rectal stump; remove the anvil shaft from the sigmoid colon stump (Figure 3-1-10). Insert a circular stapler through the anus and complete the end-to-end anastomosis of the sigmoid colon and rectum (Figure 3-1-11, Figure 3-1-12).

CRC-NOSES I, Method B (Video 3-2)

1. Specimen extraction

Use a linear cutting stapler to resect and close the sigmoid colon at the pre-cut line (Figure 3-1-13). Disinfect the stump with the iodoform gauze. The assistant inserts the oval forceps through the anus to the rectal stump, grasping the mesenteric remnant and bowel wall. Gently evert the rectum and pull it outside the anus at an even pace (Figure 3-1-14). After eversion, make an incision on the rectal wall (Figure 3-1-15), and introduce the anvil through the everted rectal wall into the pelvic cavity (Figure 3-1-16). Flush the specimen with iodine solution. Transect the rectum 1-2cm below the lower tumor margin (Figure 3-1-17, Figure 3-1-18). Remove the specimen.

2. Digestive tract reconstruction

A small incision is made on the wall of the sigmoid colon, and it is disinfected with the iodoform gauze (Figure 3-1-19). The anvil is then placed into the lumen of the sigmoid colon (Figure 3-1-20), and the incision of the sigmoid colon is closed using a linear cutting stapler (Figure 3-1-21). The anvil shaft is removed from the sigmoid colon stump (Figure 3-1-22). A circular stapler is introduced transanally, the puncture needle is rotated out, and an end-to-end anastomosis between the sigmoid colon and rectum is performed (Figure 3-1-23). The anastomosis is then tested for patency without leakage through air and water injection test. The surgical area is irrigated with saline, and hemostasis is confirmed. Drainage tubes are placed through the left and right lower abdominal trocar sites (Figure 3-1-24, Figure 3-1-25). For patients undergoing ultralow sphincter-preserving procedures, the anastomosis can also be reinforced and sutured through the anus (Figure 3-1-26).

# 2 Laparoscopic Radical Surgery for Lower Rectal Cancer with Transanal Specimen Extraction and Auxiliary Incision-Free Abdomen (CRC-NOSES IC, Parks Method)

## [Introduction]

The special anatomical location of lower rectal cancer makes anus-preserving surgery more challenging. Although the double stapling technique increases the chance of anus preservation, it is still difficult to transect and close the rectum at the level of the pelvic floor muscle surface for obese patients or patients with a narrow pelvis. Parks proposed transabdominal resection for rectal cancer with transanal coloanal anastomosis in 1982. This approach provides anus preserving opportunity for more rectal cancer patients without affecting the long-term efficacy. It also makes up for the deficiency of double stapling technique in anus-preserving surgery for lower rectal cancer. CRC-NOSES IC, i.e., laparoscopic lower rectal cancer resection with transanal specimen extraction and single-layer coloanal anastomosis (Figure 3-2-1, Video 3-3), is not only a

sublimation of the traditional Parks method but also an improvement of the theoretical system of NOSES for the lower rectum. The characteristics of this procedure are distinct: ①While ensuring the radical resection of rectal cancer, the advantages of NOSES are fully utilized, resulting in minimal postoperative trauma, reduced pain, and rapid recovery. ②In the transanal specimen extraction and manual single-layer coloanal anastomosis, both ends are sutured with absorbable sutures. The use of absorbable sutures is preferred due to their excellent tissue compatibility, which reduces the disadvantages associated with stapler-tissue incompatibility, thereby decreasing the risk of anastomotic inflammation and potential stenosis. ③This procedure can protect the internal and external anal sphincter to the greatest extent to preserve the anal function and ensure the postoperative bowel control function.

## 2.1    Indications and contraindications

### [Indications]

1. Lower rectal tumor or benign tumor.
2. The extent of invasion is more than 1/2 of the rectal circumference, which makes it hard for the specimen to be everted out of the anus.
3. Protuberant-type tumors with a circumferential diameter less than 3cm.
4. The distance from the distal edge of the tumor to the dentate line should be 2-3cm.

### [Contraindications]

1. Patients with severe local tumor infiltration.
2. Tumors with a circumferential diameter greater than 3cm.
3. Mucinous adenocarcinoma or signet ring cell carcinoma, where the status of the distal resection margin is uncertain.
4. Severely obese patients (BMI>35kg/m²).

## 2.2    Surgical procedures, techniques, and key points

### [Trocar Placement]

1. The camera trocar (10mm trocar) is positioned 1-2cm above the umbilicus.

2. The surgeon's main trocar (12mm trocar) is placed below the McBurney's point.
3. The surgeon's auxiliary trocar (5mm trocar) is located approximately 10cm to the right of the umbilicus.
4. The assistant's auxiliary trocar (5mm trocar) is placed opposite to the McBurney's point.
5. The assistant's main trocar (5mm trocar) is situated on the left at the upper umbilical level, near the lateral edge of the rectus abdominis (Figure 3-2-2).

### [Exploration]

1. General exploration

Explore the liver, gallbladder, stomach, spleen, greater omentum, colon, small intestine, rectum, and pelvic cavity.

2. Tumor exploration

The surgeon can determine the location and size of the tumor through digital rectal examination and assess the feasibility of performing this surgery.

3. Evaluation of anatomical structures

This includes evaluating the thickness of the sigmoid colon and rectal mesentery, the length of the vascular arch, and determining the range for the proposed resection.

### [Dissection and separation]

1. First incision point

The incision starts 3-5cm below the sacral promontory, often at a thin spot, using an ultrasonic scalpel to open the mesentery and enter the Toldt's space.

2. Mobilization and division of inferior mesenteric vessels

Expanding the Toldt's space, dissection continues headward to the root of the inferior mesenteric artery and laterally to the left gonadal vessels. Lymph nodes around the root of the inferior mesenteric artery are dissected, and the inferior mesenteric vessels are ligated and transected.

3. Mobilization of the posterior rectum

Proceeding dissection distally along the Toldt's space into the presacral space, the rectosacral fascia is incised, entering the superior musculus levator ani. The dissection continues distally to the hiatus of musculus levator ani.

4. Mobilization of the right side of the rectum

Dissection is carried out along the boundary between

the mesorectum and the right pelvic wall to the peritoneal reflection, which is then transversely incised on the right side.

5. Mobilization of the sigmoid colon and the left rectal wall

Open the adhesions between the sigmoid colon and the left abdominal wall, connect with the medial Toldt's space, and proceed cephalad in dissection. If necessary, mobilize the splenic flexure of colon. Continue the dissection caudally along the boundary to the peritoneal reflection, where it meets with the right side.

6. Mobilization of the anterior rectal wall

Incise the peritoneal reflection and proceed dissection distally to the anterior rectal space, ensuring to preserve the integrity of Denonvillier's fascia. Continue to dissect distally to the level of the musculus levator ani. Dissection to this level marks the endpoint of TME, where the rectum typically has no mesentery and does not require isolation of the rectum.

7. Trimming the sigmoid mesocolon

Divide the mesocolon reversely, starting at the horizontal pre-cut line and dissect the sigmoid mesocolon retrograde from distal to proximal.

## [Specimen resection and digestive tract reconstruction]

1. Specimen resection

After the rectum is fully mobilized laparoscopically, the sigmoid colon is transected at the pre-cut line above the tumor using a linear cutting stapler (Figure 3-2-3). The abdominal operation is then followed by the perineal procedure. An anal retractor or bladder retractor is used to fully expose the rectum through the anus, and the rectal lumen is thoroughly disinfected with the iodoform gauze (Figure 3-2-4). The rectum is incised 0.5cm above the dentate line, and the rectum is completely transected using an electrocautery (taking care to avoid damaging the internal anal sphincter) (Figure 3-2-5). During the transection of the rectal wall, the location of the lower resection margin can be directly visualized to ensure its safety (Figure 3-2-6). The proximal bowel and mesentery are pulled out through the anus (Figure 3-2-7), and the specimen is removed for postoperative pathological examination.

2. Digestive tract reconstruction

After irrigating the pelvic cavity with iodine solution and ensuring no bleeding, digestive tract reconstruction begins with a manual single-layer anastomosis between the sigmoid colon and the anal canal. The reserved sutures (Figure 3-2-8) are respectively sutured at the 3, 6, 9, and 12 o'clock positions on the anal canal, and the reserved sutures are expanded in four directions (Figure 3-2-9). The sigmoid colon is pulled out through the anus with oval forceps under laparoscopic guidance. After checking that the mesentery is not twisted, the sigmoid colon stump is opened outside the anus and prepared for anastomosis. Using the four reserved sutures, full-thickness sutures are applied to attach the sigmoid colon to the anus. After gently retracting the sigmoid colon back into the anal canal, the reserved sutures are tied to secure the anastomosis. Additional full-thickness sutures (2-3 stitches) are placed between each adjacent pair of reserved sutures for reinforcement (Figure 3-2-10). Once all four quadrants are sutured, check the density of the anastomotic sutures, whether the anastomotic stoma is unobstructed, and whether there is any bleeding. The end-to-end anastomosis of the sigmoid colon and the anal canal is completed (Figure 3-2-11).

# 3　Laparoscopic Ultralow Anterior Resection with Intersphincteric Dissection and Transanal Specimen Extraction without Auxiliary Abdominal Incision Method (CRC-NOSES ID)

## [Introduction]

CRC-NOSES ID is mainly applicable to patients with small tumors located at the lower and ultralow rectum. As with conventional laparoscopic radical resection of rectal cancer, the laparoscopic operation should strictly follow the TME principle. Anatomy and dissection should be performed in the correct plane, and the dissection of the pelvic floor should be more adequate to facilitate transperineal operation in the intersphincteric space, which is the key to the accurate completion of the procedure. The operating characteristics of CRC-NOSES ID are intersphincteric transection of bowel in the anal canal after adequate laparoscopic dissection, extraction of the specimen through a natural orifice, and anastomosis of the proximal sigmoid colon to the anal canal. CRC-NOSES ID can not only ensure the radical resection of small tumors located at the lower and ultralow rectum, but also preserve the anal function to the maximum extent, and avoid the auxiliary incision in the abdominal wall. Therefore, this procedure fully satisfies the requirements of functional surgery and minimally invasive surgery (Figure 3-3-1, Video 3-4).

## 3.1　Indications and contraindications

### [Indications] (Figure 3-3-2-Figure 3-3-4)

1. Ultralow rectal cancer.
2. Infiltrative or ulcerated tumor with good mobility.
3. The protuberant-type tumor and the thickness of tumor should be less than 2cm.
4. The depth of local invasion should be $T_1$ or $T_2$.
5. The pathological type should be moderately-well differentiated adenocarcinoma.

## [Contraindications]

1. The inferior margin of tumor is within 3cm above the dentate line.
2. The thickness of tumor is more than 3cm.
3. The depth of the rectal cancer invasion reaches $T_3$.
4. Poorly differentiated or mucinous adenocarcinoma, with distal resection edge status which cannot be determined by intraoperative frozen section examination.
5. Severely obese patients.

## 3.2　Surgical procedures, techniques, and key points

### [Trocar placement]

1. The camera trocar (10mm trocar) is located just above the umbilicus.
2. The surgeon's main trocar (12mm trocar) is located below the McBurney's point, which will make the ultralow rectal operation easier, especially when the lower rectal wall being isolated, and will form a vertical angle to transect the mesentery.
3. The surgeon's auxiliary trocar (5mm trocar) is located at about 10cm from the right side of the umbilicus, so as to reduce the interference of laparoscopy when operating in the lower rectum.
4. The assistant's auxiliary trocar (5mm trocar) is located opposite the McBurney's point, which is mainly used for lifting and retracting, in the meantime, facilitate placing the drainage tube.
5. The assistant's main trocar (5mm trocar) is located at the left side of upper umbilical level adjacent to the lateral edge of the rectus abdominis (Figure 3-3-5).

## [Surgical team position]

Abdominal operation: The surgeon stands on the right side of the patient, the assistant stands on the left side of the patient, and the camera holder stands on the same side of the surgeon. Perineal operation: The surgeon stands between the patient's legs, and the assistants separately stand on the left and right side of the patient (Figure 3-3-6).

## [Special surgical instruments]

Ultrasonic scalpel, electric scalpel with needle electrode, anal retractor.

## [Exploration]

1. General exploration

Observe for any lesions such as metastatic implants on the surfaces of various organs and the peritoneum.

2. Tumor exploration

Determine the feasibility of surgery based on the tumor's location, size, and depth of invasion.

3. Evaluation of anatomical structures

The surgeon needs to evaluate the length of sigmoid colon, the length of mesenteric marginal vessels, and the thickness of mesentery to determine the feasibility of transanal specimen extraction. Tumor location determines whether to preserve inferior mesenteric vessels and superior rectal artery.

## [Dissection and separation]

1. First incision point

The incision starts 3-5cm below the sacral promontory, often at a thin spot, using an ultrasonic scalpel to open the mesentery and enter the Toldt's space.

2. Mobilization and division of inferior mesenteric vessels

Expanding the Toldt's space, dissection continues headward to the root of the inferior mesenteric artery and laterally to the left gonadal vessels. Lymph nodes around the root of the inferior mesenteric artery are dissected, and the inferior mesenteric vessels are ligated and transected.

3. Mobilization of the posterior rectum

Proceeding dissection distally along the Toldt's space into the presacral space, the rectosacral fascia is incised, entering the superior musculus levator ani. The dissection continues distally to the hiatus of musculus levator ani.

4. Mobilization of the right side of the rectum

Dissection is carried out along the boundary between the mesorectum and the right pelvic wall to the peritoneal reflection, which is then transversely incised on the right side.

5. Mobilization of the sigmoid colon and the left rectal wall

Open the adhesions between the sigmoid colon and the left abdominal wall, connect with the medial Toldt's space, and proceed cephalad in dissection. If necessary, mobilize the splenic flexure of colon. Continue the dissection caudally along the boundary to the peritoneal reflection, where it meets with the right side.

6. Mobilization of the anterior rectal wall

Incise the peritoneal reflection and proceed dissection distally to the anterior rectal space, ensuring to preserve the integrity of Denonvillier's fascia. Continue to dissect distally to the level of the musculus levator ani. Dissection to this level marks the endpoint of TME, where the rectum typically has no mesentery and does not require isolation of the rectum.

7. Trimming the sigmoid mesocolon

Divide the mesocolon reversely, starting at the horizontal pre-cut line and dissect the sigmoid mesocolon retrograde from distal to proximal.

## [Specimen resection and digestive tract reconstruction]

1. Specimen resection

After adequate dilation of the anus, the distal resection edge is determined at about 1-2cm distal to the tumor, then the rectal wall is incised circumferentially (Figure 3-3-7). Afterward, dissection is performed upwards to the pelvic cavity within the intersphincteric space from the posterior wall to the lateral wall, eventually to the anterior wall (Figure 3-3-8, Figure 3-3-9). The rectum and mesentery are then transanally extracted to confirm the integrity of the resection margin (Figure 3-3-10). The oval forceps is inserted into the anus to pull the proximal sigmoid colon out of the body, during which attention should be paid to the prevention of mesenteric volvulus. The operation should be gentle to protect the

sphincter from being damaged by excessive retraction tension.

2. Digestive tract reconstruction

The extracted proximal sigmoid colon stump is opened (Figure 3-3-11), and intermittent sutures of the sigmoid colon stump to the anal canal are performed to complete the anastomosis (Figure 3-3-12). Check the anastomosis to confirm that there is no bleeding and perform local disinfection (Figure 3-3-13). Place two drainage tubes in the pelvic cavity and close the trocar incisions.

# 4  Laparoscopic Radical Surgery for Low Rectal Cancer with Transanal Specimen Extraction and Auxiliary Incision-Free Abdomen (CRC-NOSES ⅠE, Bacon Method)

## [Introduction]

CRC-NOSES ⅠE is the combination of laparoscopy surgery and improved Bacon method, mainly applicable to patients with lower rectal cancer who have a large circumference of invasion. The main differences between conventional laparoscopic surgery and CRC-NOSES ⅠE are digestive tract reconstruction and specimen extraction (Figure 3-4-1, Video 3-5). The operation characteristics of CRC-NOSES ⅠE are as follows: ①The rectum is dissected into the internal and external space of the sphincter according to the TME principle; ②The anus is annularly sutured from 1-2cm below the tumor and above the intersphincteric sulcus; ③The rectal wall is circularly incised and then dissected upward into the abdominal plane; ④The rectum is extracted from the anus and the normal rectum is retained at 3-5cm, then cutting off the rectum at 5-7cm above the upper edge of tumor; ⑤The anoplasty is conducted after 2-3 weeks. This technique requires excellent skills and tacit cooperation between the surgeon and assistant. In addition, the aseptic principle and tumor-free principle must be strictly practiced. The CRC-NOSES ⅠE can not only ensure the R0 resection but also achieve anal function preservation in lower rectal cancer, which is an ideal operation in line with the requirements of functional surgery.

## 4.1  Indications and contraindications

### [Indications] (Figure 3-4-2-Figure 3-4-4)

1. Lower rectal cancer or benign tumor that cannot be excised under endoscopy.

2. Tumor involving over 1/2 or all of the rectal circumference is suitable for Bacon method. The flat-type tumor is the best.

3. The tumor should not invade the internal and external anal sphincters.

4. Patients with lower rectal cancer who are in need of additional radical resection after transanal local excision, but anastomosis cannot be performed with conventional laparoscopic instruments.

### [Contraindications]

1. The tumor is too large to be extracted out of the anus.

2. Patients with an insufficient length of the sigmoid colon and its mesentery, rendering transanal specimen extraction unfeasible.

3. The mesorectum is too thick to be extracted out of the anus.

4. Severely obese patients (BMI>30kg/m$^2$).

5. Local inflammation is serious in patients with rectovaginal fistula.

## 4.2  Surgical procedures, techniques, and key points

### [Anesthesia]

General anesthesia with or without epidural anesthesia.

### [Patient position]

The patient is placed in a modified lithotomy

position, with the head lowered and tilted to the right, and the right thigh slightly flattened, which facilitates performing the operation for the surgeon. (Figure 3-4-5).

## [Trocar placement]

1. The camera trocar (10mm trocar) is located within 2cm of the umbilicus or on the umbilicus.

2. The surgeon's main trocar (12mm trocar) is located at the McBurney's point.

3. The surgeon's auxiliary trocar (5mm trocar) is located at 5cm above the right paramedian of the umbilicus.

4 The assistant's auxiliary trocar (5mm trocar) is located opposite the McBurney's point.

5. The assistant's main trocar (5mm trocar) is located at the intersection of the umbilicus level and the outer edge of left rectus abdominis (Figure 3-4-6).

## [Surgical team position]

Abdominal operation: The surgeon stands on the right side of the patient, the assistant stands on the left side of the patient, and the camera holder stands on the same side of the surgeon. Perineal operation: The surgeon stands between the patient's legs, and the assistants separately stand on the left and right side of the patient (Figure 3-4-7).

## [Exploration]

1 General exploration

Observe for any lesions such as metastatic implants on the surfaces of various organs and the peritoneum.

2 Tumor exploration

Determine the feasibility of surgery based on the tumor's location, size, and depth of invasion.

3 Evaluation of anatomical structures

The surgeon needs to evaluate the length of sigmoid colon, the length of mesenteric marginal vessels, and the thickness of mesentery to determine the feasibility of transanal specimen extraction. Tumor location determines whether to preserve inferior mesenteric vessels and superior rectal artery.

## [Dissection and separation]

1 First incision point

The incision starts 3-5cm below the sacral promontory,

ofter at a thin spot, using an ultrasonic scalpel to open the mesentery and enter the Toldt's space.

2. Mobilization and division of inferior mesenteric vessels

Expanding the Toldt's space, dissection continues headward to the root of the inferior mesenteric artery and laterally to the left gonadal vessels. Lymph nodes around the root of the inferior mesenteric artery are dissected, and the inferior mesenteric vessels are ligated and transected.

3. Mobilization of the posterior rectum

Proceeding dissection distally along the Toldt's space into the presacral space, the rectosacral fascia is incised, entering the superior musculus levator ani. The dissection continues distally to the hiatus of musculus levator ani.

4. Mobilization of the right side of the rectum

Dissection is carried out along the boundary between the mesorectum and the right pelvic wall to the peritoneal reflection, which is then transversely incised on the right side.

5. Mobilization of the sigmoid colon and the left rectal wall

Open the adhesions between the sigmoid colon and the left abdominal wall, connect with the medial Toldt's space, and proceed cephalad in dissection. If necessary, mobilize the splenic flexure of colon. Continue the dissection caudally along the boundary to the peritoneal reflection, where it meets with the right side.

6. Mobilization of the anterior rectal wall

Incise the peritoneal reflection and proceed dissection distally to the anterior rectal space, ensuring to preserve the integrity of Denonvillier's fascia. Continue to dissect distally to the level of the musculus levator ani. Dissection to this level marks the endpoint of TME, where the rectum typically has no mesentery and does not require isolation of the rectum.

7. Trimming the sigmoid mesocolon

Divide the mesocolon reversely, starting at the horizontal pre-cut line and dissect the sigmoid mesocolon retrograde from distal to proximal.

## [Specimen resection and digestive tract reconstruction]

1. Perineal operation

The anus should be fully expanded to expose the

dentate line (Figure 3-4-8). Disinfect the anal canal with iodoform cotton ball (Figure 3-4-9) and suture the anus by purse string suture at about 1cm below the tumor (Figure 3-4-10). Purse string suture can not only effectively reduce the risk of tumor planting and intestinal contents contamination, but also ensure the distance of the distal resection margin. The surgeon should open the intestinal wall near the dentate line, preserving the internal anal sphincter, dissect upward in order to meet the mobilized bowel in the peritoneal cavity (Figure 3-4-11). To remove the specimen, the dissected colon is extracted from the anus and then transected at 7-10cm above the tumor (Figure 3-4-12). During this procedure, the surgeon should follow the asepsis and tumor-free principles, and operate gently to avoid any damage to the bowel and the mesentery. About 5-8 stitches are needed to fix the redundant bowel to the anus. In this process, the surgeon should avoid suturing mesenteric vessels so as not to affect the blood supply. Finally, rinse the pelvic cavity and place a drainage tube in the pelvic cavity (Figure 3-4-13, Figure 3-4-14). The specimen is removed and the sigmoid colon is fixed on the anus with sutures (Figure 3-4-15).

2. Secondary anoplasty

The secondary anoplasty can be performed after 2-3 weeks. The perineum is fully exposed (Figure 3-4-16), and the excess bowel is transected at the level of good blood supply at the anal margin, leaving a 0.5cm bowel (Figure 3-4-17). It should be noted that when the bowel mucosa is sutured with the anal skin, the blood vessels on the mesentery side should be fully ligated and embedded. In addition, intestinal mucosa should not be excessive eversion so as to avoid mucosa necrosis or mucosa prolapse (Figure 3-4-18).

# 5　Laparoscopic Radical Surgery for Low Rectal Cancer with Transanal Specimen Extraction and Auxiliary Incision-Free Abdomen (CRC-NOSES I F, Petr Method)

## [Introduction]

In the surgical treatment for low rectal cancer, there are a few options to extract the specimen transanally, which are united into CRC-NOSES I group. In each variation, intra-abdominal proximal colon division is followed by specimen extraction by pulling or everting the rectum through anus. The rectum is divided distally to the tumor; the rectal stump is closed with a linear cutting stapler and prepared for the anastomosis (Figure 3-5-1, Video 3-6). CRC-NOSES I F differs from the above mentioned techniques in totally extra-abdominal bowel division proximally and distally to the tumor. The main advantage of this method is the possibility of direct visual control of the distal resection margin. With no intra-abdominal bowel division, the risk of abdominal cavity contamination is minimized. The main steps of NOSES I F include lymph node dissection, vessels division, TME, mobilization of the sigmoid colon, and splenic flexure, if necessary. Also, it involves rectum eversion through the anus and colon division distally to the tumor and then proximally, installing the circular stapler anvil in the proximal colon limb, returning it back to the abdomen, closing up the rectal stump and colorectal anastomosis creation. CRC-NOSES I F is suitable for patients with a small tumor located at middle or lower rectum.

## 5.1　Indications and contraindications

### [Indications] (Figure 3-5-2)

1. Tumor is located at the lower rectum.

2. Localized tumor, preferably without serosal invasion.

3. Tumors with a circumferential diameter less than 3cm.

4. The distance from the lower tumor margin to the dentate line should be 3-5cm.

## [Contraindications]

1. Locally advanced tumor.

2. Tumors with a circumferential diameter greater than 3cm.

3. Mucinous adenocarcinoma or signet ring cell carcinoma.

4. Severely obese patients (BMI>35kg/m$^2$).

## 5.2 Anesthesia, patient position, trocar placement, and surgical team position

### [Anesthesia]

General anesthesia with or without epidural component.

### [Patient position]

The patient should assume the functional lithotomy position, with the right thigh slightly abducted (Figure 3-5-3).

### [Trocar placement] (Figure 3-5-4)

1. The camera trocar (10mm trocar) is located at the umbilicus.

2. The surgeon's main trocar (12mm trocar) is located at the external 1/3 between the right anterior superior iliac spine and the umbilicus, which facilitates deep operation in pelvic cavity and is easier to place the linear cutting stapler.

3. The surgeon's auxiliary trocar (5mm trocar) is located at the right side about 2cm lower and 10cm laterally to the umbilicus. The position of the trocar can be changed based on the patient's constitution; however, it should be at a sufficient distance from two neighboring trocars.

4. The assistant's main trocar (5mm trocar) is located at the left lateral margin of rectus abdominis at umbilical level.

5. The assistant's auxiliary trocar (5mm trocar) is located at the external 1/3 between the umbilicus and the left anterior superior iliac spine.

### [Surgical team position]

The surgeon stands on the right side of the patient, the assistant stands on the left side of the patient, and the camera holder stands on the same side of surgeon (Figure 3-5-5).

## [Special surgical instruments]

Ultrasonic scalpel, instrument for everting, circular stapler (29mm trocar), linear cutting stapler (optional), laparoscopic graspers.

## 5.3 Surgical procedure, techniques, and key points

### [Exploration]

1. General exploration

Observe for any lesions such as metastatic implants on the surfaces of various organs and the peritoneum.

2. Tumor exploration

Determine the feasibility of surgery based on the tumor's location, size, and depth of invasion.

3. Evaluation of anatomical structures

The surgeon needs to evaluate the length of sigmoid colon, the length of mesenteric marginal vessels, and the thickness of mesentery to determine the feasibility of transanal specimen extraction.

### [Dissection and separation]

1. First incision point

The incision starts 3-5cm below the sacral promontory, often at a thin spot, using an ultrasonic scalpel to open the mesentery and enter the Toldt's space.

2. Mobilization and division of inferior mesenteric vessels

Expanding the Toldt's space, dissection continues headward to the root of the inferior mesenteric artery and laterally to the left gonadal vessels. Lymph nodes around the root of the inferior mesenteric artery are dissected, and the inferior mesenteric vessels are ligated and transected.

3. Mobilization of the posterior rectum

Proceeding dissection distally along the Toldt's space into the presacral space, the rectosacral fascia is incised, entering the superior musculus levator ani. The dissection continues distally to the hiatus of musculus levator ani.

4. Mobilization of the right side of the rectum

Dissection is carried out along the boundary between

the mesorectum and the right pelvic wall to the peritoneal reflection, which is then transversely incised on the right side.

5. Mobilization of the sigmoid colon and the left rectal wall

Open the adhesions between the sigmoid colon and the left abdominal wall, connect with the medial Toldt's space, and proceed cephalad in dissection. If necessary, mobilize the splenic flexure of colon. Continue the dissection caudally along the boundary to the peritoneal reflection, where it meets with the right side.

6. Mobilization of the anterior rectal wall

Incise the peritoneal reflection and proceed dissection distally to the anterior rectal space, ensuring to preserve the integrity of Denonvillier's fascia. Continue to dissect distally to the level of the musculus levator ani. Dissection to this level marks the endpoint of TME, where the rectum typically has no mesentery and does not require isolation of the rectum.

7. Trimming the sigmoid mesocolon

Divide the mesocolon reversely, starting at the horizontal pre-cut line and dissect the sigmoid mesocolon retrograde from distal to proximal.

## [Rectal resection and digestive tract reconstruction]

1. Rectal eversion through the anus

For extra-abdominal resection of the specimen, it is important to make sure that the length of the colon is enough for transanal extraction. A rectal exteriorizer is inserted through the anus until its head is located above the tumor. A wire is used to secure the rectum around the rod below its head (Figure 3-5-6).

The rod is carefully pilled out, dragging the everted rectum outside the anus resulting in a double cylindric structure, with the rectum being as the outer cylinder and the sigmoid colon being the inner cylinder. During this eversion, it is important to laparoscopically evaluate the length of the intra-abdominal part of the colon to prevent its overtension. The rectum is everted until the tumor comes out and is under direct vision (Figure 3-5-7).

2. Specimen resection

The rectal wall is treated with an antiseptic solution. It is important to measure the distal pre-cut line, which should be located at least 2cm above the everted tumor

toward the anus. Under direct vision, the circular pre-cut line is marked by an electrosurgery instrument (Figure 3-5-8). The rectal wall is carefully divided at the marked line (Figure 3-5-9). It is important not to damage the wall of sigmoid colon located below.

Following the resection of the outer cylinder under direct vision, the distal edge of the rectal stump is grasped with Alice forceps. Importantly, if TME is performed, the pre-cut line should be as close to the bowel edge as possible, so as not to leave the fragments of mesorectal cellular tissue on the rectal stump. Then the proximal pre-cut line should be planned. The rectum is then unrolled, and the specimen acquires its usual look. The colon is divided with a linear cutting stapler. End-to-end or side-to-end anastomosis can be done (Figure 3-5-10).

For the end-to-end anastomosis, the colon is transected between a purse-string and a straight clamp, the anvil is inserted, and the lumen is closed with a purse-string suture around the anvil shaft. When forming a side-to-end anastomosis, the anvil is inserted into the lumen through the small distal incision, and the anvil shaft is pulled from the side.

The lumen is closed with a linear cutting stapler or uninterrupted suture proximally to previously made incision (Figure 3-5-11). The colonic stump with the anvil is disinfected and returned into the abdomen. The purse-string suture is performed at the rectal stump to enable the fixation of the circular stapler. A thin polymer tube is inserted transanally to the rectum, with one end being outside the anus and the other end protruding outside the purse-string to the abdominal cavity. The purse-string suture is closed around it.

3. Digestive tract reconstruction

The anastomosis is performed using a circular stapler. To ensure that the trocar of the circular stapler correctly passes through the rectal stump, it is first fixed to the polymer tube inserted previously. The tube is used as a guide to position the trocar of the circular stapler right to the center of the purse-string suture. The tube is pulled and then extracted through one of the trocar of the circular stapler (Figure 3-5-12, Figure 3-5-13).

To perform laparoscopic colorectal anastomosis (Figure 3-5-14). It is important to prevent fatty tissues or other structures from getting caught in the anastomotic site.

After the extraction of the circular stapler, the integrity of the proximal and the distal edge is verified. The air and water injection test is performed to ensure the completeness of the anastomosis (Figure 3-5-15). A drainage tube is installed into the pelvic cavity through the right lower trocar.

# 6 Laparoscopic Conformal Radical Surgery for Low Rectal Cancer with Transanal Specimen Extraction and Auxiliary Incision-Free Abdomen (CRC-NOSES ⅠG)

## [Introduction]

Laparoscopic conformal anus-preserving surgery for low rectal cancer with transanal specimen extraction could solve the problem of performing intracorporeal rectal transection in narrow surgical field, and reduce rates of local recurrence and complications, as well as significantly improve anal function. Dissection of the rectum is continued to the levator ani and stopped at the levator hiatus without entering the intersphincteric space, which is filled with nerve fibers, elastic fibers and Pacinian corpuscles. So, excessive dissection in the intersphincteric space coludinjure these fine strcutures which may damage the postoperative anal function. An analysis of 102 patients who underwent the conformal anus-preserving surgery showed that the median value of the distance between the tumor and the anal margin was 3cm (3-4cm), and the median value of the distance between the tumor and the distal resection margin was 0.5cm (0.3-0.8cm). The local recurrence and distant metastasis rates were 2% and 10.8%, respectively. The 3-year survival rate was 100%, and disease-free survival rate was 83.9%. The Wexner score and low anterior resection syndrome score at 12 months after ileostomy closure were 5.9±4.3 and 29.2±6.9, respectively. As an anus-preserving surgery, the advantage of this technique is that it can obtain a good balance between oncological safety and organ function preservation (Figure 3-6-1, Video 3-7).

## 6.1 Indications and contraindications

### [Indications] (Figure 3-6-2, Figure 3-6-3)

1. Patients with a preoperative pathological report of electronic colonoscopic biopsy indicating a highly or moderately differentiated adenocarcinoma or stromal tumor.

2. Patients with MRI or B-mode ultrasound images revealing no infiltration of the external anal sphincter or puborectalis muscle and levator ani muscle or whose examination after preoperative neoadjuvant radiochemotherapy meets these requirements.

3. The mass can be pushed during digital rectal examination, and the diameter of the tumor is less than 3cm.

4. The distance from the lower edge of the tumor to the dentate line is less than or equal to 2cm.

### [Contraindications]

1. Preoperative anal incontinence or a significantly diminished anal continence function.

2. Presence of severe abdominal adhesions.

3. Patients with poor cardiac, pulmonary, hepatic or renal function who cannot tolerate laparoscopic surgery.

4. Patients whose sigmoid colon and mesentery length precludes transanal specimen extraction.

5. Severely obese patients (BMI>35kg/m$^2$).

## 6.2　Anesthesia, patient position, trocar placement and surgical team position

### [Anesthesia]

General anesthesia with or without epidural anesthesia.

### [Patient position]

The patient is placed in the lithotomy position (Figure 3-6-4).

### [Trocar placement]

1. The camera trocar (12mm trocar) is placed at the umbilicus.

2. The surgeon's main trocar (12mm trocar) is placed at the McBurney's point.

3. The surgeon's auxiliary trocar (5mm trocar) is placed 10cm to the right of the umbilicus and parallel to it.

4. The assistant's main trocar (5mm trocar) is placed at the left lateral margin of rectus abdominis at umbilical level.

5. The assistant's auxiliary trocar (5mm trocar) is placed opposite to the McBurney's point. Forceps introduced via this port have relatively few uses and are mainly used to elevate tissues. The lateral position of the port facilitates drain placement (Figure 3-6-5).

### [Surgical team position]

The surgeon stands to the right of the patient. The assistant stands to the left of the patient. The camera-holder stands on the same side as the surgeon (Figure 3-6-6).

### [Special surgical instruments]

Ultrasonic scalpel, 60mm linear cutting stapler, 25mm circular stapler, rectal stump suture.

## 6.3　Surgical procedure, techniques and key points

### [Exploration]

1. General exploration

Observe for any lesions such as metastatic implants on the surfaces of various organs and the peritoneum.

2. Tumor exploration

Determine the feasibility of surgery based on the tumor's location, size, and depth of invasion.

3. Evaluation of anatomical structures

The surgeon needs to evaluate the length of sigmoid colon, the length of mesenteric marginal vessels, and the thickness of mesentery to determine the feasibility of transanal specimen extraction.

### [Dissection and separation]

1. First incision point

The incision starts 3-5cm below the sacral promontory, often at a thin spot, using an ultrasonic scalpel to open the mesentery and enter the Toldt's space.

2. Mobilization and division of inferior mesenteric vessels

Expanding the Toldt's space, dissection continues headward to the root of the inferior mesenteric artery and laterally to the left gonadal vessels. Lymph nodes around the root of the inferior mesenteric artery are dissected. Usually, after the left colic atery is preserved, the distal artery and the inferior mesenteric vein are ligated and transected.

3. Mobilization of the posterior rectum

Proceeding dissection distally along the Toldt's space into the presacral space, the rectosacral fascia is incised, entering the superior musculus levator ani. The dissection continues distally to the hiatus of musculus levator ani.

4. Mobilization of the right side of the rectum

Dissection is carried out along the boundary between the mesorectum and the right pelvic wall to the peritoneal reflection, which is then transversely incised on the right side.

5. Mobilization of the sigmoid colon and the left rectal wall

Open the adhesions between the sigmoid colon and the left abdominal wall, connect with the medial Toldt's space, and proceed cephalad in dissection. If necessary, mobilize the splenic flexure of the colon. Continue the dissection caudally along the boundary to the peritoneal reflection, where it meets with the right side.

6. Mobilization of the anterior rectal wall

Incise the peritoneal reflection and proceed dissection

distally to the anterior rectal space, ensuring to preserve the integrity of Denonvillier's fascia. Continue to dissect distally to the level of the musculus levator ani. Dissection to this level marks the endpoint of TME, where the rectum typically has no mesentery and does not require isolation of the rectum.

7. Trimming the sigmoid mesocolon

Divide the mesocolon reversely, starting at the pre-cut line and dissect the sigmoid mesocolon retrograde from distal to proximal.

## [Specimen resection and digestive tract reconstruction]

1. Specimen resection

The bowel is transected using a linear cutting stapler at the intended site of anastomosis. Transanal pull-through of the distal rectum is performed as follows: the rectum and anal canal are irrigated with iodoform, and the anus is dilated to accommodate 3-4 fingers to ensure that the anal sphincter is completely relaxed. Oval forceps are used to clamp the top of the rectal stump, and the bowel together with the mesentery are gradually inserted deeper into the rectal cavity and pulled out of the anus. For patients who are obese or who have a thick mesentery, the excess proximal mesorectum can first be divided. The rectum that was previously pushed out through the abdomen is clamped transanally and retracted extracorporeally via the anus in order to fully evert the rectum. The distal rectum is then thoroughly irrigated with warm water. The tumor is prevented from coming into contact with surrounding tissues, and avoid touching the tumor with both hands during the procedure.

Conformal resection and anastomosis of the distal rectum (Figure 3-6-7-Figure 3-6-9): The pre-cut line is designed according to the tumor location after the tumor is visualized. The pre-cut line is designed obliquely from the tumor side to the contralateral side and it should be at least 1cm away from the distal and lateral margins of the tumor. This conformal resection could preserve the opposite rectal wall and dentate line as more as possible. After the pre-cut line is designed, under direct vision, circumferentially incise the rectal or anal canal mucosa along the pre-cut line from the tumor side, and deepen layer by layer until full-thickness incision is achieved and the intestinal tract is transected. If there is suspicion about the safety of the specimen margin or the distal resection margin is less than 1cm due to the low position of the tumor, intraoperative frozen pathological examination should be performed before anastomosis to determine the margin status and decide the subsequent surgical procedure.

2. Digestive tract reconstruction

Once the tumor is extracted, the closed rectal stump is repeatedly irrigated with warm water. The sigmoid colon stump is then pulled out of the anus, and a stapler anvil is introduced into the sigmoid colon stump. After being rinsed and disinfected, the sigmoid colon stump is returned into the abdominal cavity. The rectal stump is closed using interrupted sutures with 3-0 absorbable suture. Much of the rectal stump is preserved on the contralateral side to the tumor (Figure 3-6-10).

Once the pneumoperitoneum is reestablished, and the stapler body is inserted transanally. A 25mm-diameter circular stapler is generally used to perform recto-sigmoid end-to-end anastomosis (Figure 3-6-11). During anastomosis, the skin of the anus is pulled outwards, and the stapler is pushed as far as possible towards the pelvic cavity to avoid excessive resection of the internal anal sphincter, rectum, and anoderm. Once anastomosis is complete, the proximal and distal anastomosiss should be evaluated to ensure that they are intact. The integrity of the anastomosis is also examined transanally. Incomplete parts of the anastomosis can be reinforced using interrupted sutures with 3-0 absorbable suture.

All patients should undergo prophylactic terminal ileal loop ostomy.

# 7 Laparoscopic Radical Surgery for Middle Rectal Cancer with Transrectal Specimen Extraction and Auxiliary Incision-Free Abdomen (CRC-NOSES IIA)

## [Introduction]

CRC-NOSES IIA is mainly applicable to patients with small tumors located at the middle rectum. As with conventional laparoscopic radical resection of rectal cancer, CRC-NOSES IIA should strictly follow the principles of TME. Anatomy and dissection should be performed in the correct plane, which is a prerequisite for the rapid and safe operation. The main operating procedures of CRC-NOSES IIA include transanal rectal extraction, removal of rectal specimen extracorporeally, and total laparoscopic end-to-end anastomosis between the sigmoid colon and rectum (Figure 3-7-1, Video 3-8). This procedure requires closer cooperation between the surgeon and assistant during the operation. In addition, the aseptic and tumor-free operation must be strictly practiced. CRC-NOSES IIA not only ensures the effect of radical cancer resection but also reduces the damage to organs and tissues. Therefore, this is an ideal procedure that is fully satisfying the requirements of functional surgery.

## 7.1 Indications and contraindications

### [Indications]

1. Middle rectal tumor or benign tumor.
2. The circumferential diameter of tumor is better less than 3cm.
3. The tumor should not invade beyond the serosa.

### [Contraindications]

1. Excessively large tumors that preclude transanal extraction.
2. Length of sigmoid colon and mesentery that precludes transanal extraction.
3. Excessively thick mesorectum that precludes transanal extraction.
4. Severe obese patients (BMI>35kg/m$^2$).

## 7.2 Surgical procedure, techniques and key points

### [Trocar placement]

1. The camera port (10mm trocar) is placed at the umbilicus.
2. The surgeon's main trocar (12mm trocar) is placed at the McBurney's point.
3. The surgeon's auxiliary trocar (5mm trocar) is placed at 5cm superior to the intersection between the umbilicus level and the right midline.
4. The assistant's auxiliary trocar (5mm trocar) is placed opposite to the McBurney's point.
5. The assistant's main trocar (5mm trocar) is placed at the umbilicus level on the lateral edge of the left rectus abdominus (Figure 3-7-2).

### [Exploration]

1. General exploration

Observe for any lesions such as metastatic implants on the surfaces of various organs and the peritoneum.

2. Tumor exploration

Determine the feasibility of surgery based on the tumor's location, size, and depth of invasion.

3. Evaluation of anatomical structures

The surgeon needs to evaluate the length of sigmoid colon, the length of mesenteric vessels, as well as the thickness of the middle mesorectum, to determine whether transrectal extraction is feasible.

### [Dissection and division]

1. First incision point

The incision starts 3-5cm below the sacral promontory,

often at a thin spot, using an ultrasonic scalpel to open the mesentery and enter the Toldt's space.

2. Mobilization and division of the roots of the inferior mesenteric vessels

Dissect and skeletonize the inferior mesenteric vessels layer by layer. After sufficient skeletonization, ligate and transect them. The lymph node dissection at the root of the mesentery should be performed by en bloc resection, with attention to protecting the hypogastric plexus.

3. Mobilization of the mesorectum

After the avascular area of the sigmoid mesocolon has been partially opened, mobilization is continued in an inferolateral direction up to the bifurcation of the left common iliac artery. Subsequently, dissection is performed inferiorly along the presacral space up to a point approximately 5cm inferior to the tumor. At this point, the left ureter and left gonadal vessels should be identified and protected.

4. Mobilization of the right side of the rectum

The right peritoneal reflection is mobilized in a horizontal direction, generally until 5cm inferior to the tumor.

5. Mobilization of the sigmoid colon and the left side of the rectum

Divide the lateral adhesions of the sigmoid colon. Mobilization is performed medially along Toldt's fascia to open the mesentery and is continued superiorly. Mobilization of the left side of the rectum is then continued in an inferior direction until the peritoneal reflection, where the left side of the rectum joins the right side.

6. Isolation of the bowel inferior to the tumor

Approximately 3cm of the bowel wall 5cm inferior to the tumor is isolated. The mesorectum should be completely isolated, as the rectal wall should be dissected twice at this point.

7. Trimming the sigmoid mesocolon

The pre-cut line for anastomosis should be determined. The course of the inferior mesenteric vessels can be visualized by elevating the mesentery, and division is performed along this course. Dissection is performed gradually towards the pre-cut line, and 2cm of the bowel wall is isolated. The length of the mobilized sigmoid colon is evaluated to determine if it is sufficient for transanal extraction.

## [Specimen resection and digestive tract reconstruction]

1. Specimen resection

After anal dilation, the iodoform gauze is introduced through the anus below the tumor (Figure 3-7-3). The surgeon applies the ultrasonic scalpel to open the rectal wall transversely 2cm below the tumor under the guidance of the gauze in the lumen (Figure 3-7-4). The assistant holds the suction in the right hand at 2cm below the tumor to avoid the intestinal content entering into the abdominal cavity when the bowel is incised transversely. The assistant inserts the oval forceps through the anus to remove the iodoform gauze. Then, a protective sleeve is placed in the abdominal cavity through the trocar (Figure 3-7-5). The assistant pulls one end of the protective sleeve out through the anus and places the proximal rectal stump into the protective sleeve (Figure 3-7-6). The assistant clamps the proximal rectal stump with the oval forceps and slowly pulls the rectum out of the anus. The purse-string forceps is applied extracorporeally at the pre-cut line above the tumor. Finally, the bowel is transected to remove the specimen (Figure 3-7-7).

2. Digestive tract reconstruction

The anvil is introduced into the sigmoid colon stump and closed with a purse-string suture, and then the sigmoid colon is reintroduced into the abdominal cavity with the oval forceps after being rinsed and disinfected (Figure 3-7-8). Inject 1000ml of iodine solution into the abdominal cavity to irrigate the abdominal cavity and perform anal dilation. The rectal stump is closed by a linear cutting stapler (Figure 3-7-9), whereafter a circular stapler is inserted transanally to complete the end-to-end anastomosis (Figure 3-7-10, Figure 3-7-11). Air and water injection test is performed to confirm the integrity of the anastomosis (Figure 3-7-12). Two drainage tubes are placed in the pelvic cavity (Figure 3-7-13).

# 8　Modified Laparoscopic Radical Surgery for Middle Rectal Cancer with Transrectal Specimen Extraction and Auxiliary Incision-Free Abdomen (CRC-NOSES ⅡB)

## [Introduction]

CRC-NOSES ⅡB is mainly applicable to patients with middle rectal cancer. Compared to CRC-NOSES ⅡA, CRC-NOSES ⅡB requires the complete transection of the rectal specimen, followed by its transanal extraction (Figure 3-8-1). Using this procedure helps to completely avoid the risk of blood-borne metastasis caused by anal compression of the tumor during specimen extraction. Dissection is performed towards the pre-cut line of sigmoid colon, and more bowel wall need to be isolated. The length of the mobilized sigmoid colon is evaluated to determine if it is sufficient for transanal extraction. Thus, this procedure is more aligned with the tumor-free principle than CRC-NOSES ⅡA.

## 8.1　Indications and contraindications

### [Indications]

1. Middle rectal cancer or benign tumors.
2. The circumferential diameter of tumor is better less than 3cm.
3. The tumor should not invade beyond the serosa.

### [Contraindications]

1. Excessively large tumors that preclude transanal extraction.
2. Length of sigmoid colon and mesentery that precludes transanal extraction.
3. Excessively thick mesorectum that precludes transanal extraction.
4. Severe obese patients (BMI>35kg/m$^2$).

## 8.2　Surgical procedure, techniques and key points

### [Trocar placement]

1. The camera port (10mm trocar) is placed at the umbilicus.
2. The surgeon's main trocar (12mm trocar) is placed at the McBurney's point.
3. The surgeon's auxiliary trocar (5mm trocar) is placed at 5cm superior to the intersection between the umbilicus level and the right midline.
4. The assistant's auxiliary trocar (5mm trocar) is placed opposite to the McBurney's point.
5. The assistant's main trocar (5mm trocar) is placed at the umbilicus level on the lateral edge of the left rectus abdominus (Figure 3-8-2).

### [Exploration]

1. General exploration

Observe for any lesions such as metastatic implants on the surfaces of various organs and the peritoneum.

2. Tumor exploration

Determine the feasibility of surgery based on the tumor's location, size, and depth of invasion.

3. Evaluation of anatomical structures

The surgeon needs to evaluate the length of the sigmoid colon, the length of mesenteric vessels, as well as the thickness of the middle mesorectum, to determine whether transrectal extraction is feasible.

### [Dissection and division]

1. First incision point

The incision starts 3-5cm below the sacral promontory, often at a thin spot, using an ultrasonic scalpel to open the mesentery and enter the Toldt's space.

2. Mobilization and division of the roots of the inferior mesenteric vessels

Dissect and skeletonize the inferior mesenteric vessels layer by layer. After sufficient skeletonization, ligate and transect them. The lymph node dissection at the root of the mesentery should be performed by en bloc resection, with attention to protecting the hypogastric plexus.

3. Mobilization of the mesorectum

After the avascular area of the sigmoid mesocolon have been partially opened, Mobilization is continued in an inferolateral direction up to the bifurcation of the left common iliac artery. Subsequently, dissection is performed inferiorly along the presacral space up to a point approximately 5cm inferior to the tumor. At this point, the left ureter and left gonadal vessels should be identified and protected.

4. Mobilization of the right side of the rectum

The right peritoneal reflection is mobilized in a horizontal direction, generally until 5cm inferior to the tumor.

5 Mobilization of the sigmoid colon and the left side of the rectum

The attachments of the sigmoid colon and left abdominal wall are released. Mobilization is performed medially along Toldt's fascia to open the mesentery and is continued superiorly. Mobilization of the left side of the rectum is then continued in an inferior direction until the peritoneal reflection, where the left side of the rectum joins the right side.

6 Isolation of the bowel inferior to the tumor

Approximately 3cm of the bowel wall 5cm inferior to the tumor is isolated. The mesorectum should be completely isolated, as the rectal wall should be dissected twice at this point.

7 Trimming the sigmoid mesocolon

The pre-cut line for anastomosis should be determined. The course of the inferior mesenteric vessels can be visualized by elevating the mesentery, and division is performed along this course. Dissection is performed gradually towards the pre-cut line, and 2cm of the bowel wall is isolated. The length of the mobilized sigmoid colon is evaluated to determine if it is sufficient for transanal extraction.

## [Specimen resection and digestive tract reconstruction]

1. Specimen resection

The distal rectal wall is transected using the linear cutting stapler at a point 2cm inferior to the tumor (Figure 3-8-3), and the iodoform gauze is used to sterilize the rectal stumps on both sides. Subsequently, the distal sigmoid colon is transected using the linear cutting stapler superior to the tumor and at the pre-cut line (Figure 3-8-4), and the iodoform gauze is used to sterilize the stumps (Figure 3-8-5). At this point, the specimen mobilization and resection are complete.

A protective sleeve is inserted into the abdominal cavity via the surgeon's main trocar (Figure 3-8-6), and the distal rectal stump is incised under the extracorporeal guidance of the assistant (Figure 3-8-7). The assistant pulls one end of the protective sleeve out through the anus (Figure 3-8-8) and places the resected rectal specimen into the protective sleeve (Figure 3-8-9). Subsequently, the assistant clamps the proximal rectal stump with oval forceps and slowly pulls the rectum out through the anus (Figure 3-8-10).

2. Digestive tract reconstruction

The protective sleeve is reinserted into the surgeon's main trocar, the sigmoid colon stump is pulled through the anus (Figure 3-8-11), and a purse-string clamp is applied at the pre-cut line on the sigmoid colon (Figure 3-8-12). The anvil is introduced into the sigmoid colon stump (Figure 3-8-13), which is then closed using purse string sutures and reintroduced into the abdominal cavity after irrigation and disinfection. Subsequently, inject 100ml of iodine solution into the abdominal cavity to irrigate the pelvic cavity and perform anal dilation.

The rectal stump is closed using the linear cutting stapler (Figure 3-8-14), and a protective sleeve is used to remove the rectal stump tissues (Figure 3-8-15). A circular stapler is inserted transanally, and the anvil is aligned with the stapler body to complete the end-to-end anastomosis (Figure 3-8-16).

The "dangerous triangle" of the anastomosis is reinforced with a figure-of-8 suture (Figure 3-8-17). Air and water injection test are conducted to check for anastomotic bleeding or leakage and for possible obstruction (Figure 3-8-18). Two drainage tubes are placed in the pelvic cavity (Figure 3-8-19).

# 9 Laparoscopic Radical Surgery for Middle Rectal Cancer with Transvaginal Specimen Extraction and Auxiliary Incision-Free Abdomen (CRC-NOSES IIIA)

## [Introduction]

CRC-NOSES IIIA is mainly applicable to female patients with larger middle rectal tumor. The key steps of CRC-NOSES IIIA is that the rectum is exteriorized through the vagina, the rectal specimen is resected extracorporeally, and an end-to-end sigmoidorectal anastomosis is then performed entirely under laparoscopy (Figure 3-9-1, Video 3-9). The difference from CRC-NOSES II lies in: ①There is no need to open the bowel intracorporeally, which better meets the requirements of aseptic principle; ②More stringent vaginal preparation is needed before operation; ③Because of the strong vaginal extensibility, the indications of CRC-NOSES IIIA are wider, but this procedure is limited to female patients.

## 9.1 Indications and contraindications

### [Indications]

1. Female patients with middle rectal tumor or benign tumor.
2. The circumferential diameter of tumor is 3-5cm.
3. The tumor should not invade beyond the serosa.
4. The sigmoid colon and mesentery are long enough to be pulled out.

### [Contraindications]

1. The tumor is too large to be pulled out.
2. The sigmoid colon and mesentery is too short to be pulled out through the vagina.
3. Severely obese patients (BMI>35kg/m$^2$).

## 9.2 Surgical procedure, techniques, and key points

### [Trocar placement]

1. The camera trocar (10mm trocar) is inserted through the umbilicus.
2. The surgeon's main trocar (12mm trocar) is located at the McBurney's point.
3. The surgeon's auxiliary trocar (5mm trocar) is located at the umbilical level at 10cm from the right side of the umbilicus.
4. The assistant's main trocar (5mm trocar) is located at the left lateral margin of rectus abdominis at umbilical level.
5. The assistant's auxiliary trocar (5mm trocar) is located opposite to the McBurney's point. In the meantime, the trocar should be placed more laterally in order to facilitate the placement of the drainage tube (Figure 3-9-2).

### [Exploration]

1. General exploration

Observe for any lesions such as metastatic implants on the surfaces of various organs and the peritoneum.

2. Tumor exploration

Determine the feasibility of surgery based on the tumor's location, size, and depth of invasion.

3. Evaluation of snatomical structures

It is necessary for the surgeon to check the length of sigmoid colon, the length of mesenteric vessels, as well as the thickness of middle mesorectum, so as to evaluate the feasibility of transvaginal specimen extraction.

## [Dissection and separation]

1. First incision point

The incision starts 3-5cm below the sacral promontory, often at a thin spot, using an ultrasonic scalpel to open the mesentery and enter the Toldt's space.

2. Division of inferior mesenteric vessels

Sequentially ligate the inferior mesenteric vessels, while being mindful to protect the inferior hypogastric plexus.

3. Mobilization of the mesorectum

Mobilization of the mesorectum is performed, with the extent tailored according to the tumor location; typically, a distal margin of 3-5cm below the tumor is sufficient.

4. Mobilization of the lateral side of the sigmoid colon

Cut through the adhesions on the lateral aspect of the sigmoid colon, taking care to protect the ureter and the gonadal vessels.

5. Isolation and division of the distal bowel

The mesorectum can be transected at 3-5cm below the distal edge of tumor. It is enough to isolate the bowel wall for approximately 2cm.

6. Trimming the sigmoid mesocolon

When dissecting the mesentery, the lateral blood vessels in the preserved side should be clamped with the vascular clips, while the other side can be directly cut off using an ultrasonic scalpel. By doing so, we can avoid damaging the blood vessels and rectal mucosa with the vascular clips when pulling out the specimen.

## [Specimen resection and digestive tract reconstruction]

1. Specimen resection

The surgeon transects the bowel with a linear cutting stapler at 4-5cm from the distal edge of the tumor (Figure 3-9-3). After the vaginal irrigation, the assistant introduces the bladder retractor through the vagina to indicate the posterior vaginal fornix (Figure 3-9-4). The surgeon applies the ultrasonic scalpel to make a 3cm transverse incision on the posterior vaginal fornix, and extends the incision to 5-6cm by longitudinal stretch (Figure 3-9-5), and inserts the protective sleeve into the abdominal cavity through the trocar. The assistant inserts the oval forceps through the vagina to pull the distal end of the protective sleeve out of the body (Figure 3-9-6). The surgeon places the specimen in the protective sleeve as the assistant clamps the rectal stump with the oval forceps through the vagina and pulls the stump out of the body (Figure 3-9-7). The purse-string forceps is applied extracorporeally at the pre-cut line of the sigmoid colon (Figure 3-9-8), and then the bowel is transected for specimen removal.

2. Digestive tract reconstruction

The stapler anvil is introduced into the sigmoid colon stump (Figure 3-9-9) and secured with a purse-string suture (Figure 3-9-10). After being rinsed and disinfected, the sigmoid colon is returned to the abdominal cavity with the oval forceps. A circular stapler is inserted transanally, and then the anvil is connected to the trocar of stapler to create the end-to-end anastomosis between the sigmoid colon and rectum (Figure 3-9-11-Figure 3-9-13). air and water injection test is performed to confirm the integrity of the anastomosis, and then perform an 8-figure suture on the "danger triangle" with absorbable suture for reinforcement.

3. Closure of trocar and suture of vaginal incision

Intraperitoneal gas is expelled. The vaginal incision can be sutured under laparoscopy (Figure 3-9-14). Then the pelvic cavity is irrigated with normal saline or distilled water, and drainage tubes are indwelled (Figure 3-9-15, Figure 3-9-16). Close the trocar and count the gauze and all instruments before the completion of surgery.

# 10   Modified Laparoscopic Radical Surgery for Middle Rectal Cancer with Transvaginal Specimen Extraction and Auxiliary Incision-Free Abdomen (CRC-NOSES ⅢB)

## [Introduction]

CRC-NOSES ⅢB, slightly different from CRC-NOSES ⅢA, is mainly applicable to female patients with relatively large middle rectal tumors (Figure 3-10-1). According to the latest research, extracting specimen via vagina would not increase short-term complications and decrease long term survival. In addition, the vaginal incision has limited effect on women's postoperative sexual life.

## 10.1   Indications and contraindications

### [Indications]

1. Female patients with middle rectal tumor or benign tumor.

2. The circumferential diameter of tumor is 3-5cm.

3. The tumor should not invade beyond the serosa.

4. The sigmoid colon and mesentery are long enough to be pulled out.

### [Contraindications]

1. The tumor is too large to be pulled out.

2. The sigmoid colon and mesentery is too short to be pulled out through the vagina.

3. Severely obese patients (BMI>35kg/m$^2$).

## 10.2   Surgical procedure, techniques, and key points

### [Trocar placement]

1. The camera trocar (10mm trocar) is located at the center of the umbilicus or 1cm above it.

2. The surgeon's main trocar (12mm trocar) is located at the McBurney's point.

3. The surgeon's auxiliary trocar (5mm trocar) is located at the umbilical level at 10cm from the right side of the umbilicus.

4. The assistant's main trocar (5mm trocar) is located at the left lateral margin of rectus abdominis at umbilical level.

5. The assistant's auxiliary trocar (5mm trocar) is located opposite to the McBurney's point. In the meantime, the trocar should be placed more laterally in order to facilitate the placement of the drainage tube (Figure 3-10-2).

### [Exploration]

1. General exploration

Observe for any lesions such as metastatic implants on the surfaces of various organs and the peritoneum.

2. Tumor exploration

Determine the feasibility of surgery based on the tumor's location, size, and depth of invasion.

3. Evaluation of anatomical structures

It is necessary for the surgeon to check the length of sigmoid colon, the length of mesenteric vessels as well as the thickness of middle mesorectum, so as to evaluate the feasibility of transvaginal specimen extraction.

### [Dissection and separation]

1. First incision point

The incision starts 3-5cm below the sacral promontory, often at a thin spot, using an ultrasonic scalpel to open the mesentery and enter the Toldt's space.

2. Division of inferior mesenteric vessels

Sequentially ligate the inferior mesenteric vessels, while being mindful to protect the inferior hypogastric plexus.

3. Mobilization of the mesorectum

The extent of mobilization is determined based on the tumor location; generally, a margin of 3-5cm distal to

the tumor is sufficient.

4. Mobilization of the lateral aspect of the sigmoid colon

Cut through the adhesions on the lateral aspect of the sigmoid colon, taking care to protect the ureter and the gonadal vessels.

5. Isolation and transection of the distal bowel below the tumor

The mesorectum can be transected at 3-5cm below the distal edge of tumor. It is enough to isolate the bowel wall for approximately 2cm.

6. Trimming the sigmoid mesocolon

Along with the ligation and transection of 2-3 sigmoid colon vessels, the mesentery is then dissected up to the pre-cut line of anastomosis. Approximately 2cm of the sigmoid colon should be isolated; excessive isolation is not required.

## [Specimen resection and digestive tract reconstruction]

1. Specimen resection

The rectum is transected using a linear cutting stapler at a point 4-5cm inferior to the tumor (Figure 3-10-3), followed by transection of the sigmoid colon at a point 5-10cm superior to the tumor (Figure 3-10-4). The assistant disinfects the vagina again and introduces a bladder retractor to indicate the position of the posterior vaginal fornix (Figure 3-10-5). The surgeon then makes a transverse incision, approximately 3-4cm long, at the posterior fornix using an electrocautery hook or ultrasonic scalpel (Figure 3-10-6), and a protective sleeve is introduced into the abdominal cavity via the 10mm trocar (Figure 3-10-7). The surgeon places the specimen into the protective sleeve. The assistant then clamps the opening of the protective sleeve transvaginally and pulls the sleeve out of the body (Figure 3-10-8). Purse string forceps are applied extracorporeally to the pre-cut line on the sigmoid colon (Figure 3-10-9).

2. Digestive tract reconstruction

The stapler anvil is inserted into the sigmoid colon stump (Figure 3-10-10) and secured with a purse-string suture. After irrigation and disinfection, the sigmoid colon is returned to the abdominal cavity with the oval forceps. A circular stapler is inserted transanally. Once the anvil is connected to the stapler trocar, end-to-end anastomosis can be created between the sigmoid colon and rectum (Figure 3-10-11-Figure 3-10-13). The integrity of the anastomosis should be evaluated. Perform an 8-figure suture on the "danger triangle" with absorbable suture. Air and water injection tests are performed to check for obstruction, bleeding, and leakage (Figure 3-10-14, Figure 3-10-15).

3. Closure of trocar and suture of vaginal incision

The vaginal incision can be closed laparoscopically with continuous sutures using barbed thread (Figure 3-10-16). The pelvic cavity is irrigated again using normal saline or distilled water, and indwelling drainage tubes are placed (Figure 3-10-17, Figure 3-10-18). The trocar port is closed, and a count of all the gauze and surgical instruments is performed before completion of the surgery.

# 11 Laparoscopic Radical Surgery for Upper Rectal Cancer with Transanal Specimen Extraction and Auxiliary Incision-Free Abdomen (CRC-NOSES IV)

## [Introduction]

CRC-NOSES IV is a novel surgical procedure for small tumors located at the upper rectum, rectosigmoid colon, and distal sigmoid colon. The main features of this procedure include: complete dissection and transection of specimen in abdominal cavity, transanal specimen extraction, and total laparoscopic end-to-end anastomosis between sigmoid colon and rectum (Figure 3-11-1, Video 3-10). The technological difficulty of this procedure is to introduce the anvil into the abdominal cavity transanally and insert the anvil into the proximal bowel lumen under

strict aseptic and tumor-free conditions.

## 11.1    Indications and contraindications

### [Indications]

1. Tumor is located at the upper rectum (≥10cm above the dentate line), rectosigmoid colon, and distal sigmoid colon.

2. The circumferential diameter of tumor is better less than 3cm.

3. The tumor should not invade beyond the serosa.

### [Contraindications]

1. Tumor location or staging does not comply with the indications above.

2. Tumors are too large or sigmoid mesentery is too thick, making it difficult to remove the specimen transanally.

3. Severely obese patients (BMI>35kg/m$^2$).

## 11.2    Surgical procedure, techniques, and key points

### [Trocar placement]

1. The camera trocar (10mm trocar) is located 3-5cm above the umbilicus.

2. The surgeon's main trocar (12mm trocar) is located above the McBurney's point.

3. The surgeon's auxiliary trocar (5mm trocar) is located at the umbilical level beside the right rectus abdominis.

4. The assistant's main trocar (5mm trocar) is located at the umbilical level beside the left rectus abdominis.

5. The assistant's auxiliary trocar (5mm trocar) is located opposite the McBurney's point, which facilitate placing the drainage tube (Figure 3-11-2).

### [Exploration]

1. General exploration

Observe for any lesions such as metastatic implants on the surfaces of various organs and the peritoneum.

2. Tumor exploration

Determine the feasibility of surgery based on the tumor's location, size, and depth of invasion.

3. Evaluation of anatomical structures

Determines whether to preserve the left colic artery and superior rectal artery based on the tumor location. The surgeon needs to evaluate the length of sigmoid colon, the length of mesenteric marginal vessels, and the thickness of mesentery to determine the feasibility of transanal specimen extraction.

### [Dissection and separation]

1. First incision point

The incision starts 3-5cm below the sacral promontory, often at a thin spot, using an ultrasonic scalpel to open the mesentery and enter the Toldt's space.

2. Division of inferior mesenteric vessels

Sequentially ligate the inferior mesenteric vessels, while being mindful to protect the inferior hypogastric plexus.

3. Mobilization of the upper mesorectum

Note that the distal end of the rectal mesentery needs to be dissected to 5cm below the tumor.

4. Mobilization of the lateral side of the sigmoid colon

Cut through the adhesions on the lateral aspect of the sigmoid colon, taking care to protect the ureter and the gonadal vessels.

5. Isolation and division of the distal bowel below the tumor

Since it is necessary to perform two separate transections on the bowel distal to the tumor, it is recommended that the extent of bowel skeletonization be somewhat wider than usual—approximately 3 to 5cm.

6. Trimming the sigmoid mesocolon

When dissecting the mesentery, the lateral blood vessels in the preserved side should be clamped with vascular clips, while the other side can be directly cut off using an ultrasonic scalpel. By doing so, we can avoid damaging the blood vessels and rectal mucosa with the vascular clips when pulling out the specimen.

### [Specimen resection and digestive tract reconstruction]

1. Specimen resection

The protective sleeve is inserted into the abdominal cavity through the surgeon's main trocar (Figure 3-11-3). Next, a window is opened at the top of the rectal stump

by the ultrasonic scalpel, insert the oval forceps through the anus to pull the protective sleeve out of the anus (Figure 3-11-4), then apply oval forceps to hold the anvil, and slide it into the abdominal cavity through the protective sleeve (Figure 3-11-5).

The distal bowel stump can be put into the protective sleeve, and a small longitudinal incision is made on the bowel wall above the tumor (Figure 3-11-6). The iodoform gauze is inserted into the sigmoid colon lumen through the longitudinal incision to disinfect the bowel lumen (Figure 3-11-7). The anvil is introduced into the sigmoid colon lumen through the longitudinal incision (Figure 3-11-8). The isolated bowel is transected with a linear cutting stapler above the longitudinal incision (Figure 3-11-9), and the sigmoid colon stump is disinfected with the iodoform gauze (Figure 3-11-10). At this point, the specimen is completely resected and placed into the protective sleeve (Figure 3-11-11).

Place the gauze and specimen in the protective sleeve (Figure 3-11-12). Afterward, the surgeon tightens the drawstring on the protective sleeve and slowly pulls out the protective sleeve containing the specimen through the anus to the outside (Figure 3-11-13).

2. Digestive tract reconstruction

The rectal stump is re-stapled with a linear cutting stapler (Figure 3-11-14). The resected rectal stump is placed in a retrieval bag or a self-made finger cot (resected from a rubber glove), and removed through the 12mm trocar (Figure 3-11-15).

The surgeon grabs the anvil from the outside of the bowel and takes the anvil shaft out of the sigmoid colon stump through one corner of it (Figure 3-11-16, Figure 3-11-17). The assistant inserts the circular stapler transanally, positions it near the left lateral angle of the rectal stump, and rotates out the piercing needle (Figure 3-11-18). The anvil shaft is connected, and the direction of mesocolon should be adjusted before completing the end-to-end anastomosis between the sigmoid colon and rectum (Figure 3-11-19).

Remove the stapler and check the integrity of the anastomosis. If necessary, reinforced suturing of the "danger triangle" area is performed laparoscopically. (Figure 3-11-20, Figure 3-11-21). air and water injection test is performed to confirm the integrity of the anastomosis and check for any leakage or bleeding. After irrigating the abdominal cavity and confirming that everything is in order, two drainage tubes are placed in the left and right lower abdomen, respectively.

# 12 Laparoscopic Radical Surgery for Upper Rectal Cancer with Transvaginal Specimen Extraction and Auxiliary Incision-Free Abdomen (CRC-NOSES V)

## [Introduction]

CRC-NOSES V is mainly applicable to female patients with larger tumor in the upper rectum, rectosigmoid colon, and distal sigmoid colon. The main operating procedures of CRC-NOSES V include complete dissection and transection of specimen in abdominal cavity, transvaginal specimen extraction, and laparoscopic end-to-end anastomosis between the sigmoid colon and rectum (Figure 3-12-1, Video 3-11). The differences between CRC-NOSES V and CRC-NOSES IV are: ①Since the specimen is removed through

the ductile vagina, CRC-NOSES V can be applied to larger tumors, but is limited to female patients; ②Only a small opening in the intestinal wall above the tumor is needed to place the anvil, so there is less chance of contamination of the abdominal cavity, and the aseptic operation is easier to control.

## 12.1 Indications and contraindications

### [Indications]

1. Tumor is located at the upper rectum (≥10cm above the dentate line), rectosigmoid colon, and distal

sigmoid colon.

2. The circumferential diameter of tumor is 3-5cm.

3. The tumor should not invade beyond the serosa.

## [Contraindications]

1. Tumor location or staging does not comply with the indications above;

2. Tumors are too large or sigmoid mesentery is too thick, making it difficult to remove the specimen transvaginally.

3. Severely obese patients (BMI>35kg/m$^2$).

## 12.2　Surgical procedure, techniques, and key points

### [Trocar placement]

1. The camera trocar (10mm trocar) is located 3-5cm above the umbilicus.

2. The surgeon's main trocar (12mm trocar) is located above the McBurney's point.

3. The surgeon's auxiliary trocar (5mm trocar) is located at the umbilical level beside the right rectus abdominis.

4. The assistant's main trocar (5mm trocar) is located at the umbilical level beside the left rectus abdominis.

5. The assistant's auxiliary trocar (5mm trocar) is located opposite the McBurney's point, which facilitate placing the drainage tube (Figure 3-12-2).

### [Exploration]

1. General exploration

Observe for any lesions such as metastatic implants on the surfaces of various organs and the peritoneum.

2. Tumor exploration

Determine the feasibility of surgery based on the tumor's location, size, and depth of invasion.

3. Evaluation of anatomical structures

Determines whether to preserve left colic artery and superior rectal artery based on the tumor location. The surgeon needs to evaluate the length of sigmoid colon, the length of mesenteric marginal vessels, and the thickness of mesentery to determine the feasibility of transvaginal specimen extraction.

### [Dissection and separation]

1. First incision point

The incision starts 3-5cm below the sacral promontory, often at a thin spot, using an ultrasonic scalpel to open the mesentery and enter the Toldt's space.

2. Division of inferior mesenteric vessels

Sequentially ligate the inferior mesenteric vessels, while being mindful to protect the inferior hypogastric plexus.

3. Mobilization of the upper mesorectum

Note that the distal end of the rectal mesentery needs to be dissected to 5cm below the tumor.

4. Mobilization of the lateral sigmoid colon and rectosigmoid colon

Cut through the adhesions on the lateral aspect of the sigmoid colon, taking care to protect the ureter and the gonadal vessels.

5. Isolation and division of the diatal bowel below the tumor

The extent of bowel isolation is usually about 2cm.

6. Trimming the sigmoid mesocolon

When dissecting the mesentery, the lateral blood vessels in the preserved side should be clamped with vascular clips, while the other side can be directly cut off using an ultrasonic scalpel. By doing so, we can avoid damaging the blood vessels and vagina with the vascular clips when pulling out the specimen.

### [Specimen resection and digestive tract reconstruction]

1. Specimen resection

The surgeon inserts the protective sleeve into the pelvic cavity through the main trocar (Figure 3-12-3). The assistant introduces the bladder retractor through the vagina to indicate the posterior vaginal fornix (Figure 3-12-4), and the surgeon applies the ultrasonic scalpel to open the vagina transversely for approximately 3cm and extends the incision to 5-6cm by longitudinal stretch (Figure 3-12-5). The assistant inserts the oval forceps through the vagina to pull the protective sleeve out of the body and open it (Figure 3-12-6). Subsequently, the anvil is introduced into the abdominal cavity through the protective sleeve (Figure 3-12-7).

A small longitudinal incision is made in the bowel

wall 1cm below the proximal pre-cut line (Figure 3-12-8). Through the incision, the surgeon inserts the iodoform gauze into the colon lumen for disinfection and lubrication; the assistant applies the suction to remove any bowel contents and pushs the iodoform gauze into the distal bowel lumen of the incision (Figure 3-12-9, Figure 3-12-10). The anvil is introduced into the proximal sigmoid colon lumen (Figure 3-12-11) and the proximal bowel is transected with the linear cutting stapler (Figure 3-12-12). Following this, the isolated bowel below the tumor is transected with a linear cutting stapler (Figure 3-12-13). At this point, the rectal tumor and the bowel segment are completely resected.

The surgeon and an assistant place the specimen and the used gauze into the protective sleeve, and another assistant applies the oval forceps to clamp the bowel wall stump below the tumor in the protective sleeve. The protective sleeve is tightened, and the assistant slowly pulls out the sleeve along with the specimen and the gauze (Figure 3-12-14).

2. Digestive tract reconstruction

The anvil shaft is protruded from one corner of the proximal colon stump (Figure 3-12-15). The assistant inserts a circular stapler transanally and extends the trocar to pierce the rectal stump (Figure 3-12-16). The anvil is connected to the trocar of stapler (Figure 3-12-17), and the direction of mesocolon should be adjusted before complete the end-to-end anastomosis between the sigmoid colon and rectum (Figure 3-12-18).

After the stapler is removed, the integrity of the anastomosis is checked. If necessary, reinforced suturing of the "danger triangle" area is performed laparoscopically. (Figure 3-12-19). Lastly, air and water injection test is performed to confirm the integrity of the anastomosis and check for any leakage or bleeding (Figure 3-12-20). After irrigating the abdominal cavity and confirming that everything is in order, drainage tubes are placed transabdominally or transvaginally (Figure 3-12-21).

3. Suture the vaginal incision.

After the drainage tubes are in place, the pneumo-peritoneum is released. The vaginal incision is exposed by lifting its anterior and posterior walls with two Allis forceps, and the incision is closed with an interrupted suture using absorbable sutures. The vaginal incision can also be closed with a continuous barbed suture through the abdominal cavity.

# 13   Laparoscopic Radical Surgery for Left-Sided Colon Cancer with Transanal Specimen Extraction and Auxiliary Incision-Free Abdomen (CRC-NOSES VIA)

## [Introduction]

CRC-NOSES VIA includes complete dissection and transection of left-sided colon in abdominal cavity, specimen extraction from the rectum and anus, and laparoscopic end-to-end anastomosis between transverse colon and rectum (Figure 3-13-1, Video 3-12). The laparoscopic technical difficulties of CRC-NOSES VIA include the complete mesocolon resection of left-sided colon, dissection of lymph nodes at the root of mesentery, and the mobilization of splenic flexure. The NOSES technical difficulties of CRC-NOSES VIA include the specimen extraction from the rectum and anus, laparoscopic digestive tract reconstruction, and application of asepsis and tumor-free operation.

## 13.1   Indications and contraindications

### [Indications]

1. Tumor is located at the descending colon and proximal sigmoid colon.

2. The circumferential diameter of tumor is preferably less than 3cm.

3. The tumor should not invade beyond the serosa.

## [Contraindications]

1. Tumor is located at the splenic flexure and transverse colon near the splenic flexure.

2. Circumferential diameter of tumor is more than 3cm.

3. Tumor invades beyond the serosa.

4. Severely obese patients (BMI>35kg/m$^2$).

## 13.2 Surgical procedure, techniques, and key points

### [Trocar placement]

1. The camera trocar (10mm trocar) is located 2-3cm below the umbilicus.

2. The surgeon's main trocar (12mm trocar) is located at the McBurney's point.

3. The surgeon's auxiliary trocar (5mm trocar) is located at the intersection of 10cm above the umbilicus and the lateral edge of the right rectus abdominis.

4. The assistant's main trocar (5mm trocar) is located at the intersection of 10cm above the umbilicus and the left midclavicular line.

5. The assistant's auxiliary trocar (5mm trocar) is located opposite to the McBurney's point, which facilitate placing the drainage tube (Figure 3-13-2).

### [Exploration]

1. General exploration

Observe for any lesions such as metastatic implants on the surfaces of various organs and the peritoneum.

2. Tumor exploration

Determine the feasibility of surgery based on the tumor's location, size, and depth of invasion.

3. Evaluation of anatomical structure

Firstly, the anatomic structure of colon and mesocolon is evaluated, i.e., whether the length of the dissected bowel and the course of the marginal vessels facilitate the anastomosis; secondly, the surgeon should determine whether the thickness of mesentery and the circumferential diameter of tumor facilitate the transrectal specimen extraction.

### [Dissection and separation]

1. Management of the root of the inferior mesenteric vessels

The root of the inferior mesenteric artery is isolated, double ligated, and transected. The vascular stump is lifted for the dissection under it with a medial to lateral fashion. The surgeon then dissects upward to the lateral side of the Treitz ligament and transect the inferior mesenteric vein at the inferior boarder of pancreas.

2. Mobilization of left mesocolon with medial approach

Elevate the stumps of the inferior mesenteric vein and the inferior mesenteric artery, and using an ultrasonic scalpel, mobilize Toldt's fascia with a combined approach of sharp and blunt dissection in the lateral, inferior, and superior directions.

3. Management of the sigmoid mesocolon and mesorectum

The mesentery is lifted along the course of the inferior mesenteric artery, dissection is performed downward to the level of the sacral promontory. Attention should be paid to protect the nerves anterior to the abdominal aorta.

4. Management of the left-sided transverse colon and splenic flexure

As the transverse colon is lifted, the surgeon transects the transverse mesocolon from the inferior mesenteric vein stump, which lies lateral to the Treitz ligament, to give direct access to the omental bursa. Then the dissection proceeds to the left to lower pole of spleen along the inferior boarder of the pancreas.

5. Mobilization of the left paracolic sulcus

The sigmoid colon is pulled to the right, while the left side of the rectum is dissected upward along the Toldt's fascia. The left paracolic sulcus is incised upward to the lower pole of spleen as indicated by the gauze.

6. Dividing and isolating the mesocolon above the tumor

The surgeon divides the transverse mesocolon and then ligates and transects the marginal vascular arcade. Dissection is continued to the bowel wall, and 2cm of the bowel is isolated.

### [Specimen resection and digestive tract reconstruction]

1. Specimen resection

A small transverse window is opened on the isolated

bowel of the sigmoid colon below the tumor (Figure 3-13-3). The anvil is held by oval forceps and introduced into the abdominal cavity through the protective sleeve (Figure 3-13-4). A small longitudinal incision is made in the bowel wall proximal to the tumor (Figure 3-13-5). The anvil is introduced into the proximal colon (Figure 3-13-6). The colon is transected with a linear cutting stapler (Figure 3-13-7). At this point, the anvil is left in the proximal bowel, and the bowel stump should be disinfected again with the iodoform gauze (Figure 3-13-8). The rectum is transected by extending the transverse incision below the tumor (Figure 3-13-9), then the left-sided colon is completely resected. A protective sleeve is introduced into the abdominal cavity through the main trocar port. The surgeon and assistant cooperate to smoothly place the specimen into the protective sleeve. The assistant applies the oval forceps to clamp oneend of the bowel extra-corporeally and slowly pulls the specimen out of the rectum and anus (Figure 3-13-10).

2. Digestive tract reconstruction

The opened rectal stump is closed with a linear cutting stapler (Figure 3-13-11), and the resected stump is placed into the specimen retrieval bag and extracted through the 12mm trocar. The abdominal cavity is irrigated with saline or distilled water. to reduce the risk of intraperitoneal infection. The anvil shaft is taken out from one corner of the pre-cut line on the proximal colon (Figure 3-13-12). The assistant inserts a circular stapler transanally and extends the trocar to pierce the left corner of rectal stump (Figure 3-13-13). The anvil is connected to the trocar of stapler, and the direction of mesocolon is adjusted (Figure 3-13-14), then the stapler is fired to complete the anastomosis (Figure 3-13-15). The surgeon should check the integrity of the anastomosis and suture the "danger triangle" with 8-figure suture for reinforcement (Figure 3-13-16). The air and water injection test is performed to check the patency of the anastomosis and ensure its accuracy (Figure 3-13-17). After irrigating the abdominal cavity and confirming that everything is in order, two drainage tubes are placed close to the anastomosis (Figure 3-13-18, Figure 3-13-19). Finally, pneumoperitoneum is released, and the trocar sites are closed.

# 14 Laparoscopic Radical Surgery for Left-Sided Colon Cancer with Transrectal Specimen Extraction and Auxiliary Incision-Free Abdomen (CRC-NOSES VIB)

## [Introduction]

CRC-NOSES VIB is characterized by its applicability to cases with tumors located relatively higher and further from the peritoneal reflection; the specimen is extracted via an incision on the anterior wall of the rectum rather than through the rectal stump; and gastrointestinal reconstruction is performed using total laparoscopic functional side-to-side anastomosis. (Figure 3-14-1, Video 3-13). The operating difficulties of this procedure mainly involve laparoscopic technical difficulties and the challenges of NOSES. Specifically, the laparoscopic technical difficulties include the complete mesocolon resection of the left-sided colon, dissection of lymph nodes at the root of the mesentery, and the mobilization of the splenic flexure. The NOSES technical difficulties include the specimen extraction after opening the rectum, total laparoscopic digestive tract reconstruction, and application of asepsis and tumor-free operation. These are the challenges the surgeons need to face and overcome.

## 14.1 Indications and contraindications

### [Indications]

1. The tumor is located in the transverse colon near the splenic flexure, the splenic flexure of the colon, the descending colon, and the proximal sigmoid colon.

2. The circumferential diameter of the tumor is preferably less than 3cm.

3. The tumor should not invade beyond the serosa.

## [Contraindications]

1. The circumferential diameter of tumor is more than 3cm.

2. Tumor invades beyond the serosa.

3. Severely obese patients (BMI>35kg/m$^2$).

## 14.2  Surgical procedure, techniques, and key points

### [Trocar placement]

1. The camera trocar (10mm trocar) is located 2-3cm below the umbilicus.

2. The surgeon's main trocar (12mm trocar) is located at the McBurney's point.

3. The surgeon's auxiliary trocar (5mm trocar) is located at the intersection of 10cm above the umbilicus and the lateral edge of the right rectus abdominis.

4. The assistant's main trocar (5mm trocar) is located at the intersection of 10cm above the umbilicus and the anterior axillary line.

5. The assistant's auxiliary trocar (5mm trocar) is located opposite to the McBurney's point, which facilitates placing the drainage tube (Figure 3-14-2).

### [Exploration]

1. General exploration

Observe for any lesions such as metastatic implants on the surfaces of various organs and the peritoneum.

2. Tumor exploration

Determine the feasibility of surgery based on the tumor's location, size, and depth of invasion.

3. Evaluation of anatomical structures

Firstly, evaluate the anatomic structure of colon and mesocolon, i.e., whether the length of the dissected bowel and the course of the marginal vessels facilitate the anastomosis; Secondly, evaluate whether the thickness of mesentery and the circumferential diameter of the tumor facilitate the transrectal specimen extraction.

### [Dissection and separation]

1. Management of the root of the inferior mesenteric vessels

The root of the inferior mesenteric artery is isolated, double ligated, and transected. The surgeon then dissects upward to the lateral side of the Treitz ligament and transect the inferior mesenteric vein at the inferior boarder of pancreas.

2. Mobilization of left mesocolon with medial approach

The inferior mesenteric vessels stumps are lifted as the surgeon applies the ultrasonic scalpel to perform sharp and blunt dissection of the Toldt's fascia downward and upward in a medial to lateral fashion.

3. Management of the sigmoid mesocolon

The surgeon lifts the sigmoid mesocolon and dissects along the predetermined pre-cut line to the marginal vascular arcade, then ligate and transect the marginal vessels. Dissection is continued to the bowel wall, and 3-4cm of the bowel is isolated.

4. Management of the left-sided transverse colon and splenic flexure

As the transverse colon is lifted, the surgeon transects the transverse mesocolon from the inferior mesenteric vein stump, which lies lateral to the Treitz ligament, to give direct access to the omental bursa. Then the dissection proceeds to the left to lower pole of spleen along the inferior boarder of the pancreas.

5. Mobilization of the left paracolic sulcus

The sigmoid colon is pulled to the right, while the left side of the rectum is dissected upward along the Toldt's fascia. The left paracolic sulcus is incised upward to the lower pole of spleen as indicated by the gauze.

6. Dividing and isolating the mesocolon above the tumor

Pull down the splenic flexure of the colon and determine the predetermined pre-cut line. The surgeon mobilizes the transverse mesocolon to the marginal vascular arcade, then divides and ligates the arcade. Dissection is continued to the bowel wall, and 2cm of the bowel is isolated.

### [Specimen resection and digestive tract reconstruction]

1. Specimen resection

The transverse colon is dissected at the bare end of the transverse colon (Figure 3-14-3), and the sigmoid colon is dissected at the bare end of the sigmoid colon (Figure 3-14-4), and the diseased intestinal tubes are

completed free to the point of completing the resection of the specimen.

2. Digestive tract reconstruction

The two severed ends are pulled close and placed parallel to each other, the tension of the proposed anastomosis is judged, and the severed ends are fixed with absorbable sutures (Figure 3-14-5). The intestinal wall is incised against the mesenteric side at both severed ends on both sides of the preanastomosis (Figure 3-14-6), and a functional side-to-side anastomosis is performed (Figure 3-14-7). Inspects the anastomosis for active bleeding, and the public openings are closed (Figure 3-14-8), and the anastomosis is reinforced with interrupted sutures (Figure 3-14-9), completing transverse-sigmoid anastomosis (Figure 3-14-10).

3. Specimen extraction

The assistant injects diluted povidone-iodine solution through the anus for irrigation and places an the iodoform gauze through the anus. The surgeon then opens the rectal wall at the site of the iodoform gauze by making an incision of approximately 5cm longitudinally on the upper rectum (Figure 3-14-11). The protective sleeve is inserted through the 12mm trocar (Figure 3-14-12), then the assistant applies the oval forceps through the incision in the upper rectum to pull the end of the protective sleeve out through the anus (Figsure3-14-13). All the used gauzes in the abdominal cavity are placed into the protective sleeve and removed through it. One end of the specimen is smoothly placed into the protective sleeve with the cooperation between the surgeon and the assistant. The assistant applies the oval forceps to clamp the end of the specimen (Figure 3-14-14, Figure 3-14-15) and slowly pulls the specimen out of the rectum and anus. Continuous suture is performed longitudinally to close the incision on the rectum under laparoscopy (Figure 3-14-16), followed by seromuscular layer embedding (Figure 3-14-17). The abdominal cavity is irrigated with distilled water (Figure 3-14-18), and the drainage tube is indwelled in to the abdominal cavity through a 5mm trocar (Figure 3-14-19). Pneumoperitoneum is released, and the trocar sites are closed.

# 15　Laparoscopic Radical Surgery for Left-Sided Colon Cancer with Transvaginal Specimen Extraction and Auxiliary Incision-Free Abdomen (CRC-NOSES Ⅶ)

## [Introduction]

CRC-NOSES Ⅶ is mainly applicable to female patients with larger tumors located at the left-sided colon. The main operating features of this procedure include laparoscopic dissection and transection of the left-sided colon, specimen extraction from the vagina, and total laparoscopic end-to-end anastomosis between the transverse colon and rectum (Figure 3-15-1, Video 3-14). Compared with CRC-NOSES Ⅵ, this procedure has a broader indication because the specimen extraction from the vagina is easier to be performed, however the vaginal incision should be sutured properly. The operating difficulties of CRC-NOSES Ⅶ mainly involve laparoscopic technical difficulties and the challenges of NOSES. Specifically, the laparoscopic technical difficulties include the complete mesocolon excision of left-sided colon, dissection of lymph nodes at the root of mesenteric vessels, and the mobilization of the splenic flexure. The NOSES technical difficulties include the transvaginal specimen extraction, total laparoscopic digestive tract reconstruction, the suturing of vaginal incision, and the strict maintenance of asepsis and tumor-free operation, etc.

## 15.1　Indications and contraindications

### [Indications]

1. The tumor is located in the transverse colon near the splenic flexure, the splenic flexure of the colon, the descending colon, and the proximal sigmoid colon.

2. The circumferential diameter of the tumor is preferably less than 5cm.

3. The tumor should not invade beyond the serosa.

## [Contraindications]

1. The circumferential diameter of tumor is more than 5cm.

2. Tumor invades beyond the serosa.

3. Severely obese patients (BMI>35kg/m$^2$).

## 15.2　Surgical procedure, techniques, and key points

### [Trocar placement]

1. The camera trocar (10mm trocar) is located 2-3cm below the umbilicus.

2. The surgeon's main trocar (12mm trocar) is located at the McBurney's point.

3. The surgeon's auxiliary trocar (5mm trocar) is located at the intersection of 10cm above the level of the umbilicus and the lateral edge of the right rectus abdominis.

4. The assistant's main trocar (5mm trocar) is located at the intersection of 10cm above the level of the umbilicus and the left midclavicular line.

5. The assistant's auxiliary trocar (5mm trocar) is located opposite to the McBurney's point (Figure 3-15-2).

### [Exploration]

1. General exploration

Observe for any lesions such as metastatic implants on the surfaces of various organs and the peritoneum.

2. Tumor exploration

Determine the feasibility of surgery based on the tumor's location, size, and depth of invasion.

3. Evaluation of anatomical structures

①Evaluate the anatomical structure of the colon, i.e., the length of the pulled down transverse colon after the dissection of the splenic flexure. Evaluate the feasibility of laparoscopic anastomosis based on the status of mesenteric marginal vessels. ②Perform digital vaginal examination to determine whether the status of the posterior vaginal fornix is suitable for incision and specimen extraction.

### [Dissection and separation]

1. Management of the root of the inferior mesenteric vessel

Ultrasonic scalpel is applied to expand the space above, below, and to the left of the inferior mesenteric artery. Double ligation and transection of the inferior mesenteric artery are performed.

2. Mobilization of left mesocolon with medial approach

Elevate the stumps of the inferior mesenteric vein and inferior mesenteric artery, and dissect along Toldt's fascia upward, downward, and laterally.

3. Management of the sigmoid mesocolon and mesorectum

The sigmoid mesocolon or mesorectum is transected. The distal superior rectal vessels are better ligated with vascular clips.

4. Management of the left-sided transverse colon and splenic flexure

The transverse colon is lifted to expose the transverse mesocolon. From the inferior mesenteric vein stump, which lies lateral to the Treitz ligament, the transverse mesocolon is divided into the bowel wall. Dissection is continued toward the left paracolic sulcus.

5. Opening the left paracolic sulcus

With the indication of the gauze, dissection is continued cephalad to open the left paracolic sulcus along Toldt's fascia.

6. Dividing and isolating the mesocolon above the tumor

The mesentery is further divided into the bowel wall, and the marginal vascular arcade is ligated and transected. The transverse colon wall should be isolated for approximately 2cm.

### [Specimen resection and digestive tract reconstruction]

1. Specimen resection

The surgeon inserts the protective sleeve into the pelvic cavity through the main trocar (Figure 3-15-3). The assistant introduces the bladder retractor through the vagina to indicate the posterior vaginal fornix (Figure 3-15-4). The surgeon uses the ultrasonic scalpel to make a 3cm transverse incision on the posterior vaginal fornix and extends the incision to 5-6cm by longitudinal stretch (Figure 3-15-5). The assistant inserts the oval forceps through the vagina to pull the distal end

of the protective sleeve out of the body. Subsequently, the anvil is introduced into the abdominal cavity through the protective sleeve (Figure 3-15-6). A small longitudinal incision is made in the bowel wall between the tumor and the proximal pre-cut line. Through the incision, the surgeon inserts the iodoform gauze into the colon lumen for disinfection and lubrication (Figure 3-15-7, Figure 3-15-8), and the surgeon applies the suction to push the iodoform gauze into the distal bowel lumen of the incision. Then, the anvil is placed in the proximal bowel lumen through the incision (Figure 3-15-9), and the proximal bowel is transected with the linear cutting stapler (Figure 3-15-10). At this point, the left-sided colon is completely resected. The assistant applies the oval forceps to clamp one end of the specimen to slowly pull out the specimen through the vagina (Figure 3-15-11).

2. Digestive tract reconstruction

The anvil shaft is protruded from one corner of the proximal colon stump (Figure 3-15-12). The assistant inserts a circular stapler through the anus and rectum and extends the trocar to pierce the rectal stump from left side of the staple line (Figure 3-15-13) to complete the end-to-end anastomosis between colon and rectum (Figure 3-15-14). The integrity of the anastomosis is checked before the 8-Figure suture is performed on the "danger triangle" (Figure 3-15-15). air and water injection test is performed to confirm the integrity of the anastomosis (Figure 3-15-16). After irrigating the abdominal cavity, two drainage tubes are placed through the trocars on the abdominal wall (Figure 3-15-17).

3. Closure of trocar and suture of vaginal incision

After the drainage tubes are in place, intraperitoneal gas is expelled and the trocar sites are closed. The vaginal incision can be sutured under laparoscopy or by extracorporeal suture. The steps of the extracorporeal suture are: fully expose the vaginal incision, lift the anterior and posterior wall of the incision with two Allis forceps, and perform interrupted suture with absorbable sutures (Figure 3-15-18).

## 16    Laparoscopic Radical Surgery for Right-Sided Colon Cancer with Transvaginal Specimen Extraction and Auxiliary Incision-Free Abdomen (CRC-NOSES VIII A)

### [Introduction]

The right hemicolon has many adjacent organs, complicated vasculature, and large anatomical variations. Therefore, CRC-NOSES VIII is one of the most difficult techniques in NOSES. The route of removal of the right hemicolon specimen is mostly applied to the vagina. The main operating features of CRC-NOSES VIIIA include complete dissection and transection of the right-sided colon in the abdominal cavity, specimen extraction from the vagina, and laparoscopic functional end-to-end anastomosis between the terminal ileum and transverse colon (Figure 3-16-1, Video 3-15). The laparoscopic digestive tract reconstruction in CRC-NOSES VIIIA is more difficult than other procedures, and requires the surgeon and assistant to be more skillful. In the process of transvaginal specimen extraction, the application of asepsis and tumor-free operation is crucial.

## 16.1    Indications and contraindications

### [Indications]

1. Female patients with right-sided colon tumor.

2. The circumferential diameter of the tumor is better less than 5cm.

3. The tumor should not invade beyond the serosa.

### [Contraindications]

1. The circumferential diameter of tumor is more than 5cm.

2. Tumor invades adjacent tissues and organs.

3. Severely obese patients (BMI>35kg/m$^2$).

4. Male patients with right-sided colon cancer.

## 16.2　Surgical procedure, techniques, and key points

### [Trocar placement]

1. The camera trocar (10mm trocar) is located at any point from the umbilicus to 5cm below the umbilicus.

2. The surgeon's main trocar (12mm trocar) is located at the middle of the left upper quadrant at the lateral edge of the rectus abdominis.

3. The surgeon's auxiliary trocar (5mm trocar) is located at the left lower quadrant, not in the same horizontal level as the camera trocar site.

4. The assistant's main trocar (12mm trocar) is located at the McBurney's point, which facilitates the insertion of linear cutting stapler during digestive tract reconstruction.

5. The assistant's auxiliary trocar (5mm trocar) is located at the right upper quadrant at the intersection between the right midclavicular line and the transverse colon projection (Figure 3-16-2).

### [Exploration]

1. General exploration

After the laparoscope is placed into the umbilical port, the liver, gallbladder, stomach, spleen, colon, small intestine, greater omentum, and pelvic cavity are routinely examined for the presence of tumor seeding or ascites.

2. Tumor exploration

The tumor is located at the right-sided colon without invading beyond the serosa. The circumferential diameter of the tumor is better to be less than 5cm.

3. Evaluation of anatomical structures

The right hemicolectomy is complicated since the right-sided colon has many adjacent organs. It is necessary to identify the anatomical location and branching relationships of the ileocolic vessels, the right colic vessels, and the middle colic vessels. In particular, the middle colic artery and vein have many vascular branches. It is recommended to ligate and transect the root of the middle colic vessels if the operation is difficult. In addition, it is necessary to evaluate the feasibility of laparoscopic functional end-to-end anastomosis between the ileum and transverse colon after the dissection of the transverse colon. Laparoscopic end-to-end or end-to-side anastomosis between the ileum and transverse colon with circular stapler is not feasible due to the limitation of the current equipment and technical conditions. For the patients whose transverse mesocolon is too short in length, CRC-NOSES VIIIA should not be performed.

### [Dissection and separation]

1. Management of the root of ileocolic artery and vein

The surgeon applies the forceps in the left hand to adequately expose the mesenteric surface along the superior mesenteric vein. A depressed and thin area at the angle between the ileocolic vessels and superior mesenteric vein can be seen. The ultrasonic scalpel is applied to open the mesentery, and the vessels are dissected and isolated gently. Along the Toldt's space, dissection is performed upwards from medial to lateral in a cavernous manner. While dissecting upwards, the identification of the duodenum proves that the correct space has been entered. The sheath of the superior mesenteric vein is opened as far as possible at the root of the ileocolic artery and vein, then dissection is continued upwards to give direct access to the rear on the right side. Following this, the root of the ileocolic artery and vein is isolated, surrounding fibrous connective tissue are removed, and vessels are double ligated and transected.

2. Management of the root of right colic artery and vein

The surgeon dissects the surface of the duodenum along the Toldt's fascia, then the right colic vein, the right gastroepiploic vein, and Henle's trunk, which converge into the superior mesenteric vein, are identified. The right colic vein is ligated and transected, where after the dissection is continued upwards along the superior mesenteric vein to expose the right colic artery. Double ligation and transection are performed at the root of it.

3. Management of the root of the middle colic artery and vein

After the isolation of the right colic vessels, dissection is performed upwards until the posterior wall of the gastric antrum is seen through a thin membrane on the surface of the pancreatic neck. A small gauze should

be placed here. Subsequently, dissection is continued upwards along the superior mesenteric vein. The middle colic artery and vein are double ligated and transected at the inferior border of the pancreas. At this point, all vessels supplying the right-sided colon have been transected.

4. Mobilization of the mesocolon

Continuing to separate further outward, upward and downward along the Toldt's space, the entire free surface was seen to be smooth, flat and clean.

5. Management of the mesoileum

When the peritoneum below the cecum is penetrated, the surgeon opens the fascia attached to its root as much as possible to extend the degree of dissection of the ileum, so as to facilitate the laparoscopic anastomosis of the bowel. The assistant lifts the terminal ileum and the surgeon applies the ultrasonic scalpel to divide the mesoileum. Attention should be paid to the course and direction of the mesenteric blood supply. The division is performed toward the wall of the terminal ileum, and approximately 2cm of the bowel is isolated.

6. Management of the greater omentum and group 6 lymph nodes

The surgeon determines the pre-cut line of the transverse colon and dissects the greater omentum. The ultrasonic scalpel is used to free the right greater omentum to the transverse colon wall, then it is pulled to the right abdominal cavity. The assistant lifts the gastric wall with the forceps in the left hand, and the course of the right gastroepiploic artery and vein can be seen. Divide the gastrocolic ligament from the transverse colon to enter the omental bursa. Dissect and divide along the lateral margin of the vascular arcade of the right gastroepiploic artery and vein toward the right side. With the dissection to the head of the pancreas, the right gastroepiploic vein and Henle's trunk can be seen, and this dissection plane is connected with the previous dissection plane.

7. Management of the transverse mesocolon

After dissecting the duodenopancreatic head region of the gastric antrum, the gauze is visualized behind the mesentery, and the mesentery is incised transversely and separated in the avascular direction of the transverse colonic mesentery. Ligation of the dissecting marginal vessels, further separation towards the transverse colon

in a pre-cut line, and nudification of the bowel wall by 1cm.

## [Specimen resection and digestive tract reconstruction]

1. Specimen resection

The mobilized transverse colon is isolated using a linear cutting stapler at the pre-cut line (Figure 3-16-3). The proximal bowel stump is pulled to the right lower abdomen. The attachment of the transverse colon at the right paracolic gutter and beneath the liver is clearly visible, and the gauze placed at the back can be seen. The ultrasonic scalpel is applied to dissect along the right paracolic sulcus to the right iliac fossa, as indicated and protected by the gauze until the dissection plane is connected with the dissection plane below (Figure 3-16-4). In the isolated area of ileum, the blood supply line is clearly visible (Figure 3-16-5). Following this, the surgeon transects the ileum medial to the blood supply line with a linear cutting stapler (Figure 3-16-6). At this point, the right hemicolectomy is completed and the specimen is placed in the pelvic cavity.

2. Digestive tract reconstruction

The transverse colon is straightened, and the terminal ileum is pulled up to the upper abdomen to be placed parallel with the transverse colon (Figure 3-16-7). The surgeon makes an incision of 5mm in one corner of the pre-cut line of the ileum with ultrasonic scalpel (Figure 3-16-8). The assistant inserts the 60mm linear cutting stapler through the 12mm trocar in the right lower quadrant and places the anvil into the ileum lumen (Figure 3-16-9). Similarly, another incision of 10mm is made in one corner of the transverse colon stump by the surgeon (Figure 3-16-10). Then, the assistant and the surgeon lift the colon and place the cartridge jaw into the colon lumen (Figure 3-16-11). The stapler is fired to complete the functional end-to-end anastomosis between the ileum and the transverse colon (Figure 3-16-12).

The presence of anastomotic bleeding in the bowel lumen is checked (Figure 3-16-13). After confirming that there is no active bleeding, the bowel stump is lifted, the linear cutting stapler is inserted through the 12mm trocar in the left upper quadrant to close the stump transversely, then the functional end-to-end anastomosis is completed (Figure 3-16-14). The resected stump tissue

is placed into the protective sleeve and extracted through the 12mm trocar. Then, Plasma-muscle layer suture of the ileo-transverse colon anastomotic union to reduce anastomotic tension (Figure 3-16-15). The digestive tract reconstruction after right hemicolectomy is completed.

3. Specimen extraction

The protective sleeve is inserted through the 12mm trocar in the left upper quadrant (Figure 3-16-16). The opening of the protective sleeve is expended, the gauze and specimen in the abdominal cavity are placed into the protective sleeve (Figure 3-16-17), then the opening of the protective sleeve is closed with Hem-Lock (Figure 3-16-18). Prior to incision of the vagina, the surgeon is required to change position on the patient's right side while switching the position of the laparoscopic monitor, and the patient's position is changed from a head-high, foot-low position to a foot-high, head-low position. The assistant lifts the uterus extracorporeally with a uterine manipulator to fully expose the posterior vaginal fornix (Figure 3-16-19). The surgeon applies the ultrasonic scalpel to open the vagina transversely for approximately 3cm (Figure 3-16-20), and extends the incision to 5-6cm by longitudinal stretch. With the cooperation of the surgeon, the assistant applies the oval forceps to clamp one end of the specimen extracorporeally (Figure 3-16-21), then slowly pulls the specimen and the protective sleeve out of the body (Figure 3-16-22).

4. Suture of vaginal incision and closure of trocar sites

The assistant fully exposes the vaginal incision by lifting the anterior and posterior wall of the incision with two Allis forceps. Interrupted suture is performed with absorbable sutures to close the incision (Figure 3-16-23). Two drainage tubes are placed in the right upper quadrant through the two trocar on the right side (Figure 3-16-24).

# 17    Laparoscopic Radical Surgery for Right-sided Colon Cancer with Transrectal Specimen Extraction via Rectal Incision and Auxiliary Incision-Free Abdomen (CRC-NOSES VIIIB)

## [Introduction]

For women patients with right-sided colon cancer, CRC-NOSES VIIIA, can be operated. However, for male patients, CRC-NOSES VIIIB is possible (Figure 3-17-1, Video 3-16). The right-sided colon has many adjacent organs, complicated vasculature, and major anatomical variations. In addition, the specimens need to be extracted through the incision on the upper rectum, and the closure of this incision needs to be completed under the laparoscopy. Therefore, this procedure is a difficult, risky technique with high damage-benefit ratio in NOSES. The main operating features of this procedure include complete dissection and transection of the right-sided colon in the abdominal cavity, laparoscopic digestive tract reconstruction of the terminal ileum and transverse colon, and right-sided colon specimen extraction through the incision on the rectum. Therefore, in the process of transrectal specimen extraction, the application of asepsis and tumor-free operation and the accurate understanding of indications of this procedure is crucial. Compared with NOSES-VIIIA, this procedure requires more accurate understanding of indications, clear surgical thinking and proficient skills.

## 17.1    Indications and contraindications

### [Indications]

1. Male patients with right-sided colon cancer or benign tumor.

2. The circumferential diameter of tumor less than 3cm is more suitable.

3. The tumor should not invade beyond the serosa.

### [Contraindications]

1. The circumferential diameter of tumor is more

than 3cm.

2. Tumor invades adjacent tissues and organs.

3. Patients who have undergone rectal or anal surgery and patients with middle and lower rectal and anal stenosis caused by rectal or anal diseases.

4. Severely obese patients (BMI>35kg/m$^2$).

## 17.2 Surgical procedure, techniques, and key points

### [Trocar placement]

1. The camera trocar (10mm trocar) is located at any point from the umbilicus to 5cm below the umbilicus.

2. The surgeon's main trocar (12mm trocar) is located at the middle of the left upper quadrant at the lateral edge of the rectus abdominis.

3. The surgeon's auxiliary trocar (5mm trocar) is located at the left lower quadrant, not in the same horizontal level as the camera trocar site.

4. The assistant's main trocar (12mm trocar) is located at the McBurney's point.

5. The assistant's auxiliary trocar (5mm trocar) is located at the right upper quadrant at the intersection between the right midclavicular line and the transverse colon projection (Figure 3-17-2).

### [Exploration]

1. General exploration

After the laparoscope is placed into the umbilical port, the liver, gallbladder, stomach, spleen, colon, small intestine, greater omentum, and pelvic cavity are routinely examined for the presence of tumor seeding or ascites.

2. Tumor exploration

Determine the feasibility of surgery based on the tumor's location, size, and depth of invasion.

3. Evaluation of anatomical structures

The right-sided colon has many adjacent organs, complicated vasculature, and major anatomical variations. It is necessary to identify the anatomical locations and relationships of the ileocolic vessels, the right colic vessels, and the middle colic vessels. In particular, the middle colic artery and vein have many vascular branches. It is recommended to ligate and transect the root of the middle colic vessels if the operation is difficult. In addition, it

is necessary to evaluate the feasibility of laparoscopic overlapped delta-shaped anastomosis after the dissection of the transverse colon.

### [Dissection and separation]

1. Anatomy and division of the root of ileocolic artery and vein

The assistant lifts the ileocolic artery and vein. The thin fossa between the "bow-stringing" of ileocolic artery and vein and superior mesenteric vein will be seen. An ultrasonic scalpel is used to incise the peritoneum of the ileal mesentery, and slowly dissect and isolate the vessels. Separate upward and outward along Toldt's space , which is cave-like, and free the duodenum upward to show that the hiatus is correct. The superior mesenteric vein sheath is opened as far as possible at the root of the ileocolic artery, separated upward, and connected to the posterior on its right side. The roots of ileocolic vessels are cleared of lymphatic and adipose tissues. The ileocolic artery and vein are clipped.

2. Management of the root of right colic artery

The right colic artery is then separated with the dissection upwards along the superior mesenteric vein, then the right colic artery is isolated and clipped. The dissection continued in the surface of the duodenum and head of the pancreas along the Toldt's fascia, reaching the accessory right colic vein, the right gastroepiploic vein, and anterior superior pancreaticoduodenal vein which formed Henle's trunk, then drained into the superior mesenteric vein. The accessory right colic vein is isolated and clipped.

3. Management of the right branch of the middle colic artery and vein

After isolating the right colonic artery and the collateral right colonic vein, the isolation was continued upward to isolate the middle colonic artery and vein at the inferior border of the pancreas, and continued along the middle colonic artery and vein to isolate the right branch of the middle colonic artery and vein, which was ligated and severed. At this point, all the vessels supplying the right-sided colon have been transected.

4. Mobilization of the mesocolon

Dissection is performed from medial to lateral along the Toldt's fascia to the right paracolic sulcus. Attention should be paid to protect the right gonadal vessels, head

of the pancreas, and duodenum. Mobilization of the terminal mesoileum, ascending mesocolon, and the right transverse mesocolon is completed by medial-to-lateral dissection.

5. Management of the mesoileum

When the peritoneum below the cecum is penetrated, lyse the physiological adhesions between the cecum and the lateral abdominal wall, and mobilize cephalad. The assistant lifts the terminal ileum and the surgeon applies the ultrasonic scalpel to divide the mesoileum. Attention should be paid to the course and direction of the mesenteric blood supply. The division is performed toward the wall of the terminal ileum, and approximately 2cm of bowel is isolated.

6. Management of the greater omentum and group 6 lymph nodes

The surgeon determines the pre-cut line of the transverse colon and dissects the greater omentum. The ultrasonic scalpel is used to free the right greater omentum to the transverse colon wall, then it is pulled to the right abdominal cavity. The assistant lifts the gastric wall with the forceps in the left hand, and the course of the right gastroepiploic artery and vein can be seen. Dissection is performed from the transverse colon to the gastroepiploic vessels, the gastrocolic ligament is transected, and the omental sac is entered. Dissect and divide along the lateral margin of the vascular arcade of the right gastroepiploic artery and vein toward the right side. With the dissection to the head of the pancreas, the right gastroepiploic vein and Henle's trunk can be seen, and this dissection plane is connected with the previous dissection plane.

7. Management of the transverse mesocolon

After dissecting the mesentery in the region of the gastric sinus duodenopancreatic head, the mesentery was dissected transversely and separated toward the avascular direction of the transverse colonic mesentery. Subsequently, the surgeon ligates and transects the marginal vessels, then dissects to the pre-cut line of the transverse colon. The bowel wall is isolated for 1cm.

## [Specimen resection and digestive tract reconstruction]

1. Specimen resection

The mobilized transverse colon is isolated using a linear cutting stapler at the pre-cut line (Figure 3-17-3). The proximal end is turned toward the right lower abdomen, at which point its transverse colon is clearly visible in the right paracolic groove and subhepatic attachment. The ultrasonic scalpel is applied to dissect along the right paracolic sulcus to the right iliac fossa until connecting with space below. In the isolated area of ileum, the blood supply line is clearly visible (Figure 3-17-4). Following this, the surgeon transects the ileum medial to the blood supply line with a linear cutting stapler (Figure 3-17-5). At this point, the right hemicolectomy is completed. Putting the specimen in the specimen bag and place it in the pelvic cavity.

2. Digestive tract reconstruction

The transverse colon is straightened, and the terminal ileum is pulled up to the upper abdomen to be placed overlapped with the transverse colon (Figure 3-17-6). The surgeon then checks the blood supply of both sides of the bowel, and estimates the tension of the anastomosis. The transverse colon and terminal ileal stumps are opened with two incisions (1cm for each) close to staple lines on the antimesenteric border (Figure 3-17-7, Figure 3-17-8), then both bowel lumens are disinfected with the iodoform gauze. The right lower abdominal trocar port was replaced with a 12mm trocar, and a linear cutting stapler was inserted, and a linear cutting stapler was inserted into the nail compartment in one side of the intestinal lumen, and the clamp mouth was temporarily closed, the surgeon and the assistant grasped the other side of the intestinal lumen, loosened the clamp mouth, and put the intestinal tube onto the anvil, made the necessary adjustments, and confirmed that there was no error, then struck the hair to complete the ileo-transverse colon functional end-to-end anastomosis. (Figure 3-17-9).

The bowel lumen is disinfected with the iodoform gauze, and the integrity of the anastomosis is confirmed. After confirming that there is no bleeding, the surgeon and the assistant pull the tail end of the suture, so that the severed end of the intestinal tube is away from the opposite side of the intestinal wall and in a straight line, and then close the common opening of the intestinal tubes of the two sides with a linear cutting stapler to complete the ileo-transverse colon functional end-to-end anastomosis. Reinforce the anastomosis with absorbable sutures (Figure 3-17-10).

3. Specimen extraction

The protective sleeve is inserted through the 12mm trocar (Figure 3-17-11). The specimen is smoothly placed into the protective sleeve (Figure 3-17-12). Before making the incision in the rectal wall, the surgeon should change to the right side of the patient and change the position of the laparoscopic display. The patient's position has changed from the anti-Trendelenburg position to the Trendelenburg position. After the assistant had fully flushed the rectum with diluted povidone-iodine solution through the anus, a longitudinal opening of about 3cm in the upper part of the rectum was selected.

(Figure 3-17-13). The second assistant used oval forceps to drag the protective sleeve and specimen through the anus to the opening of the upper rectum with oval forceps (Figure 3-17-14-Figure 3-17-16).

The assistant wipes the bowel lumen with the iodoform gauze as the surgeon confirms that there is no active bleeding. Laparoscopic seromuscular layer embedding of the anastomosis is performed (Figure 3-17-17). The abdominal cavity is irrigated with distilled water, and one drainage tube is indwelled in the abdominal cavity through the 12mm trocar on the right side. Pneumoperitoneum is released, and the trocar sites are closed.

# 18 Laparoscopic Radical Surgery for Right-sided Colon Cancer with transcolonic dragging out of the specimen and Auxiliary Incision-Free Abdomen (CRC-NOSES VIIIC)

## [Introduction]

CRC-NOSES VIIIC method is mainly suitable for right hemicolectomy patients with small tumors, including early tumors of ileocecum, ascending colon, hepatic curvature of colon and right-sided colon. The main operation procedures of CRC-NOSES VIIIC included: ①Laparoscopic resection of the right-sided colon; ②Colonoscopy-assisted removal of specimens from the left-sided transverse colon, splenic curvature of the colon, descending colon, sigmoid colon, rectum and anus; ③Laparoscopic functional side-to-side anastomosis of the transverse colon and ileum (Figure 3-18-1, Video 3-17). For strictly screened patients with right-sided colon tumor, the CRC-NOSES VIIIC is safe and feasible.

## 18.1 Indications and contraindications

### [Indications]

1. Tumors of ileocecum, ascending colon, hepatic flexure of colon and right-sided transverse colon.
2. The circumferential diameter of the tumor should be less than 5cm.
3. The tumor should not invade beyond the serosa.

### [Contraindications]

1. The tumor is too big to be extracted.
2. Tumor invades adjacent organs and structures.
3. Severely obese patients (BMI>30kg/m$^2$).

## 18.2 Surgical procedure, techniques, and key points

### [Trocar placement]

1. The camera trocar (10mm trocar) is located at any point from the umbilicus to 5cm below the umbilicus.
2. The surgeon's main trocar (12mm trocar) is located at the middle of the left upper quadrant at the lateral edge of the rectus abdominis.
3. The surgeon's auxiliary trocar (5mm trocar) is located at the left lower quadrant, not in the same horizontal level as the camera trocar site.
4. The assistant's main trocar (12mm trocar) is located at the McBurney's point, taking into account the placement of a drain at the end of the operation.
5. The assistant's auxiliary trocar (5mm trocar) is located at the right upper quadrant at the intersection between the right midclavicular line and the transverse

colon projection (Figure 3-18-2).

## [Surgical team position]

For right hemicolectomy, the surgeon stands on the patient's left side, the assistant stands on the patient's right side, and the scopist stands between the patient's legs. For specimen removal and digestive tract reconstruction, the surgeon stands on the patient's right side, the assistant stands on the patient's left side, the scopist stands on the same side as the surgeon, and the endoscopist and assistant stand between the patient's legs.

## [Exploration]

1. General exploration

After the laparoscope is placed into the umbilical port, the liver, gallbladder, stomach, spleen, colon, small intestine, greater omentum, and pelvic cavity are routinely examined for the presence of tumor seeding.

2. Exploration of tumor

The surgeon should examine the tumor location and size.

3. Exploration of anatomical structure

The degree of hypertrophy of the right hemicolonic mesentery, greater omentum, and epiploic appendages, and the caliber of the colonic lumen are examined to determine the suitability for extracorporeal evacuation via the colon, rectum, or anus.

## [Dissection and separation]

1. Marking the scope of resection of the right-sided colon

Lifting the ileocecal arteriovenous mesentery and see that there is a recessed weak spot below the angle of intersection with the superior mesenteric vein. Use the ultrasonic scalpel to perform the first cut at the weak spot, and then incise the mesentery superficially toward the end of the ileum to the pre-cut lineof the ileum (about 15cm away from the ileocecal portion), and incise the mesentery superficially upward to the place where the midpoint of the transverse colon is to be severed, and mark the scope of the right hemicolon resection in this way. This marks the extent of right hemicolectomy.

2. Anatomy and division of the roots of the arteries and veins of the ileocecal

Ultrasonic scalpel is used to separate the duodenum upward and laterally along the Toldt's space, and the duodenum is seperated upward to remove fat, connective tissue and lymph nodes around the vascular root of the ileocolon, and then Hem-Lock ligated and severed the ileal artery and vein respectively.

3. Anatomy of right colic and middle colic vessels

Continue cephalad separation along the anterior wall of the superior mesenteric vein After dissecting the fat and lymph nodes surrounding the root of the middle colic vessels, the right branch of the middle colic artery and vein are ligated and divided separately. Henle's trunk is fused of the right gastroepiploic vein with the right colic vein. The right colic vein is ligated and divided. The right colic artery has variable origin, and it is originated from the superior mesenteric artery in 41% of patients. There is not the right colic artery in 18% of patients.

4. Anatomy of right mesocolon and transverse mesocolon

The right colonic mesentery was freed from medial to lateral according to the CME principle , and separated along the surface of the duodenum and the head of the pancreas. The transverse colon is lifted up ventrally by the assistant using a bowel grasper. Under the clear exposure of transverse mesocolon, the surgeon makes an incision in the avascular area of the transverse mesocolon as well as vessels toward the bowel wall of the middle transverse colon. The exposed length of the bowel wall should be appropriately 2-3cm.

5. Anatomy of greater omentum and hepatocolic ligament

The greater omentum is incised toward the midpoint of the transverse colon with an ultrasonic scalpel. The assistant lifts the anterior wall of the stomach ventrally. In this way, the gastrocolic ligament is placed under tension and thus could be divided more easily. Initial dissection of the gastrocolic ligament starts in the middle of the transverse colon with subsequent entry into the lesser sac. The dissection can be continued from the middle to right along the outer margin of the right gastroepiploic vein. The hepatocolic ligament and the lateral ligament of the right-sided colon are dissected.

6. Trimming of the ileocolic mesentery and free ileocecal peritoneum

The terminal ileum is lifted up by the assistant using

grasper forceps. The distance between the proximal tumor edge and the pre-cut line is about 15cm. The exposed length of the bowel wall should be appropriately 1-2cm on the terminal ileum. Lifting the ileocecal portion, to the left and upward, incise the lateral peritoneum under the ileocecal portion, and free it upward and inward along the lateral aspect of the ascending colon to join with the superior and medial aspect, whereupon the right-sided colon is completely free.

7. Division of the terminal ileum and right-sided transverse colon

The protective sleeve was inserted into the abdominal cavity through a 12mm trocar port. After the right half of the colon was completely freed, a clear ischemic line was seen at the end of the ileum, and the end ileum was closed by cutting the proximal part of the ischemic line proximal to the proposed resection using a 60mm linear cutting stapler. The terminal ileal stump is sterilized with a small piece of povidone gauze, which is then placed in the protective sleeve. The endoscopist inserts the colonoscope through the anus, reaches the ascending colon to confirm the ascending colon lesion, and then cuts the middle part of the closed transverse colon with a 60mm linear cutting stapler in the ischemic line lateral to the pre-cut line, and then disinfects the transverse colon stump with a small piece of povidone gauze.

## [Specimen extraction and digestive tract reconstruction]

1. Specimen extraction

The right-sided colon specimen is packed into a protective sleeve (Figure 3-18-3). Under the guidance of laparoscopy, colonoscopy reaches the closed transverse colon through the anus (Figure 3-18-4). After bowel irrigation with normal saline in colonoscopy, the stump is cut open with ultrasonic scalpel and disinfected with a small piece of povidone gauze. After extending the tip of

the colonoscope, then disinfected with a small piece of povidone gauze (Figure 3-18-5). Excess fluid is removed with the suction. The protective sleeve containing the specimen is clamped by endoscopic foreign body retrieval (Figure 3-18-6), With the help of laparoscopic non-invasive forceps, the protective sleeve containing the right half of the colon was moved into the left half of the colon and slowly passed through the left half of the transverse colon, the splenic flexure of the colon, the descending colon, the sigmoid colon, the rectum, and finally removed through the anus. (Figure 3-18-7-Figure 3-18-11).

2. Digestive tract reconstruction

The opened stump of the transverse colon is closed with a 60mm linear cutting stapler (Figure 3-18-12). The resected stump tissue is put into a protective sleeve. The terminal ileum is pulled to the upper abdomen to be placed parallel to the transverse colon. The antimesenteric border of the terminal ileum stump is cut open with an ultrasonic scalpel, and the bowel lumen is disinfected with a small piece of povidone gauze (Figure 3-18-13). Similarly, a small incision is made on the antimesenteric bowel wall of the transverse colon about 6cm from the stump (Figure 3-18-14). The povidone gauze is also put into the opened bowel lumen for disinfection (Figure 3-18-15). The terminal ileum and the transverse colon are functional side-to-side anastomosed with a 60mm linear cutting stapler (Figure 3-18-16). After carefully inspecting the common opening in the bowel lumen to confirm the absence of bleeding, the area is disinfected again with a small piece of povidone gauze (Figure 3-18-17), the common opening of the anastomosis is closed with an absorbable suture (Figure 3-18-18). The anastomotic seromuscular layer is sutured to reinforce and reduce anastomotic tension. Ileocolic mesentery is sutured to avoid internal abdominal hernia (Figure 3-18-19).

# 19 Laparoscopic Total Colectomy with Transanal Specimen Extraction and Auxiliary Incision-Free Abdomen

## (CRC-NOSES IX )

## [Introduction]

CRC-NOSES IX is completed on the basis of laparoscopic total colectomy combined with unique digestive tract reconstruction and transanal specimen extraction. Operative features of this procedure: total laparoscopic freeing of the whole colon and its mesentery, removal of the whole colon specimen through the anus, and total laparoscopic side-to-end ileo-rectal anastomosis. (Figure 3-19-1, Figure 3-19-2, Video 3-18). From the technical point of view, total colectomy is one of the most difficult and complex surgical procedures in colorectal cancer resection. This procedure has a wide range of surgical resection, involving all technical difficulties regarding right hemicolectomy, left hemicolectomy, and rectal resection. These difficulties put forward high requirements to the surgeons, especially young surgeons' operating skills. Theoretically, most surgeons believe that total colectomy with transanal specimen extraction is very difficult or even impossible. As a result, total colectomy with transanal specimen extraction is very rare in the surgical field. We propose the adoption of radical resection of colon cancer with greater omentum preserved in this procedure, so as to reduce the difficulty of transanal specimen extraction. As long as the indications for this surgical procedure are strictly mastered, and as long as there is a clear and meticulous surgical strategy combined with appropriate surgical techniques, this technique can be fully achieved.

## 19.1 Indications and contraindications

### [Indications] (Figure 3-19-3)

1. Familial adenomatous polyposis.
2. Lynch syndrome-associated colorectal cancer.
3. Multiple primary colorectal cancer and the circumferential diameter of the largest tumor is better less than 3cm.
4. Ulcerative colitis which is not sensitive to medical treatment.
5. Patients with constipation or other benign diseases that need total colectomy.

### [Contraindications]

1. Multiple primary colorectal cancer and the circumferential diameter of the tumor is more than 3cm.
2. Severely obese patients (BMI>35kg/m$^2$), or patients with mesenteric thickening.
3. Tumor invades beyond the serosa.

## 19.2 Surgical procedure, techniques, and key points

### [Anesthesia method]

General anesthesia with or without epidural anesthesia.

### [Patient position]

The patient is placed in the functional lithotomy position. The bilateral thighs are abducted as much as possible, with the upward elevation angle less than 15 degrees, to facilitate the surgeon's operation (Figure 3-19-4).

### [Trocar placement]

1. The camera trocar (10mm trocar) is located at the umbilicus, which takes the right and left colic and rectal field of vision into consideration.
2. The surgeon's main trocar 1 (12mm trocar) is located at the left upper quadrant, which facilitates the mobilization of the right-sided colon.
3. The surgeon's main trocar 2 (12mm trocar) is

located at the McBurney's point, which facilitates the mobilization of the left-sided colon and rectum.

4. The auxiliary trocar 1 (5mm trocar) is located opposite to the McBurney's point.

5. The auxiliary trocar 2 (5mm trocar) is located at the intersection between the transverse colon projection and the right midclavicular line (Figure 3-19-5).

## [Surgical team position]

The right hemicolectomy: the surgeon stands on the left side of the patient, the assistant stands on the right side of the patient. The left hemicolectomy and rectal resection: the surgeon stands on the right side of the patient, the assistant stands on the left side of the patient, the camera holder stands on the same side of the surgeon or between two legs of the patient (Figure 3-19-6, Figure 3-19-7).

## [Special surgical instruments]

Ultrasonic scalpel, 60mm linear cutting stapler, 25mm circular stapler, protective sleeve.

## [Exploration]

1. General exploration

After the laparoscope is placed into the umbilical port, the liver, gallbladder, stomach, spleen, colon, small intestine, greater omentum, and pelvic cavity are routinely examined for the presence of tumor seeding or ascites.

2. Exploration of the tumor

For multiple primary tumors or polyposis with cancerization, the circumferential diameter of the largest tumor should be less than 3cm.

3. Evaluation of anatomical structures

Total colectomy is a highly challenging procedure due to the complex adjacency of organs. It is necessary to observe the structure of the entire colon and any abnormalities in blood vessels, the presence of abnormalities in the rectal ampulla, and whether the mesentery is hypertrophic, so as to comprehensively determine the feasibility of adopting this surgical procedure.

## [Dissection and separation]

1. Management of the root of the ileocolic artery and vein

The surgeon stands on the left side of the patient, while the patient is placed in the anti-Trendelenburg position and slightly tilted to the left. The ileocolic vessels are lifted to expose the angle between the ileocolic vessels and the course of superior mesenteric vein (Figure 3-19-8). After opening the mesentery at the root of the ileocolic vessels, dissection is performed along the Toldt's space upwards from medial to lateral, then the horizontal part of the duodenum can be identified (Figure 3-19-9, Figure 3-19-10). Following this, the lymph nodes are dissected at the root of the ileocolic vessels along the surface of the superior mesenteric vein. After adequate isolation (Figure 3-19-11), the ileocolic vessels are ligated and transected at the root (Figure 3-19-12, Figure 3-19-13).

2. Management of the root of right colic artery and vein

By lifting the stump of ileocolic vessels, dissection is performed the surface of the duodenum along the Toldt's fascia gradually. After that, dissection is continued along the right colic vein to the head of the pancreas and the superior mesenteric vein. Ligation and transection can be performed at the root of the right colic vein (Figure 3-19-14). Subsequently, the surgeon dissects upwards along the surgical trunk of the superior mesenteric vein to expose the right colic artery, then ligates and transects it at the root (Figure 3-19-15).

3. Management of the root of the middle colic vessels

After the dissection of the right colic artery and vein, the inferior border of the pancreatic neck and the posterior wall of the gastric antrum can be identified. Then, the surgeon dissects upwards toward the area above the root of the right colic artery to expose the middle colic artery and vein. Dissection in this area should be performed extremely carefully before double ligate and transect the middle colic vessels. Then, the dissection is continued along the pancreatic neck to the left, to dissect the transverse mesocolon toward the Treitz ligament.

4. Management of the terminal ileum

While cropping the terminal ileal mesentery, the posterior peritoneal attachment of the cecum is simultaneously opened to pass through Toldt's fascia. Freeing the ileal mesentery to the ileal bowel wall

(Figure 3-19-16). Approximately 2cm of the wall of the ileum is isolated (Figure 3-19-17). The blood supply line should be checked carefully to ensure the blood supply of the anastomosis.

5. Management of the greater omentum

In the middle of the transverse colon, the surgeon detaches the greater omentum from the wall of the transverse colon along the taeniae coli to enter the omental cavity (Figure 3-19-18). The assistant then flips the greater omentum, and the gauze on the surface of the pancreatic body is visible. On the right side of the stomach and colon, the gastrocolic ligament and transverse mesocolon are mostly fused, but there is a space between them. Dissection is performed along the right gastroepiploic artery and vein to the right to give direct access to the mesentery at the inferior border of the pancreas, as indicated by the gauze placed before. Dissection is further continued to the surface of the duodenum to give direct access to the previous dissection space, then the right greater omentum is separated completely. Subsequently, the attachment of the greater omentum is detached along the taeniae coli to the splenic flexure until the lower pole of the spleen is exposed. A gauze is placed on the surface of the pancreatic tail for protection and indication (Figure 3-19-19).

6. Mobilization of the right paracolic sulcus and its mesentery

Dissect and transect the mesentery step by step along the surface of the duodenum and Toldt's fascia, starting from the hepatic flexure of the colon and moving downward and laterally (Figure 3-19-20, Figure 3-19-21) until reaching the cecum. At this point, the right-sided colon is completely mobilized.

7. Management of the root of the inferior mesenteric artery

The surgeon stands on the right side of the patient, and the patient is placed in the right-tilted anti-Trendelenburg position. Then the surgeon opens the mesorectum below the sacral promontory to enter the presacral space and dissects upwards to the left (Figure 3-19-22, Figure 3-19-23) to identify the inferior hypogastric nerves. The dissection is continued upwards to the root of the inferior mesenteric artery (Figure 3-19-24). Approximately 1cm of the vessel is isolated before double ligation and transection is performed at its origin

(Figure 3-19-25, Figure 3-19-26).

8. Management of the inferior mesenteric vein

The root of the inferior mesenteric artery is lifted, and the posterior peritoneum is incised along the lateral side of the abdominal aorta toward the Treitz ligament. As the space anterior to Toldt's fascia is further expanded, the course of the inferior mesenteric vein can be identified (Figure 3-19-27). On the left side of the Treitz ligament, the inferior mesenteric vein is ligated and transected at the inferior border of the pancreas (Figure 3-19-28). After the dissection of the mesentery, the surgeon places a gauze underneath the dissected mesentery for protection and indication (Figure 3-19-29). At this point, all vessels supplying the left-sided colon have been transected.

9. Management of left mesocolon and left paracolic sulcus

The mesentery is lifted for the dissection along the Toldt's fascia from medial to lateral, then the peristalsis and course of the left ureter can be identified (Figure 3-19-30), as well as the left gonadal vessels and left adipose capsule of the kidney (Figure 3-19-31). The correct dissection plane should be smooth, flat, and clean. At the ligament of Treitz, it meets the transverse mesocolon resected during right hemicolectomy. Along the inferior margin of the pancreas, under the guidance and protection of a gauze strip, the mesocolon of the splenic flexure of the colon is dissected to the left until reaching the inferior pole of the spleen (Figure 3-19-32). Afterward, the dissection proceeds downwards along the left paracolic sulcus to the sigmoid colon (Figure 3-19-33).

10. Mobilization of the mesorectum

The surgeon should determine the extent of rectal resection according to the nature of the lesion. If the rectal lesion is malignant, the extent of resection may be 3-5cm below the lesion. If the rectal lesion is benign, the rectal ampulla may be preserved, and polyps in the rectum may be resected under colonoscopy. The posterior and right wall of the mesorectum is dissected along the presacral space according to the principle of TME (Figure 3-19-34, Figure 3-19-35). Detailed operation is the same as before. Subsequently, the adhesion between the sigmoid colon and the left abdominal wall is detached (Figure 3-19-36), the peritoneum on the left of the rectum is separated to the pre-cut line.

11. Isolation of rectum from the pre-cut line

On the right side of the pre-cut line, the rectum is isolated layer by layer. Following this, the surgeon transects the mesorectum at the same level on the left side of the rectum, and the assistant lifts the rectum to further isolate the posterior rectal wall and get both sides connected (Figure 3-19-37). The peritoneal reflection is incised to perform dissection around the anterior rectal wall and get both sides connected (Figure 3-19-38).

## [Specimen resection and digestive tract reconstruction]

1. Specimen resection

The ileum is transected with a linear cutting stapler at the isolated area of the ileum (Figure 3-19-39) and a window is made on the rectal wall above the pre-cut line of the rectum (Figure 3-19-40). The distal rectum is transected after sufficient safe distal resection margin is double-checked. At this point, the dissection and resection of the total colon are completed.

2. Specimen extraction

The protective sleeve is inserted into the abdominal cavity through the 12mm trocar port (Figure 3-19-41). The assistant and surgeon place the specimen into the protective sleeve (Figure 3-19-42), then the assistant applies the oval forceps to clamp the rectal stump and slowly pulls the total colon specimen out of the body through the protective sleeve inside the rectum (Figure 3-19-43, Figure 3-19-44).

3. Digestive tract reconstruction

Abdominal and pelvic lavage is performed by sufficient iodine solution and inspected for bleeding before digestive tract reconstruction (Figure 3-19-45). The assistant inserts the anvil into the abdominal cavity through the protective sleeve inside the rectal stump (Figure 3-19-46). The distance between the terminal ileum and the rectal stump is checked to select the anastomosis site in the ileum. The surgeon then makes an incision of approximately 2cm on the ileum stump along the staple line (Figure 3-19-47) and places the anvil into the intended anastomosis site in the ileal cavity (Figure 3-19-48). The ileum stump is closed with a linear cutting stapler (Figure 3-19-49). Then a small incision is made in the intended anastomosis site of the ileum to take cut the anvil shaft. After confirming no errors, set them aside for use (Figure 3-19-50).

The rectal stump is closed with a linear cutting stapler (Figure 3-19-51), and the resected stump tissue is extracted with a specimen retrieval bag through the 12mm trocar port (Figure 3-19-52). The assistant inserts the circular stapler through the anus and extends the trocar to pierce one corner of the rectal stump (Figure 3-19-53). Align and connect with the stapler trocar (Figure 3-19-54), and the stapler is fired to complete the side-to-end anastomosis between the ileum and the rectum (Figure 3-19-55).

Check the integrity of the anastomosis carefully. Air and water injection test is also performed to confirm the integrity of the anastomosis (Figure 3-19-56). After excluding active bleeding, two drainage tubes are placed in the two sides of the pelvic cavity through the trocars on the left and right lower quadrant (Figure 3-19-57, Figure 3-19-58). Finally, the pneumoperitoneum is released and the trocar sites are closed to complete the surgery.

# 20 Laparoscopic Total Colectomy with Transvaginal Specimen Extraction and Auxiliary Incision-Free Abdomen
## (CRC-NOSES X)

### [Introduction]

Total colectomy is one of the most difficult and complex techniques in colorectal surgery involving complex surgical procedures and a wide resection range. Compared with conventional laparoscopic total colectomy, the main differences of CRC-NOSES X lie in the digestive tract reconstruction and the route

of specimen extraction. The technical features of this procedure include total laparoscopic mobilization of the entire colon and its mesentery, transvaginal extraction of the total colectomy specimen, followed by a laparoscopic side-to-end anastomosis between the terminal ileum and the rectum (Figure 3-20-1). Compared with CRC-NOSES IX, the procedure of CRC-NOSES X has a wider indication. In addition, this technique reduces the exposure of bowel within the abdominal cavity, which may reduce the risk of infection (Figure 3-20-2).

## 20.1　Indications and contraindications

### [Indications]

1. Multiple colorectal cancer, and the circumferential diameter of tumor, is better at 3-5cm.

2. Familial adenomatous polyposis, which is hard to be extracted through the anus.

3. Lynch syndrome-associated colorectal cancer.

4. Ulcerative colitis which is not sensitive to medical treatment and local mesenteric thickening, which makes it hard for specimen to be extracted from the anus.

5. This procedure is suitable for total colectomy with complete resection of the greater omentum.

### [Contraindications]

1. Multiple primary colorectal cancer, and the circumferential diameter of tumor, is more than 5cm.

2. Severely obese patients (BMI>35kg/m$^2$), or patients with mesenteric thickening.

3. Tumor invades beyond the serosa.

## 20.2　Surgical procedure, techniques, and key points

### [Anesthesia method]

General anesthesia with or without epidural anesthesia.

### [Patient position]

The patient is placed in functional lithotomy position with both thighs slightly elevated to under 15 degrees, which facilitates performing the operation for the surgeon (Figure 3-20-3).

### [Trocar placement]

1. The camera trocar (10mm trocar) is located at the umbilicus, which takes the right and left colic and rectal field of vision into consideration.

2. The surgeon's main trocar 1 (12mm trocar) is located at the left upper quadrant, which facilitates the mobilization of right-sided colon.

3. The surgeon's main trocar 2 (12mm trocar) is located at the McBurney's point, which facilitates the left hemicolectomy and rectal resection.

4. The auxiliary trocar 1 (5mm trocar) is located opposite to the McBurney's point.

5. The auxiliary trocar 2 (5mm trocar) is located at the intersection between the transverse colon projection and the right midclavicular line (Figure 3-20-4).

### [Surgical team position]

The right hemicolectomy: the surgeon stands on the left side of the patient; the assistant stands on the right side of the patient. The left hemicolectomy and rectal resection: the surgeon stands on the right side of the patient; the assistant stands on the left side of the patient. The camera holder stands on the same side of the surgeon or between two legs of the patient (Figure 3-20-5, Figure 3-20-6).

### [Special surgical instruments]

Ultrasonic scalpel, 60mm linear cutting stapler, 25mm circular stapler, vaginal suture line, uterine manipulator, sterile protective sleeve.

### [Exploration]

1. General exploration

After the laparoscope is placed into the umbilical port, the liver, gallbladder, stomach, spleen, colon, small intestine, greater omentum, and pelvic cavity are routinely examined for the presence of tumor seeding or ascites.

2. Exploration of the tumor

For multiple primary tumors, the evaluation of the largest tumor is most critical, and the circumferential diameter of the largest tumor is the most important factor for determining whether this NOSES procedure can be performed.

3. Evaluation of anatomical structures

Total colectomy is very complex. It is necessary to observe the adjacent organs thoroughly. Assess whether there are abnormalities in the blood supply vessels of the entire colon, the degree of mesenteric hypertrophy, and any abnormal changes in the pelvis and posterior vaginal fornix, and re-evaluate the feasibility of the surgery.

## [Dissection and separation]

1. Management of the root of the ileocolic vessels

The surgeon stands on the left side of the patient, and the patient is placed in the anti-Trendelenburg position slightly tilted to the left. After the surgical field is fully exposed, the surgeon opens the *mesentery* of blood vessels below the root of the ileocolic vessels (Figure 3-20-7) and on the surface of the superior mesenteric vein (Figure 3-20-8, Figure 3-20-9). Dissection is continued upward on the surface of the superior mesenteric vein. The ileocolic artery is often accompanied by the ileocolic vein, and the ileocolic artery crosses the superior mesenteric vein to join the course of the ileocolic vein. Occasionally, they are separated, and the ileocolic artery is derived from the posterior of the superior mesenteric vein. After adequate isolation, the ileocolic vessels are ligated and transected at the root (Figure 3-20-10, Figure 3-20-11).

2. Management of the root of right colic artery and vein

Dissect upward along the superior mesenteric vein (Figure 3-20-12), then open the sheath of blood vessels to expose the right colic artery firstly (Figure 3-20-13). In most cases, the right colic artery is not accompanied by the vein, and they need to be managed separately. However, in rare cases, the right colic artery is accompanied by the vein and can be managed simultaneously (Figure 3-20-14, Figure 3-20-15). The stump of the right colic artery is lifted, and dissection is performed upward in a medial to the right lateral pattern. During the dissection, the pancreatic capsule is visible and the Toldt's space should be dissected on the surface of the pancreas (Figure 3-20-16, Figure 3-20-17). Henle's trunk is usually located at the surface of pancreas. There are two smaller veins that drain into the Henle's trunk, respectively. The vein from the right is the right colic vein, which can be ligated at the root, and the vein from

the superior is connected with the right gastroepiploic vein.

3. Management of the root of the middle colic artery and vein

After the dissection of the right colic vessels, the inferior border of the pancreatic neck can be exposed. The mesentery is opened, then the middle colic vessels are isolated and double ligated with hemoclip at the root (Figure 3-20-18). At this point, all vessels supplying the right-sided colon have been managed.

4. Mobilization of the right mesocolon

Firstly, the root of the blood vessel is dissected, and the stumps of right colic vessels are lifted. Blunt and sharp dissection is performed along the Toldt's fascia downward and upward in a medial to lateral fashion. Dissection is then continued to the surface of duodenum, and the correct dissection plane should be smooth, flat, and clean. The identification of right ureter and the right gonadal vessels also indicates the correct space for dissection (Figure 3-20-19).

5. Management of the terminal ileum

The surgeon grasps the terminal ileum and carefully divides the mesentery according to the status of the vascular arcade. End-to-end anastomosis between the ileum and rectum can be performed if the colon specimen can be completely extracted through the vagina. If it is difficult, side-to-end anastomosis between the ileum and rectum can be performed. The mesentery of the ileum is divided to the pre-cut line, and approximately 3cm of the wall of ileum is isolated. The blood supply line should be checked carefully to ensure the blood supply of the anastomosis (Figure 3-20-20).

6. Mobilization of the right paracolic sulcus and greater omentum

The greater curvature is lifted to expose the course of the gastroepiploic vessels. In the transparent thin area of the gastrocolic ligament, the ultrasonic scalpel is applied to open the gastrocolic ligament to enter the omental bursa (Figure 3-20-21-Figure 3-20-23), and the course of the pancreas can be seen. Along the course of the right gastroepiploic artery and vein, the gastrocolic ligament is dissected and transected (Figure 3-20-24, Figure 3-20-25), whereafter the dissection is continued to the right to Henle's trunk (Figure 3-20-26). Subsequently, the posterior gastric wall and the right transverse

mesocolon are dissected, and the dissection planes are connected. After the hepatocolic ligament is transected (Figure 3-20-27), the surgeon incises downward along the right paracolic sulcus to the attachment of cecum (Figure 3-20-28) and gives direct access to the dissected mesentery of the terminal ileum. At this point, the dissection of the right-sided colon has been completed.

7. Management of the root of the inferior mesenteric artery

The surgeon stands on the right side of the patient, and the patient is placed in the anti-Trendelenburg position with right side tilted. The surgical field is adequately exposed. At this point, since the dissection of the mesentery of the terminal ileum is completed, the abdominal aorta and its bifurcation are visible (Figure 3-20-29). The posterior peritoneum is incised at the angle between the abdominal aorta and the inferior mesenteric artery. The lymphatic and adipose tissues are dissected at the root of the inferior mesenteric artery, and double ligation and division are performed at the root of vessels (Figure 3-20-30, Figure 3-20-31).

8. Management of the root of the inferior mesenteric vein

Dissection is performed along the left side of the abdominal aorta from the root of the inferior mesenteric artery to the Treitz ligament in a medial to lateral fashion. The left mesocolon is lifted (Figure 3-20-32) to transect the inferior mesenteric vein at the inferior border of the pancreas lateral to the Treitz ligament (Figure 3-20-33).

9. Mobilization of the left mesocolon

The surgeon lifts the left mesocolon and the inferior mesenteric artery stump and continues dissecting along the Toldt's fascia downward and upward in a medial to lateral fashion. The correct dissection plane should be smooth, flat, and clean (Figure 3-20-34). The course and peristalsis of the left ureter can be observed, and the left gonadal vessels and the left adipose capsule of kidney are identified. A gauze is placed underneath the mesentery for protection and indication (Figure 3-20-35).

10. Management of the left greater omentum and the left transverse mesocolon

The surgeon lifts the gastroomental vascular arch with the left hand and dissects along the gastroomental vascular arch to the left (Figure 3-20-36). Gradually, dissection is continued to the gastrocolic ligament, then to the lower pole of spleen (Figure 3-20-37). The assistant pulls down the greater omentum to expose the left transverse mesocolon and the pancreatic tail. In most cases, this is the avascular area of mesentery. Occasionally, vascular branches can be seen running from the left side of the Treitz ligament and near the tail of the pancreas to the splenic flexure of the colon. The surgeon applies the ultrasonic scalpel to dissect along the inferior border of pancreas, from the Treitz ligament and inferior mesenteric vein stump to the spleen and the paracolic sulcus lateral to the splenic flexure (Figure 3-20-38-Figure 3-20-40). When the dissection reaches the gauze underneath the left mesocolon, the left-sided colon is mobilized completely (Figure 3-20-41).

11. Mobilization of mesorectum and the isolation of rectum

The extent of rectal resection depends on the nature of the lesion, and the rectal ampulla should be preserved if possible. The defecation reflex receptors are located at the rectal ampulla. Therefore, the preservation of rectal ampulla can maintain the integrity of defecation reflex pathway, which facilitates the maintenance and recovery of bowel function. After the dissection of posterior and right rectal wall according to the principle of TME (Figure 3-20-42), the surgeon detaches the physiological sigmoid adhesions and dissects the peritoneum on the left of the rectum to the pre-cut line (Figure 3-20-43). The mesorectum on the right side of pre-cut line on the rectum is transected. Occasionally, the diameters of the superior rectal vessels are too big, and the distal side of vessels can be ligated with vascular clips to avoid bleeding. Following this, the surgeon transects the mesorectum at the same level on the left side of the rectum, and the assistant lifts the rectum. The surgeon further isolates the posterior rectal wall and gets both sides connected.

## [Specimen resection and digestive tract reconstruction]

1. Specimen resection

With a linear cutting stapler, the rectum is transected at the pre-cut line on the isolated area of rectum (Figure 3-20-44), as well as the ileum (Figure 3-20-45).

2. Specimen extraction

The vagina has also been considered another ideal option to remove more bulky colorectal specimen when

compared with anus, which presents several properties involving good elasticity, adequate blood supply, healing ability, and easy access. After the vaginal irrigation, the assistant introduces the bladder retractor through the vagina to indicate the posterior vaginal fornix. Under its indication, the surgeon applies the ultrasonic scalpel to open the posterior vaginal fornix transversely for approximately 3cm and extends the incision to 5-6cm by longitudinal stretch (Figure 3-20-46). The protective sleeve is introduced into the abdominal cavity through the vagina. The assistant applies the oval forceps to clamp the distal end of protective sleeve and pull it out through the vagina (Figure 3-20-47). At the same time, the surgeon and the assistant place the whole colon into the protective sleeve step by step (Figure 3-20-48), and the assistant gently pulls the specimen out of the body through the protective sleeve inside the vagina (Figure 3-20-49).

3. Digestive tract reconstruction

The assistant inserts the anvil into the abdominal cavity through the vagina, evaluates the distance between the terminal ileum and the rectal stump, and selects the site of anastomosis in the ileum. An incision of approximately 2cm is made on the ileum stump along the staple line (Figure 3-20-50), through which the anvil is placed in the ileal cavity (Figure 3-20-51). After the adjustment of position, the ileum stump is transected with the linear cutting stapler (Figure 3-20-52), and the resected stump can be extracted through the vagina. A small incision in the intended anastomosis site of the ileum is made to take out the anvil shaft (Figure 3-20-53). The assistant inserts the circular stapler through the anus and extends the trocar to pierce one corner of the rectal stump (Figure 3-20-54). The anvil is connected to the trocar of stapler (Figure 3-20-55) to complete the side-to-end anastomosis between the ileum and the rectum, then the anastomosis is sutured to be reinforced (Figure 3-20-56). Check the integrity of the anastomosis carefully. Air and water injection test is performed to confirm the integrity of the anastomosis (Figure 3-20-57), and active bleeding should be excluded. Two drainage tubes are placed in the pelvic cavity through the trocars on the left and right lower quadrant (Figure 3-20-58, Figure 3-20-59). Finally, the pneumoperitoneum is released and trocar sites are closed.

4. Suturing of the vaginal incision

Fully expose the vaginal incision, clamp the anterior and posterior wall of the vaginal incision with two Allis forceps, and perform interrupted suture with absorbable sutures (Figure 3-20-60). After making sure that there is no leakage or bleeding, an iodoform gauze can be indwelled in the vagina to compress the posterior vaginal fornix, and the gauze should be extracted 48 hours after operation.

# 21 Laparoscopic Radical Surgery for Transverse Colon Cancer with Transvaginal Specimen Extraction and Auxiliary Incision-Free Abdomen

## [Introduction]

Transverse colectomy can be selected for female patients with transverse colon cancer who undergo laparoscopic radical transverse colon cancer resection with transvaginal specimen extraction. This technique has stricter requirements for vaginal preoperative preparation. Transvaginal specimen extraction has broader indications due to the strong extensibility of the vagina, but is limited to female patients. The difficulty of this technique is mainly reflected in the complete endoscopic gastrointestinal reconstruction unique to the NOSES operation, that is, the overlapping triangular anastomosis using the laparoscopic linear cutting stapler.

## 21.1 Indications and contraindications

### [Indications]

1. Female transverse colon cancer or benign tumor.
2. Tumors with a circumferential diameter of

3-5cm.

3. Tumors without extra-serosal invasion.

## [Contraindications]

1. Excessively large tumors that preclude transvaginal extraction.

2. Tumor invasion of adjacent tissues and organs.

3. Severely obese patients (BMI>35kg/m$^2$).

## 21.2　Surgical procedure, techniques, and key points

### [Trocar placement]

1. The camera port (10mm trocar) can be placed between the umbilicus and a point 5cm inferior to the umbilicus.

2. The surgeon's main trocar (12mm trocar) is placed in the middle of the left upper quadrant, on the lateral edge of the rectus abdominis.

3. The surgeon's auxiliary trocar (5mm trocar) is placed at the lower left abdomen on a different level than that of the camera port.

4. The assistant's main trocar (5mm trocar) is placed at the McBurney's point.

5. The assistant's auxiliary trocar (5mm trocar) is placed at the upper right abdomen on the intersection between the right midclavicular line and transverse colon projection (Figure 3-21-1).

### [Exploration]

1. General exploration

Observe for any lesions such as metastatic implants on the surfaces of various organs and the peritoneum.

2. Tumor exploration

Determine the feasibility of surgery based on the tumor's location, size, and depth of invasion.

3. Evaluation of anatomical structures

The transverse colon has many adjacent organs, complex vasculature, and large anatomical variations. It is necessary to identify the ileocolic vessels, the right colic vessels, and the middle colic vessels. In addition, it is also necessary to evaluate the feasibility of laparoscopic overlapped triangle anastomosis between the ascending and transverse colon after the dissection of the transverse colon and the ascending colon.

### [Dissection and separation]

1. Management of the root of right colic vessels

The first incision is made using the ultrasonic scalpel at the weak area of the transverse mesocolon at the inferior margin of the pancreatic neck. And the space can then be expanded superiorly and to the right. The right colic artery is isolated and clipped at the root.

2. Management of the middle colic vessels

The middle colic vessels are separated from the inferior edge of pancreas, and then ligated and amputated.

3. Management of the Henle's truck

Continue to dissect along the duodenum and the surface of pancreatic head in the anterior pancreatic fascia. After careful dissection, it can be seen that the accessory right colonic vein, the right gastroepiploic vein, and the anterior superior pancreaticoduodenal vein join into the Henle's truck and then enter the superior mesenteric vein. Ligate and divide at the root of each vascular branch.

4. Management of the greater omentum and group 6 lymph nodes

Dissection and transection are then continued toward the right along the lateral edge of the right gastroepiploic arcade, and group 6 lymph nodes lateral to the arcade are removed.

5. Mobilization and management of the ascending mesocolon

The right genital vessels, pancreatic head and duodenum should be protected. The pre-cut line is determined 10cm from the proximal edge of the tumor. Then dissect the ascending mesocolon and isolate the bowel wall.

6. Management of the transverse mesocolon

The mesentery at the distal edge of the transverse colon is dissected and transected along the distal pre-cut line of the transverse colon. Subsequently, the surgeon ligates and transects the marginal vascular arch, then dissects to the pre-cut line of the transverse colon. The bowel wall is isolated.

### [Specimen resection and digestive tract reconstruction]

1. Specimen resection

The bowel is closed and transected at the pre-cut line

on the transverse colon using the linear cutting stapler (Figure 3-21-2). Subsequently, the ascending colon is closed and transected using a linear cutting stapler along the proximal pre-cut line on the transverse colon (Figure 3-21-3). This marks the completion of radical resection of the transverse colon tumor. The specimen is placed in a protective sleeve, and the bag is placed within the pelvic cavity (Figure 3-21-4).

2. Digestive tract reconstruction

The terminal transverse colon is pulled to the right, and the terminal ascending colon is pulled up to the upper abdomen to be placed overlapped with the transverse colon (Figure 3-21-5). Suture for fixation is performed between the transverse colon stump and the bowel wall at 7cm from the terminal ascending colon (Figure 3-21-6). The surgeon then checks the blood supply of both sides of the bowel, and estimates the tension of the anastomosis. After the examination, the transverse colon and terminal ascending colon are opened with two incisions (1cm for each) on the antimesenteric border (Figure 3-21-7, Figure 3-21-8). Then both bowel lumens are disinfected with alcoholic or the iodoform gauze. The linear cutting stapler is introduced through the surgeon's main trocar, where after the cartridge jaw and the anvil are inserted into the two bowel lumens separately. With the necessary adjustment, the stapler is fired to complete the side-to-side anastomosis between the transverse and ascending colon (Figure 3-21-9, Figure 3-21-10).

The bowel lumen is disinfected with alcoholic or the iodoform gauze again, and the integrity of the anastomosis is confirmed. If there is bleeding, suture to stop bleeding (Figure 3-21-11). After confirming no active bleeding, suture one needle at each of the two ends and the middle of the common opening of the intestinal tubes on both sides for traction and fixation (Figure 3-21-12). The surgeon and assistant grasp the tail of traction sutures to keep the side-to-side anastomosis V-shaped and close the enterotomies with a linear cutting stapler. The overlapped delta-shaped anastomosis between the transverse colon and ileum is completed (Figure 3-21-13, Figure 3-21-14).

3. Specimen extraction

After the assistant fully disinfects the vagina, place the oval forceps in the posterior vaginal fornix and open them upwards for indication. (Figure 3-21-15). The surgeon uses an ultrasonic scalpel to cut the posterior fornix horizontally about 3-5cm (Figure 3-21-16). The assistant applies the oval forceps into the abdominal cavity through the incision, and holds the specimen protective sleeve and one end of the intestinal tube (Figure 3-21-17, Figure 3-21-18). Then slowly pulls the specimen and the protective sleeve out of the body (Figure 3-21-19).

The surgeon uses V-loc suture to continuously suture the posterior vaginal fornix incision (Figure 3-21-20, Figure 3-21-21). The abdominal cavity was rinsed with distilled water, and the instruments were checked for complete. After confirming that there was no active bleeding, an abdominal drainage tube was indwelled through the right 12mm Trocar hole. Stop pneumoperitoneum, expel gas from abdominal cavity, and close the puncture hole.

## 22　Laparoscopic Radical Surgery for Transverse Colon Cancer with Transrectal Specimen Extraction via Rectal Incision and Auxiliary Incision-Free Abdomen

### [Introduction]

The key operative feature of this procedure occurs during laparoscopic digestive tract reconstruction; in these cases, the laparoscopic creation of an overlapped delta-shaped anastomosis using a linear cutting stapler is required, which is more technically challenging than other anastomosis procedures. Therefore, this procedure requires strict adherence to the indications, clear surgical thinking, and proficiency in surgical skills.

## 22.1    Indications and contraindications

### [Indications]

1. Transverse colon cancer or benign tumors.

2. Tumors with a circumferential diameter of 3-5cm.

3. Tumors without extra-serosal invasion.

### [Contraindications]

1. Excessively large tumors that preclude transanal extraction.

2. Tumor invasion of adjacent tissues and organs.

3. Severely obese patients (BMI>35kg/m$^2$).

## 22.2    Surgical procedure, techniques, and key points

### [Trocar placement]

1. The camera port (10mm trocar) can be placed between the umbilicus and a point 5cm inferior to the umbilicus.

2. The surgeon's main trocar (12mm trocar) is placed in the middle of the left upper quadrant, on the lateral edge of the rectus abdominis.

3. The surgeon's auxiliary trocar (5mm trocar) is placed at the lower left abdomen on a different level than that of the camera port.

4. The assistant's main trocar (12mm trocar) is placed at the McBurney's point.

5. The assistant's auxiliary trocar (5mm trocar) is placed at the upper right abdomen on the intersection between the right midclavicular line and transverse colon projection (Figure 3-22-1).

### [Exploration]

1. General exploration

Observe for any lesions such as metastatic implants on the surfaces of various organs and the peritoneum.

2. Tumor exploration

Determine the feasibility of surgery based on the tumor's location, size, and depth of invasion.

3. Evaluation of anatomical structures

The transverse colon has many adjacent organs, complex vasculature, and large anatomical variations. It is necessary to identify the ileocolic vessels, the right colic vessels, and the middle colic vessels. In addition, it is also necessary to evaluate the feasibility of laparoscopic overlapped triangle anastomosis between the ascending and transverse colon after the dissection of the transverse and ascending colon.

### [Dissection and separation]

1. Management of the root of right colic vessels

The first incision is made using the ultrasonic scalpel at the weak area of the transverse mesocolon at the inferior margin of the pancreatic neck. And the space can then be expanded superiorly and to the right. The right colic vessels is isolated and clipped at the root.

2. Management of the middle colic vessels

The middle colic vessels are separated from the inferior edge of pancreas, and then ligated and amputated.

3. Management of the Henle's truck

Continue to dissect along the duodenum and the surface of pancreatic head in the anterior pancreatic fascia. After careful dissection, it can be seen that the accessory right colonic vein, the right gastroepiploic vein, and the anterior superior pancreaticoduodenal vein join into the Henle's truck and then enter the superior mesenteric vein. Ligate and divide at the root of each vascular branch.

4. Management of the greater omentum and group 6 lymph nodes

Dissection and transection are then continued toward the right along the lateral edge of the right gastroepiploic arcade, and group 6 lymph nodes lateral to the arcade are removed.

5. Mobilization and management of the ascending mesocolon

The right genital vessels, pancreatic head and duodenum should be protected. The pre-cut line is determined 10cm from the proximal edge of the tumor. Then dissect the ascending mesocolon and isolate the bowel wall.

6. Management of the transverse mesocolon

The mesentery at the distal edge of the transverse colon is dissected and transected along the distal pre-cut line of the transverse colon. Subsequently, the surgeon ligates and transects the marginal vascular arch, then dissects to the pre-cut line of the transverse colon. The

bowel wall is isolated.

## [Specimen resection and digestive tract reconstruction]

### 1. Specimen resection

The bowel is closed and transected at the pre-cut line on the transverse colon using the linear cutting stapler (Figure 3-22-2). Subsequently, the ascending colon is closed and transected using a linear cutting stapler along the proximal pre-cut line on the transverse colon (Figure 3-22-3). This marks the completion of radical resection of the transverse colon tumor. The specimen is placed in a protective sleeve, and placed within the pelvic cavity (Figure 3-22-4).

### 2. Digestive tract reconstruction

The two stumps of the transverse colon are overlapped and placed (Figure 3-22-5). The proximal and distal transverse colon stumps are secured with a suture at an overlap of 7cm (Figure 3-22-6). Adequate blood supply to the bilateral bowels and a tension-free anastomosis are ensured, and 1cm incisions are made on the antimesenteric border of the proximal stump and the corresponding antimesenteric border of the distal transverse colon (Figure 3-22-7, Figure 3-22-8). The incision of the bowel wall is disinfected using alcohol or the iodoform gauze. The linear cutting stapler is introduced via the surgeon's main trocar port. The two sides of the cartridge are placed within the respective lumens of the proximal and distal transverse colon stumps, and adjustments are made where necessary. The stapler is fired after inspection to complete side-to-side anastomosis of the transverse colon (Figure 3-22-9-Figure 3-22-11).

The common opening of the two stumps is disinfected using alcohol or the iodoform gauze, and the side-to-side anastomosis is inspected for intra-luminal bleeding, which can be sutured for hemostasis. When no active bleeding is observed, the common opening of the two bowel stumps is closed with continuous sutures using the V-Loc barbed thread.

### 3. Specimen extraction

The rectum is transanally disinfected and the assistant uses oval forceps to place an the iodoform gauze at the rectum and opens the forceps toward the left and right to indicate the position for incision (Figure 3-22-12). The surgeon uses the ultrasonic scalpel to create a longitudinal incision of 3-5cm at the anterior rectal wall (Figure 3-22-13). Subsequently, the assistant inserts the oval forceps into the abdominal cavity via the incision on the anterior rectal wall and clamps the specimen protective sleeve at one end of the bowel (Figure 3-22-14, Figure 3-22-15). The specimen and protective sleeve are gradually pulled through the rectal incision and extracted extracorporeally (Figure 3-22-16).

The anterior rectal wall is then closed laparoscopically with continuous sutures using the V-Loc barbed thread (Figure 3-22-17, Figure 3-22-18). The abdominal cavity is irrigated with distilled water, the instruments are inspected, the patient is checked for active bleeding, and one indwelling abdominal drainage tube is inserted via the right 12mm trocar port. The pneumoperitoneum is deflated by exsufflating the gas from the abdominal cavity, and the trocar port are closed.

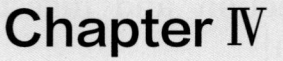

# Chapter IV
# Standardized Procedures of Laparoscopic Gastric NOSES

## 1 Laparoscopic Distal Gastrectomy with Transrectal Specimen Extraction and Auxiliary Incision-Free Abdomen
### (GC-NOSES I, Billroth I Anastomosis)

### [Introduction]

GC-NOSES I is a novel surgical procedure for tumor located at the middle and lower third of the stomach, $T_3$ or below, and the largest diameter of the tumor is less than 5cm, which is mostly applicable to male patients. The main feature of this procedure include: after the perigastric lymph node dissection is completed, the specimen is placed in the protective sleeve and can be extracted through the rectum. This procedure does not require auxiliary incisions in the abdominal wall to extract the specimen out of the body. After the surgery, only a few tiny trocar scars are left on the abdominal wall, which makes this procedure a truly laparoscopic radical gastrectomy for gastric cancer.

## 1.1 Indications and contraindications

### [Indications]

1. Gastric cancer, stage $cT_{1-3}N_{0-1}M_0$, with lesions in the distal part of stomach.
2. The largest diameter of tumor ≤ 5cm.
3. BMI ≤ 30kg/m².

### [Contraindications]

1. The tumor is too large to be pulled out through the rectum.

2. It is suspected that the tumor invades beyond the serosa or involves adjacent organs.
3. Patients with acute gastrointestinal obstruction or tumor perforation requiring emergency surgery.
4. Severely obese patients (BMI>30kg/m²), especially those with high visceral fat content.
5. Patients with history of pelvic surgery or rectal and anal deformities.

## 1.2 Surgical procedure, techniques, and key points

### [Trocar placement]

1. The camera trocar (10mm trocar) is located at the umbilicus or 1cm above or below the umbilicus according to the abdominal type of the patient.
2. The surgeon's main trocar (12mm trocar) is located 1-2cm below the costal margin of the left anterior axillary line.
3. The surgeon's auxiliary trocar (5mm trocar) is located at the umbilical level of the left midclavicular line.
4. The assistant's auxiliary trocar (5mm trocar) is located 1-2cm under the costal margin of the right anterior axillary line.
5. The assistant's main trocar (10mm trocar) is located at the umbilical level of the right midclavicular line (Figure 4-1-1).

## [Exploration]

1. General exploration

Observe for any lesions such as metastatic implants on the surfaces of various organs and the peritoneum.

2. Tumor exploration

Determine the feasibility of surgery based on the tumor's location, size, and depth of invasion.

3. Evaluation of anatomical structures

Determine the surgical plan based on the tumor's location, and anatomical structures, and evaluate the feasibility of transrectal extraction.

## [Dissection and separation]

1. Mobilization of the greater omentum and dissection of lymph nodes of the subpyloric region

During the dissection, under the premise of ensuring the safety of distal resection margin, preserving the duodenum long enough for Billroth I gastroduodenal anastomosis.

2. Dissection of lymph nodes in the superior pancreatic region

Move the stomach to the right upper quadrant to fully expose the superior plane of the pancreas, and complete the dissection of lymph nodes in the corresponding region.

3. Dissection of lymph nodes in the lesser curvature of stomach

Adopt the posterior approach to lift the stomach cephalad ventrally, and complete the dissection of group 1 and 3 lymph nodes.

4. Dissection of group 4sb lymph nodes

Gradually dissect the anterior fascia plane of the pancreas at the lower pole of spleen and the tail of pancreas cephalad to the splenic hilar region. Ligate and transect the left gastroepiploic vessels at the root to complete the dissection of group 4sb lymph nodes.

5. Transection of the distal stomach

Transect the gastric body with two 60mm linear cutting staplers with blue cartridge at 8cm on the side of the greater curvature and 5-6cm on the side of the lesser curvature from the upper edge of the tumor.

## [Specimen resection and digestive tract reconstruction]

1. Specimen resection

At 8cm from the greater curvature side and 5-6cm from the lesser curvature side of the primary cancer focus, the gastric body was transected with two 60mm linear cutting staplers.

2. Specimen extraction

The patient is placed in the Trendelenburg position. At about 5-6cm above the peritoneal reflection, make an incision about 3-5cm in length in the anterior rectal wall along the longitudinal axis of the bowel wall of the antimesenteric border of the rectum (Figure 4-1-2). The assistant inserts the grasping forceps from the anus and introduce it into the abdominal cavity through the incision in the anterior rectal wall. The surgeon hands one end of the specimen bag to the grasping forceps of the assistant. The surgeon lifts the bowel wall at the rectal incision and gently pulls it cephalad with the left hand. Meanwhile, the assistant slowly pulls the specimen bag out of the anus to complete the transanal specimen extraction (Figure 4-1-3). After the specimen extraction, irrigate the pelvic cavity repeatedly, suture the incision in the anterior rectal wall with 3-0 V-loc barbed suture in a continuous manner, and make several interrupted sutures for embedding.

3. Digestive tract reconstruction

A window is opened in the proximal greater curvature side 5cm from the stump of the stomach, and another window is opened in the duodenal stump. A 60mm linear cutting stapler with blue cartridge is inserted in the two windows to perform Billroth I anastomosis between the proximal greater curvature of the remnant stomach and the anterior wall of the duodenum (Figure 4-1-4). After firing the stapler, remove the stapler and see if there is active bleeding (Figure 4-1-5), and suture the common opening with 3-0 V-loc barbed suture in a continuous manner (Figure 4-1-6). Lift the remnant stomach ventrally, check for the presence of anastomotic tension and complete the Billroth I gastroduodenal anastomosis (Figure 4-1-7).

# 2 Laparoscopic Distal Gastrectomy with Transvaginal Specimen Extraction and Auxiliary Incision-Free Abdomen

## (GC-NOSES II, Billroth I Anastomosis)

### [Introduction]

GC-NOSES II is a novel surgical procedure for tumor located at the middle and lower third of the stomach, $T_3$ or below stage, and the largest diameter of the tumor less than 5cm, which is mostly applicable to female patients with cosmetic requirements for the abdominal wall. The main feature of this procedure include: after the perigastric lymph node dissection is completed, the greater omentum and the distal stomach is placed in the specimen bag and can be extracted through the posterior vaginal fornix. This procedure does not require auxiliary incisions in the abdominal wall to extract the specimen out of the body. After the surgery, only a few tiny trocar scars are left on the abdominal wall, which makes this procedure a truly laparoscopic radical gastrectomy for gastric cancer.

## 2.1 Indications and contraindications

### [Indications]

1. Gastric cancer, stage $cT_{1-3}N_{0-1}M_0$, with lesions in the distal part of stomach.

2. The largest diameter of tumor $\leqslant$ 5cm.

3. BMI $\leqslant$ 30kg/m$^2$.

4. Female patients.

### [Contraindications]

1. The tumor is too large to be pulled out through the vagina.

2. It is suspected that the tumor invades beyond the serosa or involves adjacent organs.

3. Patients with acute gastrointestinal obstruction or tumor perforation requiring emergency surgery.

4. Severely obese patients (BMI>30kg/m$^2$), especially those with high visceral fat content.

5. Patients with history of pelvic or gynecological surgery or vaginal deformities.

## 2.2 Surgical procedure, techniques, and key points

### [Trocar placement]

1. The camera trocar (10mm trocar) is located at the umbilicus or 1cm above or below the umbilicus according to the abdominal type of the patient.

2. The surgeon's main trocar (12mm trocar) is located 1-2cm below the costal margin of the left anterior axillary line.

3. The surgeon's auxiliary trocar (5mm trocar) is located at the umbilical level of the left midclavicular line.

4. The assistant's auxiliary trocar (5mm trocar) is located 1-2cm under the costal margin of the right anterior axillary line.

5. The assistant's main trocar (10mm trocar) is located at the umbilical level of the right midclavicular line (Figure 4-2-1).

### [Exploration]

1. General exploration

Observe for any lesions such as metastatic implants on the surfaces of various organs and the peritoneum.

2. Tumor exploration

Determine the feasibility of surgery based on the tumor's location, size, and depth of invasion.

3. Evaluation of anatomical structures

Determine the surgical plan based on the tumor's location, and anatomical structures, and evaluate the feasibility of transanal extraction.

## [Dissection and separation]

1. Mobilization of the greater omentum and dissection of lymph nodes of the subpyloric region

During the dissection, under the premise of ensuring the safety of distal resection margin, preserving duodenum long enough for Billroth I gastroduodenal anastomosis.

2. Dissection of lymph nodes in the superior pancreatic region

Move the stomach to the right upper quadrant to fully expose the superior plane of the pancreas, and complete the dissection of lymph nodes in the corresponding region.

3. Dissection of lymph nodes in the lesser curvature of stomach

Adopt the posterior approach to lift the stomach cephalad ventrally, and complete the dissection of group 1 and 3 lymph nodes.

4. Dissection of group 4sb lymph nodes

Gradually dissect the anterior fascia plane of the pancreas at the lower pole of spleen and the tail of pancreas cephalad to the splenic hilar region. Ligate and transect the left gastroepiploic vessels at the root to complete the dissection of group 4sb lymph nodes.

## [Specimen resection and digestive tract reconstruction]

1. Specimen resection

Transect the gastric body with two 60mm linear cutting staplers with blue cartridge at 8cm on the side of the greater curvature and 5-6cm on the side of the lesser curvature from the upper edge of the tumor.

2. Specimen extraction

First, after the vagina is thoroughly irrigated by the perineal assistant, the patient is placed in the Trendelenburg position. The small bowel is moved to the upper abdomen. Without any obstruction in the pelvic cavity, the uterus is suspended ventrally with the purse-string suture through the broad ligaments on both sides, so that the posterior vaginal fornix can be fully exposed. At the peritoneal reflection, the assistant lifts the cervix ventrally with a uterine manipulator, and the surgeon applies the cautery hook to make a 4-5cm incision along the posterior vaginal fornix (Figure 4-2-2), and introduces a specimen bag through the incision in the posterior vaginal fornix (Figure 4-2-3). One end of the specimen bag is introduced into the posterior vaginal fornix, and the assistant slowly pulls the specimen bag out of the body through the vagina with the grasping forceps. The operation should be gently performed to avoid bleeding of the posterior vaginal fornix (Figure 4-2-4). After the specimen extraction, the incision in the posterior vaginal fornix is continuously sutured with a 3-0 absorbable suture. Several interrupted stitches or continuous suture with V-loc barbed suture are performed for reinforcement (Figure 4-2-5, Figure 4-2-6). After the suture, the pelvic cavity is irrigated again, and the patient is placed in the reverse-Trendelenburg position again for the following digestive tract reconstruction.

3. Digestive tract reconstruction

A window is opened in the proximal greater curvature side 5cm from the gastric stump, and another window is opened in the duodenal stump. A 60mm linear cutting stapler with blue cartridge is inserted in the two windows to perform Billroth I anastomosis between the proximal greater curvature of the remnant stomach and the anterior wall of the duodenum (Figure 4-2-7). After firing the stapler, remove the linear cutting stapler and see if there is active bleeding (Figure 4-2-8), and suture the common opening with 3-0 V-loc barbed suture in a continuous manner (Figure 4-2-9). Lift the remnant stomach ventrally, check for the presence of anastomotic tension and complete the Billroth I gastroduodenal anastomosis (Figure 4-2-10).

# 3 Laparoscopic Distal Gastrectomy with Transrectal Specimen Extraction and Auxiliary Incision-Free Abdomen

## (GC-NOSES III, Billroth II Anastomosis)

### [Introduction]

GC-NOSES III is mainly applicable to male gastric cancer patients and some female patients having a small specimen size of the tumor, within stage $T_3$ and without serosal infiltrating. Except that the method of specimen extracting is different from that of conventional laparoscopic surgery, the extent of gastrointestinal resection and lymph node dissection, as well as dissecting plane during the surgery are consistent with conventional laparoscopic surgery. The operating characteristics are as follows: perform radical resection of gastric cancer and digestive tract reconstruction under laparoscope with an incision in the upper rectum, and remove the specimen through the rectum. This procedure requires the surgeon to fully understand the indications, and the doctor and patient's acceptance on the risk of surgery should be evaluated.

## 3.1 Indications and contraindications

### [Indications]

1. Gastric cancer, stage $cT_{1-3}N_{1-2}M_0$, with lesions in the distal part of stomach.

2. The maximum diameter of tumor is better $\leqslant$ 4cm.

### [Contraindications]

1. The tumor is too large to be pulled out through the anus.

2. The tumor invades the serosa or involves adjacent organs.

3. Patients with acute gastrointestinal obstruction or tumor perforation requiring emergency surgery.

4. Severely obese patients (BMI>35kg/m$^2$).

5. Patients with history of pelvic surgery or rectal and anal deformities.

## 3.2 Surgical procedure, techniques, and key points

### [Trocar placement]

Trocar sites of the operation should meet the needs of both radical gastrectomy for gastric cancer and transrectal specimen collection.

1. The camera trocar (10mm trocar) is located at 1cm below the umbilicus.

2. The surgeon's main trocar (12mm trocar) is 2cm below the costal margin of the left anterior axillary line.

3. The surgeon's auxiliary trocar (5mm trocar) is at the umbilical level of the left midclavicular line.

4. The assistant's auxiliary trocar (5mm trocar) is under the costal margin of the right anterior axillary line.

5. The assistant's main trocar (12mm trocar) is at the umbilical level of the right midclavicular line (Figure 4-3-1).

### [Exploration]

1. General exploration

Observe for any lesions such as metastatic implants on the surfaces of various organs and the peritoneum.

2. Tumor exploration

Determine the feasibility of surgery based on the tumor's location, size, and depth of invasion.

3. Evaluation of anatomical structures

Determine the surgical plan based on the tumor's location, and anatomical structures, and evaluate the feasibility of transrectal extraction.

### [Dissection and separation]

1. Dissection of the greater omentum

The greater omentum is flipped cephalad and transected from the left side of the transverse colon. After

the lesser omental sac is entered, the dissection is turned to the right to the hepatic flexure, and continued to the posterior side of the anterior lobe of mesocolon. Next, the anterior lobe of the mesocolon is resected.

2. Dissection of lymph nodes around the stomach

2.1 Dissection of group 6 lymph nodes

Using the middle colic artery and vein as a marker, enter the fused fascial space between the gastroduodenum and the mesentery of the transverse colon. Expose the Henle's trunk and dissect the right gastroepiploic vein at the root. Continue the dissection along the surface of the pancreatic head to open the gastro-pancreatic ligament and expose the gastroduodenal artery. Then, expose and dissect the right gastroepiploic artery at the root to completely clear the lymph nodes of group 6.

2.2 Dissection of group 4sb lymph nodes

Expose the pancreatic tail and locate the splenic vessels. Release the splenic flexure of the colon and separate the adhesions between the greater omentum and the middle and lower poles of the spleen. Protect the pancreatic tail and expose the root. After dissecting into the branches of the lower pole of the spleen, transect the left gastroepiploic artery and vein and clear the lymph nodes of the fourth splenic branch.

2.3 Dissection of group 11p, 7, 8, 9 lymph nodes:

The separation is performed closely along the upper edge of the pancreas to expose the proximal end of splenic artery, followed by dissection of group 11p lymph nodes. After the celiac trunk is exposed, the left gastric artery and vein are separated and transected after clipping at the root. Subsequently, group 7, 8 and 9 lymph nodes are dissected.

2.4 Dissection of group 5 and 12a lymph nodes

The surgeon then exposes the common hepatic artery by retracting the pancreas inferolaterally to the left. The right gastric artery and the proper hepatic artery are adequately exposed along the gastroduodenal artery and the common hepatic artery. The anterior and lateral sides of the proper hepatic artery are dissected upwards, and group 12a lymph nodes are dissected. The right gastric artery and vein are transected after being ligated at the root and group 5 lymph nodes are dissected. The duodenum is transected with a linear cutting stapler at the distal end of pylorus and group 5 lymph nodes are dissected.

2.5 Dissection of group 1 and 3 lymph nodes

An ultrasonic scalpel is applied to cut closely along the stomach wall of lesser curvature, and dissect the lymph nodes in lesser curvature and the right side of cardia (groups 1 and 3 lymph nodes).

## [Specimen resection and digestive tract reconstruction]

1. Specimen resection

The stomach is dissected 5cm proximal to the tumour using an intracavitary linear cutting stapler. The appropriate nail bin is selected according to the thickness of the gastric wall (Figure 4-3-2). The surgeon then places the protective sleeve into the abdominal cavity through the main trocar port and places the resected specimen into the specimen bag (Figure 4-3-3).

2. Digestive tract reconstruction

2.1 Billroth II anastomosis

Windows are opened in the antimesenteric border of the jejunum 15-20cm from the ligament of Treitz and at the point of gastric stump and greater curvature, respectively. A 60mm linear cutting stapler is applied to perform the side-to-side anastomosis between the jejunum and the proximal gastric stump in an antecolic fashion. The common opening of stomach and jejunum is ligated with a 4-0 absorbable suture in an interrupted pattern. (Figure 4-3-4-Figure 4-3-8).

2.2 Roux-en-Y anastomosis of the distal gastric jejunum

The side-to-side anastomosis of the gastric jejunum and closing of the common opening of gastric jejunum is same as those of Billroth II anastomosis. The proximal and distal jejunum are anastomosed with a 60mm linear cutting stapler in a side-to-side fashion. The location of the intragastric anastomosis was 7-10cm from the ligament of Treitz and the location of the outtragastric anastomosis was 40-45cm from the gastrojejunal anastomosis. The blocking position of afferent loop is about 3cm from the gastric jejunum anastomosis (Figure 4-3-9-Figure 4-3-11).

3. Specimen extraction

After radical resection of gastric cancer and the digestive tract reconstruction, the patient is placed in the functional lithotomy position, then the perineal area and rectal cavity is disinfected with diluted povidone-

iodine solution. The laparoscopic monitor is moved to the side of patient's foot, while the patient is placed in the right-leaning Trendelenburg position. The assistant stretches the sigmoid colon to fully expose the upper rectum, making it parallel to the longitudinal axis of the body, and then the surgeon makes an incision of 5-6cm length in the anterior wall of the upper rectum (Figure 4-3-12). The pelvis is repeatedly disinfected with diluted povidone-iodine solution and irrigated with normal saline, after which a protective sleeve is placed (Figure 4-3-13, Figure 4-3-14), and the specimen is removed from the anus through the protective sleeve (Figure 4-3-15, Figure 4-3-16). Finally, the rectum incision is sutured in continuous or intermittent pattern, and the pelvic cavity is irrigated repeatedly (Figure 4-3-17, Figure 4-3-18).

# 4 Laparoscopic Distal Gastrectomy with Transvaginal Specimen Extraction and Auxiliary Incision-Free Abdomen
## (GC-NOSES IV , Billroth II Anastomosis)

GC-NOSES IV is mainly applicable to female patients with tumors located at the middle and lower stomach. On the basis of strict adherence to the radical resection of tumor and digestive tract reconstruction in the conventional laparoscopic surgery for gastric cancer, this procedure adopts total laparoscopic operation, incision of the posterior vaginal fornix, and transvaginal specimen extraction. According to the *Expert Consensus of Natural Orifice Specimen Extraction Surgery (NOSES) in Colorectal Neoplasm (2017)*, this is a resection extraction procedure.

## 4.1 Indications and contraindications

### [Indications]

1. Female patients.
2. Gastric cancer, stage $cT_{1-3}N_{0-1}M_0$, with lesions in the distal part of stomach.
3. The maximum diameter of tumor is better ≤ 4cm.

### [Contraindications]

1. Female patients with fertility plan.
2. Locally advanced cancer ($cT_4N_{2-3}M_1$).
3. The tumor is too large to be pulled out through the posterior vaginal fornix.
4. Severely obese patients (BMI>30kg/m²).
5. Patients with history of pelvic surgery or vaginal deformities.

## 4.2 Surgical procedure, techniques, and key points

### [Trocar placement]

1. The camera trocar (10mm trocar) is located 1cm below the umbilicus.
2. The surgeon's main trocar (12mm trocar) is located below the costal margin of the left anterior axillary line.
3. The surgeon's auxiliary trocar (5mm trocar) is located at the umbilical level of the left midclavicular line.
4. The assistant's auxiliary trocar (5mm trocar) is located under the costal margin of the right anterior axillary line.
5. The assistant's main trocar (12mm trocar) is located at the umbilical level of the right midclavicular line (Figure 4-4-1).

### [Exploration]

1. General exploration

Observe for any lesions such as metastatic implants on the surfaces of various organs and the peritoneum.

2. Tumor exploration

The tumor is located at the anterior wall of gastric antrum and does not invade beyond the serosal layer.

3. Evaluation of anatomical structures

Determine the surgical plan based on the tumor's

location, and vaginal structures, and evaluate the feasibility of transvaginal extraction.

## [Dissection and separation]

1. Dissection of the greater omentum

The greater omentum is flipped cephalad and transected from the left side of the transverse colon. The lesser omental sac is entered, and the incision is extended to the hepatic flexure of colon on the right side. Dissection is performed along the posterior region of the anterior lobe of the transverse mesocolon. The anterior lobe of the mesocolon is resected.

2. Dissection of group 4sb lymph nodes

The pancreatic tail is exposed to identify the splenic vessels. The splenic flexure is mobilized, then the adhesion between the greater omentum and middle and lower pole of spleen is detached. Attention should be paid for the protection of the pancreatic tail. The left gastroepiploic artery and vein are exposed and transected at the root after they derived into the branch of the lower pole of spleen, then group 4sb lymph nodes are dissected.

3. Dissection of group 6 lymph nodes

With the guidance of middle colic vessel, the fusion fascia space between the gastroduodenum and transverse mesocolon is entered, and the right gastroepiploic vein is transected. The dissection is continued along the surface of the pancreatic head to expose the gastroduodenal artery. The right gastroepiploic artery is isolated and transected at the root, then group 6 lymph nodes are completely dissected.

4. Transection of the duodenum

The duodenum is first exposed using the Kocher method. This involves incising the peritoneum and separating it from the duodenum, which is then turned inward. The duodenum is then exposed and the surrounding tissues are cleansed, especially around the pylorus. Group 6 lymph nodes are also removed. Finally, the duodenum is closed and severed in the predetermined position using a closure device or sutures to ensure that the severed end is securely closed.

5. Dissection of group 8a and 12a lymph nodes

The surgeon then dissects along the superior border of pancreas to expose the common hepatic artery. The pancreas is gently pushed to the lower left, and group 8a lymph nodes is dissected along the anterior and superior border of the common hepatic artery. The assistant pulls the common hepatic artery downwards to the right and the surgeon facilitates the dissection of the lymphatic and adipose tissues medial to the proper hepatic artery and the portal vein, i.e., group 12a lymph nodes. The root of the right gastric vascular is ligated and transected.

6. Dissection of group 11p, 7, and 9 lymph nodes

The pancreatic capsule is opened to perform dissection along the superior border of pancreas. The proximal end of the splenic artery is exposed, and group 11p lymph nodes are dissected. From left to right, the celiac trunk is exposed and the left gastric artery and vein are dissected and transected after being ligated at the root, and group 7 and 9 lymph nodes are dissected.

7. Dissection of lymph nodes in the lesser curvature and the right side of cardia

The peritoneum is incised in layers using an ultrasonic scalpel along the stomach wall of the lesser curvature, and dissect the lymph nodes in lesser curvature and the right side of cardia (group 1 and 3 lymph nodes).

## [Specimen resection and digestive tract reconstruction]

1. Specimen resection

Dissect the stomach 5cm from the proximal end of the tumor (Figure 4-4-2), select the appropriate nail compartment according to the thickness of the gastric wall, place the protective sleeve into the abdominal cavity through the main trocar port, and place the resected specimen into the specimen bag (Figure 4-4-3).

2. Digestive tract reconstruction

2.1    Billroth II anastomosis

Windows are opened in the antimesenteric border of the jejunum 15-20cm from the ligament of Treitz (Figure 4-4-4) and at the point of gastric stump and greater curvature (Figure 4-4-5). A 60mm linear cutting stapler is applied to perform the side-to-side anastomosis between the jejunum and the proximal gastric stump in an antecolic fashion (Figure 4-4-6). The common opening is sutured with a 4-0 absorbable suture in an interrupted pattern or 3-0 barbed suture in a continuous pattern (Figure 4-4-7).

### 2.2 Roux-en-Y anastomosis of the gastric jejunum

The side-to-side anastomosis of the gastric jejunum and closing of the opening of gastric jejunum is the same as those of Billroth II anastomosis. The proximal and distal jejunum are anastomosed with a 60mm linear cutting stapler in a side-to-side fashion. The location of the intragastric anastomosis was 7-10cm from the ligament of Treitz and the location of the outtragastric anastomosis was 40-45cm from the gastrojejunal anastomosis (Figure 4-4-8, Figure 4-4-9). The blocking position of afferent loop is about 3cm from the anastomosis position of gastric jejunum (Figure 4-4-10).

3. Specimen extraction

The vagina is disinfected repeatedly. After the uterus is suspended (Figure 4-4-11), the posterior vaginal fornix is withstood with an abdominal spatula (Figure 4-4-12) to facilitate the surgeron to make incision in the posterior vaginal fornix. Attention should be paid to ensure the incision is not exceeding the bilateral sacral ligaments (Figure 4-4-13). A protective sleeve is placed transvaginally (Figure 4-4-14). The specimen is held by the oval forceps and extracted along the long axis of stomach (Figure 4-4-15-Figure 4-4-17). The pelvic cavity is irrigated repeatedly with distilled water, diluted povidone-iodine solution, and saline solution (Figure 4-4-18). The incision of the posterior vaginal fornix is closed by continuous suture with 3-0 barbed suture (Figure 4-4-19).

## 5 Laparoscopic Proximal Gastrectomy with Transanal Specimen Extraction and Auxiliary Incision-Free Abdomen
### (GC-NOSES V)

### [Abstract]

Proximal gastrectomy is a standard procedure for early gastric cancer or benign lesions in the upper stomach (eg. cardia, fundus, and partial gastric body). GC-NOSES V is mainly applicable to male and some female patients with early lesions in the upper stomach. On the basis of strict adherence to the radical resection of tumor and digestive tract reconstruction in the conventional laparoscopic surgery for gastric cancer, this procedure opens the rectum and extracts the specimen through the anus, which manifests the combination of minimally invasive surgery and function preservation surgery. This is a resection extraction NOSES procedure. The operating characteristics of this procedure are: ①Radical resection of gastric cancer, dissection of lymph nodes, and digestive tract reconstruction completely under laparoscopy. The operation is the same as that in the conventional laparoscopic surgery and the operation difficulty is not increased. ②With no auxiliary incision in the abdominal wall, the function of abdominal wall is preserved and the postoperative pain is reduced to the maximum extent.

## 5.1 Indications and contraindications

### [Indications]

1. Upper gastric cancer, stage $cT_{1-2}N_0M_0$.

2. The circumferential diameter of tumor is better $\leqslant$ 4cm.

### [Contraindications]

1. Locally advanced cancer ($cT_{3-4}N_{1-3}M_{0-1}$).

2. The tumor is too large to be pulled out through the anus.

3. Patients with acute gastrointestinal obstruction or tumor perforation requiring emergency surgery.

4. Severely obese patients (BMI>30kg/m$^2$).

5. Patients with history of pelvic surgery or rectal and anal deformities.

## 5.2   Patient position, trocar Placement and surgical team position

### [Patient position]

The patient should be placed in the horizontal supine position with legs abduction (Figure 4-5-1), which will be changed to the functional lithotomy position (Figure 4-5-2) when removing the specimen by opening the rectum.

### [Trocar placement]

1. The camera trocar (10mm trocar) is located 1cm below the umbilicus.

2. The surgeon's main trocar (12mm trocar) is located 2cm below the costal margin of the left anterior axillary line.

3. The surgeon's auxiliary trocar (5mm trocar) is located at the umbilical level of the left midclavicular line.

4. The assistant's auxiliary trocar (5mm trocar) is located under the costal margin of the right anterior axillary line.

5. The assistant's main trocar (12mm trocar) is located at the umbilical level of the right midclavicular line (Figure 4-5-3).

### [Surgical team position]

1   Abdominal exploration, anatomical dissection and lymph node dissection

The positions of the surgeon, assistant and camera holder should be on the left side, right side, and between the patient's legs, separately (Figure 4-5-4).

2.  Digestive tract reconstruction

The positions of the surgeon, assistant and camera holder should be on the right side, left side, and between the patient's legs, separately (Figure 4-5-5).

3.  Transanal specimen extraction

The positions of the surgeon, assistant and camera holder should be on the right side, left side and the left side of the patient, separately (Figure 4-5-6). In this step, the monitor should be placed on the side of the patient's foot.

### [Surgical instruments]

Ultrasonic scalpel, 60mm linear cutting stapler, 3-0 barbed suture, 4-0 absorbable suture, protective sleeve.

## 5.3   Surgical procedure, techniques, and key points

### [Exploration]

On the basis of detailed preoperative examination, the liver, gallbladder, stomach, spleen, greater omentum, colon, small intestine, mesocolic surface, and pelvic cavity are routinely examined for the presence of tumor seeding, ascites and other abnormalities.

### [Dissection and separation]

1. Dissection of the greater omentum

Elevate the greater omentum cranially, then divide it from the left side of the transverse colon to enter the lesser sac. Proceed to the right toward the hepatic flexure of the colon, dissecting behind the anterior leaf of the transverse mesocolon. Carefully remove the anterior leaf of the transverse mesocolon while preserving the right gastroepiploic vessels. The right gastroepiploic vessels provide the sole blood supply to the remnant stomach. If injured, total gastrectomy may become necessary; therefore, protecting the right gastroepiploic vessels is of critical importance.

2. Mobilize the proximal stomach and divide the blood vessels.

The greater omentum is transected from the middle of colon to the splenic flexure. The left gastroepiploic vessels are transected at the root, and group 4sb lymph nodes are dissected. Apply the ultrasonic scalpel to transect the short gastric artery close to the hilum of the spleen, then group 4sa lymph nodes are dissected.

3. Dissection of group 7, 8a, 9, 11p and 11d lymph nodes

The left gastric vessels are identified, skeletonized and transected at the origin. Group 7, 9 and 11p lymph nodes are dissected. Afterwards, the surgeon then performs dissection along the splenic artery to remove group 11d lymph nodes, then performs dissection along the common hepatic artery and the proper hepatic artery to remove group 8a lymph nodes.

4. Dissection of group 1 and 2 lymph nodes and skeletonize the esophagus

Dissection is continued to the left side of the

cardia, transects the anterior and posterior vagal trunk, and isolates the lower esophagus. Traction stitch is sutured in the esophagus proximal to the tumor to pull the esophagus downwards. The surgeon then continues to dissect the esophagus upwards adequately, until the length of isolated esophagus is enough to obtain enough resection margin and to meet the need of anastomosis.

### [Specimen resection and digestive tract reconstruction]

1. Specimen resection

The esophagus is transected with a linear cutting stapler at 2cm above the esophagogastric junction, and the stomach is transected with a linear cutting stapler at 5cm from the distal end of the tumor. The resected specimen is placed in a specimen bag (Figure 4-5-7-Figure 4-5-9).

2. Digestive tract reconstruction (Overlap method)

Stitches are made on the left and right sides of the esophageal stump with the 3-0 Polyglactin 910 Suture (3-0 Vicryl™). The ultrasonic scalpel is applied to open the middle of the esophageal stump. Subsequently, with the guidance of the gastric tube, the surgeon inserts the two jaws of the linear cutting stapler into the esophageal lumen and the gastric cavity, respectively. After the anastomosis between the posterior wall of the esophagus and the anterior wall of the remnant stomach is created, the common opening is closed with 3-0 barbed suture (Figure 4-5-10-Figure 4-5-13).

3. Transrectal specimen extraction

After radical resection of the gastric cancer and the digestive tract reconstruction, the patient is placed in the functional lithotomy position, then the perineal area and rectal cavity is disinfected with the iodophor. The laparoscopic monitor is moved to the side of patient's foot, while the patient is placed in the right-leaning Trendelenburg position. The assistant stretches the sigmoid colon to fully expose the upper rectum, and then the surgeon makes an incision of 5-6cm length in the anterior wall of the upper rectum (Figure 4-5-14). The protective sleeve is inserted into the rectum after disinfecting with diluted povidone-iodine solution (Figure 4-5-15, Figure 4-5-16), whereafter the specimen is removed from the anus through the protective sleeve (Figure 4-5-17, Figure 4-5-18). Finally, the bowel wall is sutured in continuous pattern with 3-0 barbed suture, and the pelvic cavity is irrigated repeatedly (Figure 4-5-19, Figure 4-5-20).

## 6 Laparoscopic Proximal Gastrectomy with Transvaginal Specimen Extraction and Auxiliary Incision-Free Abdomen
### (GC-NOSES VI)

### [Abstract]

GC-NOSES VI is a gastric function preserving surgery that is mainly applicable to female patients with early cancer in the upper stomach and gastroesophageal junction. Under the premise of ensuring adequate lymph node dissection and strict adherence to the radical resection of tumor and digestive tract reconstruction in the conventional laparoscopic surgery for gastric cancer, this procedure makes incision in the posterior vaginal fornix and adopts transvaginal specimen extraction, which puts forward higher requirements for the implementation of aseptic and tumor-free principles. This is a resection extraction NOSES procedure.

## 6.1 Indications and contraindications

### [Indications]

1. Female patients.

2. Upper gastric cancer or gastroesophageal junction cancer, stage $cT_{1-2}N_{0-1}M_0$.

3. The circumferential diameter of tumor is better $\leqslant$ 4cm.

## [Contraindications]

1. Unmarried women or married women with plans for future pregnancies.

2. Locally advanced cancer ($cT_{3-4}N_{1-3}M_{0-1}$), or the tumor is large.

3. Patients with acute gastrointestinal obstruction or tumor perforation.

4. Severely obese patients ($BMI > 30kg/m^2$).

5. Patients with serious pelvic adhesion or vaginal deformities.

## 6.2  Patient position, trocar placement and surgical team position

### [Patient position]

The patient should be placed in the horizontal supine position with legs abduction (Figure 4-6-1), which will be changed to the functional lithotomy position (Figure 4-6-2) when removing the specimen through the posterior vaginal fornix.

### [Trocar placement]  (Figure 4-6-3)

1. The camera trocar (10mm trocar) is located 1cm below the umbilicus.

2. The surgeon's main trocar (12mm trocar) is located below the costal margin of the left anterior axillary line.

3. The surgeon's auxiliary trocar (5mm trocar) is located at the umbilical level of the left midclavicular line.

4. The assistant's auxiliary trocar (5mm trocar) is located under the costal margin of the right anterior axillary line.

5. The assistant's main trocar (12mm trocar) is located at the umbilical level of the right midclavicular line.

### [Surgical team position]

1. Abdominal exploration, anatomical dissection and lymph node dissection

The positions of the surgeon, assistant and camera holder should be on the left side, right side, and between the patient's legs, separately (Figure 4-6-4).

2. Digestive tract reconstruction

The positions of the surgeon, assistant and camera holder should be on the right side, left side, and between the patient's legs, separately (Figure 4-6-5).

3. Transvaginal specimen extraction

The positions of the surgeon, assistant and camera holder should be on the right side, left side and the left side of the patient, separately (Figure 4-6-6). In this step, the monitor should be placed on the side of the patient's foot. The trocar function should be changed accordingly (Figure 4-6-7).

## [Surgical instruments]

Ultrasonic scalpel, 60mm linear cutting stapler, 3-0 barbed suture, 4-0 absorbable suture, protective sleeve.

## 6.3  Surgical procedure, techniques, and key points

### [Exploration]

On the basis of detailed preoperative examination, the liver, gallbladder, stomach, spleen, greater omentum, colon, small intestine, mesocolic surface, and pelvic cavity are routinely examined for the presence of tumor seeding, ascites and other abnormalities.

### [Dissection and separation]

1. Liver retraction and dissection of the gastroesophageal junction from the diaphragmatic crura.

Firstly, the surgeon opens the hepatogastric ligament, sutures the hepatic side of the hepatogastric ligament as traction stitch to suspend the left lobe of liver to fully expose the surgical field. Sharp dissection is performed between the gastroesophageal junction and the right diaphragmatic crus, then the Gerota's space is entered.

2. Dissection of the greater omentum and the gastrosplenic ligament

The greater omentum is flipped cephalad and transected from the left side of the transverse colon. The incision is extended to the hepatic flexure of colon on the right side. Dissection is performed along the posterior region of the anterior lobe of the transverse mesocolon. Afterwards, the anterior lobe of the transverse mesocolon is resected and attention should be paid to the preservation of the right gastroepiploic vessel. Then the patient is placed in the right-leaning position. The gastrosplenic ligament is exposed, and the greater

omentum is transected from the middle of colon to the splenic flexure. Subsequently, the left gastroepiploic vessels are transected at the root, and group 4sb lymph nodes are dissected. Apply the ultrasonic scalpel to transect the short gastric artery close to the hilum of the spleen, and group 4sa lymph nodes are dissected.

3. Dissection of group 7, 8a, 9, 11p, and 11d lymph nodes

The dissection is performed along the superior border of pancreas. The proximal end of the splenic artery is exposed, and group 11p lymph nodes are dissected. The celiac trunk is exposed and the left gastric vessels are dissected and transected after being ligated at the root. Group 7 and 9 lymph nodes are dissected, whereafter the dissection is continued along the common hepatic artery for the excision of group 8a lymph nodes. Group 11d lymph nodes are further dissected along the splenic artery. Whether to dissect group 10 lymph nodes is determined according to the tumor location and whether splenic hilar lymph nodes are enlarged.

4. Dissection of group 1 and 2 lymph nodes and skeletonize the esophagus

The surgeon transects the anterior and posterior gastric vagal nerves, and isolates the esophagus for enough length. When the dissected length of esophagus is insufficient, the diaphragm can be opened for 4-5cm from the fornix of the esophageal diaphragmatic hiatus anteriorly, and the bilateral diaphragmatic crura can be transected in the middle and lower part of it to push the pleura aside laterally. A traction stitch is sutured in the esophagus above the tumor to pull the esophagus downwards as much as possible. The esophagus should be adequately dissected upwards in the posterior mediastinum to ensure that there is enough resection margin.

## [Specimen resection and digestive tract reconstruction]

1. Specimen resection

The esophagus is transected with a linear cutting stapler at 2cm above the esophagogastric junction and the stomach is transected with a linear cutting stapler at 5cm from the distal end of the tumor. The resected specimen is placed in a specimen bag (Figure 4-6-8).

2. Digestive tract reconstruction

2.1   Instrumental anastomosis (Overlap method)

The two jaws of the linear cutting stapler are inserted into the windows of the posterior wall of the esophagus and the anterior wall of the remnant stomach, respectively. Then the stapler is fired to complete the side-to-side anastomosis. The common opening is sutured with 3-0 barbed suture.

2.2   Digestive tract reconstruction with hand-sewn anastomosis

The anterior wall of the remnant stomach and the posterior wall of the esophagus are sutured with 3-0 Polyglactin 910 suture for 3 stitches, whereafter the anterior wall of the remnant stomach and the posterior wall of the esophagus are opened for hand-sewn anastomosis. The anastomosis between the anterior wall of the stomach and the posterior wall of the esophagus is performed with interrupted full-thickness sutures using 3-0 Polyglactin 910 suture, and the common opening anastomosis is performed with continuous sutures using 3-0 barbed suture.

3. Specimen extraction

For transvaginal specimen extraction, the patient is placed in the functional lithotomy position, and the laparoscopic monitor is moved to the side of patient's foot. The perineal area and vagina are disinfected with the iodoform gauze. After replacing the patient in the right-leaning Trendelenburg position, the surgeon should suspend the uterus to expose the posterior vaginal fornix (Figure 4-6-9). Use the abdominal spatula to withstand the posterior vaginal fornix. An transverse incision of approximately 5cm is made with the ultrasonic scalpel. Through the incision, the protective sleeve is inserted into the vagina (Figure 4-6-10-Figure 4-6-12) to remove the specimen from it (Figure 4-6-13-Figure 4-6-15). Finally, the posterior vaginal fornix is continuously sutured with 3-0 barbed suture, and irrigation of the pelvic cavity is performed repeatedly (Figure 4-6-16-Figure 4-6-19).

# 7 Laparoscopic Total Gastrectomy with Transanal Specimen Extraction and Auxiliary Incision-Free Abdomen

## (GC-NOSES VII)

### [Abstract]

GC-NOSES VII is a resection extraction NOSES procedure. The operating characteristics are as follows: radical resection of gastric cancer and digestive tract reconstruction under laparoscopy with an incision in the upper rectum, and specimen extraction through the anus. The procedure conforms to the concept of minimally invasive surgery. While adhering to the basic principles of cancer surgery, minimizing surgical damage is achievable through optimizing the surgical approach, refining operational procedures, and preserving the structure and function of the abdominal wall. This approach aims to mitigate the impact on patients' quality of life.

## 7.1 Indications and Contraindications of NOSES

### [Indications]

1. Gastric cancer, stage $cT_{1-3}N_{1-2}M_0$, with lesions invading the body of the stomach, the upper and middle part of the stomach or the gastroesophageal junction.

2. The circumferential diameter of tumor is better ≤4cm.

3. Male patients and some female patients who are not suitable for transvaginal specimen extraction.

### [Contraindications]

1. The tumor is too large to be pulled out through the anus.

2. The tumor penetrates the serosa or involves adjacent organs.

3. Patients with acute gastrointestinal obstruction or tumor perforation.

4. Severely obese patients (BMI>30kg/m²).

5. Patients with history of pelvic surgery or rectal and anal deformities.

## 7.2 Surgical procedure, techniques, and key points

### [Trocar placement]

1. The camera trocar (10mm trocar) is located 1cm below the umbilicus.

2. The surgeon's main trocar (12mm trocar) is located 2cm below the costal margin of the left anterior axillary line.

3. The surgeon's auxiliary trocar (5mm trocar) is located at the umbilical level of the left midclavicular line.

4. The assistant's auxiliary trocar (5mm trocar) is located under the costal margin of the right anterior axillary line.

5. The assistant's main trocar (12mm trocar) is located at the umbilical level of the right midclavicular line (Figure 4-7-1).

### [Exploration]

1. General exploration

Observe for any lesions such as metastatic implants on the surfaces of various organs and the peritoneum.

2. Tumor exploration

Determine the feasibility of surgery based on the tumor's location, size, and depth of invasion.

3. Evaluation of anatomical structures

Determine the surgical plan based on the tumor's location, and anatomical structures, and evaluate the feasibility of transanal extraction.

## [Dissection and separation]

1. Dissecting the anterior lobe of the transverse mesocolon and the gastrocolic ligament

The greater omentum is flipped cephalad. Open the gastrocolic ligament and transected from the left side of the transverse colon. The lesser omental sac is entered, and the incision is extended to the hepatic flexure of colon on the right side. Dissection is performed along the posterior region of the anterior lobe of the transverse mesocolon. The anterior lobe of the mesocolon is resected.

2. Dissection of group 6 lymph nodes

The Henle's trunk is exposed and the right gastroepiploic vein is transected at the root. The dissection is continued along the surface of the pancreatic head. The gastropancreatic ligament is opened to expose the gastroduodenal artery. The right gastroepiploic artery is skeletonized and transected at the root. Group 6 lymph nodes are completely dissected.

3. Dissection of group 4sb and 10 lymph nodes

After entering the omental bursa, the pancreatic tail and the splenic vessels are exposed, the splenic vessel is located, the splenic flexure is mobilized, and the adhesion between the greater omentum and middle and lower pole of spleen is detached. The pancreatic tail is protected. The left gastroepiploic vessels are exposed and transected at the root, group 4sb lymph nodes are dissected, and the 10 lymph nodes are further dissected.

4. Dissection of group 4sa lymph nodes

After pulling the stomach and the greater omentum to the left, the dissection is continued upwards. The short gastric vessels are transect for the dissection of group 4sa lymph nodes.

5. Dissection of group 8a, 12a and 5 lymph nodes

The surgeon then exposes the common hepatic artery by retracting the pancreas inferolaterally to the left, and dissect group 8a lymph nodes along the anterior and superior border of the common hepatic artery. The right gastric artery and the proper hepatic artery are adequately exposed along the gastroduodenal artery and the common hepatic artery. The anterior and lateral sides of the proper hepatic artery are dissected upwards, and group 12a lymph nodes are dissected. The right gastric artery and vein are transected after being ligated at the root and

group 5 lymph nodes are dissected. The duodenum is transected with a linear cutting stapler at the distal end of pylorus and group 5 lymph nodes are dissected. Incise the anterior perivascular fascia of the portal vein at the junction of the common hepatic artery, gastroduodenal artery, and the superior border of the pancreas to expose the portal vein. Lift the common hepatic artery anteriorly toward the abdominal wall, dissect along the anterior aspect of the portal vein, and clear the lymph nodes between the portal vein and the proper hepatic artery. Dissect along the medial aspect of the portal vein upward toward the hepatic hilum, retract the common hepatic artery inferolaterally to the right, and clear the lymphatic and fatty tissues along the medial sides of the proper hepatic artery and portal vein.

6. Dissection of group 11p, 7, and 9 lymph nodes

The greater omentum is placed below the liver. The assistant grasps and holds the plica gastropancreatica, and turns the stomach upwards. The anterior pancreatic capsule is dissected. The dissection is performed closely along the superior border of pancreas to expose the proximal end of splenic artery, followed by dissection of group 11p lymph nodes. From left to right, the celiac trunk is exposed and the left gastric vessels are dissected and transected after being ligated at the root, and group 7 and 9 lymph nodes are dissected. Dissection along the splenic artery to the distal end to transect the posterior gastric vessels is performed, followed by the dissection of group 11p lymph nodes.

7. Dissection of lymph nodes in the lesser curvature

Using an ultrasonic scalpel, perform layered dissection closely along the lesser curvature of the stomach to clear the lymph nodes along the lesser curvature.

8. Mobilization of the lower esophagus and lymph nodes on the right and left sides of the cardia

Using an ultrasonic scalpel, perform layered dissection closely along the esophagus to expose and transect the anterior and posterior vagus nerves. Dissect the lymph nodes on both the right and left sides of the cardia (groups 1 and 2). If the mobilized length of the esophagus is insufficient, further dissection can be performed in the posterior mediastinum, or by making an anterior incision of 4-5cm in the diaphragmatic dome at the esophageal hiatus. During the dissection, carefully

retract the pleura laterally to avoid pleural injury. Gently pull the esophagus downward to achieve adequate mobilization and ensure a safe proximal resection margin.

## [Specimen extraction and digestive tract reconstruction]

1. Specimen resection

The surgeon transects the esophagus at 3cm from the proximal edge of tumor, puts the specimen in the specimen bag and temporarily places it in the left lower abdomen until the specimen is extracted through the anus (Figure 4-7-2-Figure 4-7-4).

2. Digestive tract reconstruction (laparoscopic Roux-en-Y esophagojejunostomy with the Overlap method)

The surgeon makes a stitch on the left and right sides of the esophageal stump with the 3-0 Polyglactin 910 suture. The ultrasonic scalpel is used to open the middle of the esophageal stump (Figure 4-7-5), then the jejunum is transected at 20cm from the Treitz's Ligament (Figure 4-7-6, Figure 4-7-7), so as to facilitate the creation of the overlap anastomosis between distal jejunum and esophagus (Figure 4-7-8). The common opening is closed with 3-0 barbed suture in a continuous pattern (Figure 4-7-9-Figure 4-7-11). After the esophagojejunal

anastomosis is created, a window is opened in the antimesenteric border of the jejunum 40cm from the esophagojejunal anastomosis, the proximal and distal jejunum are anastomosed with a linear cutting stapler in a side-to-side fashion, and the common opening of jejunum is closed with a 3-0 Polyglactin 910 suture in an intermittent pattern (Figure 4-7-12, Figure 4-7-13).

3. Specimen extraction

After radical resection of the gastric cancer and the digestive tract reconstruction, the patient is placed in the functional lithotomy position, then the perineal area and rectal cavity are disinfected with the iodophor. The laparoscopic monitor is moved to the side of patient's foot, while the patient is placed in the Trendelenburg position. The assistant stretches the sigmoid colon to fully expose the upper rectum, and then the surgeon makes an incision of 5-6cm in the anterior wall of the upper rectum (Figure 4-7-14). The protective sleeve is inserted into the rectum through the trocar after further disinfecting with iodoform gauze (Figure 4-7-15, Figure 4-7-16), whereafter the specimen is removed from the anus through the protective sleeve (Figure 4-7-17, Figure 4-7-18). Finally, suture the bowel wall in continuous pattern with 3-0 baebed suture and irrigate the pelvis (Figure 4-7-19-Figure 4-7-21).

---

# 8 Laparoscopic Total Gastrectomy with Transvaginal Specimen Extraction and Auxiliary Incision-Free Abdomen

## (GC-NOSES Ⅷ)

### [Abstract]

GC-NOSES Ⅷ is mainly applicable to female patients with tumors located at the middle and upper stomach and gastroesophageal junction. As with conventional laparoscopic surgery for gastric cancer, principles of radical resection and digestive tract reconstruction should be strictly followed. Except that the method of specimen extraction is different from that of conventional laparoscopic surgery, the gastrointestinal tract resection, the extent of lymph node dissection, and dissection plane of surgery are consistent with those of conventional laparoscopic surgery. This is a resection extraction NOSES procedure. The operating characteristics are as follows: radical resection of gastric cancer and digestive tract reconstruction is performed under laparoscopy, then an incision is made in the posterior vaginal fornix to extract the specimen. Laparoscopic radical resection and digestive tract reconstruction provides a broader view of operation field as to easily determine the direction of the bowel during reconstruction. In this way, common mistakes

while operating with small auxiliary incision, such as bowel torsion and over-tension of the anastomosis, can be effectively avoid. Transvaginal specimen extraction avoids the auxiliary incision in the abdominal wall, preserves the function of abdominal wall to the maximum, reduces postoperative pain, which facilitates early ambulation and shortens recovery time, so as to minimize the physical and psychological effects of surgery.

## 8.1　Indications and contraindications

### [Indications]

1. Gastric cancer, stage $cT_{1-3}N_{1-2}M_0$, with lesions in the middle and upper part of the stomach or the gastroesophageal junction.

2. The circumferential diameter of tumor is better≤4cm.

### [Contraindications]

1. The tumor is too large to be pulled out through the vagina.

2. The tumor invades beyond the serosa or invades adjacent organs.

3. Severely obese patients (BMI>30kg/m$^2$).

4. Patients with serious cardiac, pulmonary, hepatic, renal and other concomitant diseases that cannot tolerate the surgery.

## 8.2　Surgical procedure, techniques, and key points

### [Trocar placement]

1. The camera trocar (10mm trocar) is located 1cm below the umbilicus.

2. The surgeon's main trocar (12mm trocar) is located below the costal margin of the left anterior axillary line.

3. The surgeon's auxiliary trocar (5mm trocar) is located at the umbilical level of the left midclavicular line.

4. The assistant's auxiliary trocar (5mm trocar) is located under the costal margin of the right anterior axillary line.

5. The assistant's main trocar (12mm trocar) is located at the umbilical level of the right midclavicular

line (Figure 4-8-1).

### [Exploration]

1. General exploration

Observe for any lesions such as metastatic implants on the surfaces of various organs and the peritoneum.

2. Tumor exploration

Determine the feasibility of surgery based on the tumor's location, size, and depth of invasion.

3. Evaluation of anatomical structures

Determine the surgical plan based on the tumor's location, and anatomical structures, and evaluate the feasibility of transvaginal extraction.

### [Dissection and separation]

1. Open the greater omentum at its attachment to the transverse colon and dissect the anterior lobe of the transverse mesocolon

The greater omentum is flipped cephalad and transected from the left side of the transverse colon. The lesser omental sac is entered, and the incision is extended to the hepatic flexure of colon on the right side. Dissection is performed along the posterior region of the anterior lobe of the mesocolon. The anterior lobe of the transverse mesocolon is resected.

2. Dissection of group 6 lymph nodes

With the marker of middle colic vessel, the surgeon firstly enters into the fusion fascia space between the gastroduodenum and transverse mesocolon. The anterior superior pancreaticoduodenal vein is exposed, and the right gastroepiploic vein is transected above the junction between the anterior superior pancreaticoduodenal vein with the right gastroepiploic vein. The dissection is continued along the surface of the pancreatic head. The gastroduodenal artery is exposed. The right gastroepiploic artery is skeletonized and transected at the root. Group 6 lymph nodes are completely dissected.

3. Dissection of group 4sb lymph nodes

The pancreatic tail is exposed, the left gastroepiploic vessels are exposed and transected at the root, splenic hilar lymph nodes are further dissected along the splenic vessels distally until the branch vessels of splenic hilum are exposed, and group 4sb lymph nodes are dissected.

4. Dissection of group 11p, 11d, 7, and 9 lymph nodes

The dissection is performed closely along the superior border of pancreas to expose the proximal end of splenic artery, followed by dissection of group 11p lymph nodes. Group 11d lymph nodes are further dissected along the splenic artery. Whether to dissect group 10 lymph nodes is determined according to the tumor location and whether splenic hilar lymph nodes are enlarged. The celiac trunk is exposed and the left gastric vessels are dissected and transected after being ligated at the root, and group 7 and 9 lymph nodes are dissected.

5. Dissection of group 12a lymph nodes

The duodenum is transected with a linear cutting stapler at 2cm from the distal end of pylorus. The capsule of the hepatoduodenal ligament is opened and the anterior and left sides of the proper hepatic artery are skeletonized, and the root of the right gastric vessel is ligated and transected. The assistant retracts the common hepatic artery inferolaterally to the right to facilitate dissection of group 12a lymph nodes along the medial sides of the proper hepatic artery and the portal vein.

6. Skeletonization of esophagus

The ultrasonic scalpel is applied to dissect the submucosa closely along the esophagus, transect the anterior and posterior gastric vagal nerves, and dissect enough length of esophagus to dissect group 110 lymph nodes. When the dissected length of esophagus is insufficient, the dissection can be performed in the posterior mediastinum, or open the diaphragm for 4-5cm from the fornix of the esophageal diaphragmatic hiatus anteriorly. During the dissection, attention should be paid to push the pleura aside laterally to prevent damage to the pleura. The esophagus is pulled downwards to dissect the esophagus adequately to ensure the safety of the proximal resection margin.

## [Specimen resection and digestive tract reconstruction]

1. Specimen resection

After complete mobilization of the esophagus, transect the esophagus transversely at 3cm proximal to the tumor using a linear cutting stapler (Figure 4-8-2). Place the specimen into a retrieval bag and temporarily position it in the left lower abdomen for subsequent extraction through the vagina.

2. Digestive tract reconstruction

2.1    Instrumental anastomosis (Overlap method)

The jejunum is transected at 25cm from the Treitz's ligament (Figure 4-8-3). Two windows are opened in the posterior wall of esophagus and the antimesenteric border of the distal jejunum, respectively. The surgeon then inserts two jaws of the linear cutting stapler into the windows, and fires the stapler to complete the side-to-side esophagojejunal anastomosis (Figure 4-8-4-Figure 4-8-6). The common opening is closed with a 3-0 barbed suture in a continuous pattern (Figure 4-8-7).

2.2    Hand-sewn anastomosis (Roux-en-Y)

The esophagojejunal anastomosis is completed by performing anastomosis first and followed by transection, i.e., lift the bowel at 25cm from the Treitz's Ligament to esophageal hiatus to be sutured with the posterior wall of esophagus for 3 stitches, and open the lateral wall of the jejunum and the posterior wall of the esophagus for hand-sewn anastomosis (Figure 4-8-8, Figure 4-8-9). The anastomosis of the posterior wall is full-thickness sutured in an intermittent pattern with absorbable suture (Figure 4-8-10). Continuous 3-0 barbed suture closure of the common opening. (Figure 4-8-11). After completing the esophagojejunostomy, transect the proximal jejunum 3cm distal to the anastomosis. Create an enterotomy on the mesenteric side of the jejunal wall 40cm distal to the esophagojejunostomy. Perform a side-to-side anastomosis between the proximal and distal jejunum using a linear cutting stapler. Close the common opening with either interrupted sutures using 3-0 Polyglactin 910 suture or continuous sutures using 3-0 barbed sutures (Figure 4-8-12-Figure 4-8-14).

3. Specimen extraction

After radical resection of gastric cancer and the digestive tract reconstruction, the patient is placed in the functional lithotomy position, followed by the disinfection of the perineal area and vagina with the iodoform gauze. Move the laparoscopic monitor to the side of patient's foot, and replace the patient in the Trendelenburg position. After suspending the uterus to expose the posterior vaginal fornix, the surgeon makes an transverse incision of 5-6cm in the posterior vaginal fornix (Figure 4-8-15). The protective sleeve is inserted through the surgeon's main trocar port after disinfecting

with diluted povidone-iodine solution (Figure 4-8-16). The specimen is removed from the vagina through the protective sleeve (Figure 4-8-17, Figure 4-8-18). Next, the pelvic cavity is irrigated repeatedly with diluted povidone-iodine solution and normal saline (Figure 4-8-19, Figure 4-8-20). Lastly, the posterior vaginal fornix is closed with continuous suture by 3-0 barbed suture (Figure 4-8-21).

# Chapter V

# The Common Complications and Management of Gastrointestinal NOSES

NOSES has unique features in specimen extraction and reconstruction of the digestive tract, but shares similarities in terms of surgical complications with open surgery and conventional laparoscopic procedures. This chapter outlines the causes, clinical presentations, and management principles of complications related to gastrointestinal NOSES.

## 1. Abdominal infection

Most of the pathogenic bacteria of abdominal infection related to gastrointestinal surgery come from the gastrointestinal tract, of which the Gram negative bacterium are the dominant bacteria. Causes of abdominal infection of NOSES include the following: insufficient preoperative preparation, nonstandard intraoperative aseptic operation, postoperative anastomotic leakage, insufficient abdominal drainage, poor patient condition, accompanied by diabetes mellitus, advanced age, malnutrition and other factors. Therefore, the key to preventing abdominal infection lies in strengthening the management of the aforementioned steps and controlling relevant risk factors to reduce the incidence of abdominal infection.

The main clinical manifestations of abdominal infection are fever, abdominal pain, and signs of peritonitis, which are often accompanied by nausea, vomiting, abdominal distension, hypotension, tachycardia, shortness of breath, leukocytosis, and other sepsis symptoms. In the late stage, it can lead to systemic failure, resulting in severe dehydration, metabolic acidosis, or septic shock.

In addition to the medical history and clinical manifestations, the diagnosis of abdominal infection should be primarily based on the characteristics of the drainage fluid and auxiliary examinations. The characteristics of drainage fluid should be closely observed if the patient has fever, abdominal pain, and other symptoms. If the drainage fluid is yellow and purulent, the possibility of abdominal infection should be considered. If the abdominal infection is caused by anastomotic leakage, drainage fluid would contain fecal sediment with foul-smelling. Auxiliary examinations include laboratory tests (white blood cell count, neutrophil percentage, biochemical analysis), imaging examination (X-ray, ultrasound, or CT), ascitic fluid analysis, and bacterial cultures. For patients without a drainage tube or drainage tube is removed, abdominal puncture can be performed to aspirate the accumulated fluid and determine its nature.

The principles of treatment include general treatment, systemic support therapy, anti-infection therapy, abdominal drainage, and surgical treatment.

General treatment: Patients can take bed rest in the 30°-45° semi-reclining position, which facilitates the accumulation of intra-abdominal exudate in the pelvic cavity for drainage. Relaxes the abdominal musculature, and prevents diaphragm compression, which facilitates the improvement of respiration and circulation. Fasting and gastrointestinal decompression could reduce bowel distention, improve the blood circulation of the bowel wall, reduce bowel content exudation when bowel perforation occurs, and promote the recovery of intestinal peristalsis.

Systemic support therapy: If systemic symptoms are prominent, blood transfusion and fluid supplementation may be necessary to correct electrolyte and acid-base imbalances. Parenteral and enteral nutrition therapy could be given to improve the patient's physical status and enhance immunity.

Anti-infective therapy mainly aims at Gram negative bacterium, for which beta-lactam and aminoglycoside

drugs can be applied. Necessary adjustments should be made according to the results of bacterial culture and drug sensitivity tests.

The drainage of the abdominal cavity is critical in the presence of anastomotic leakage. The open drainage is prone to causing retrograde or exogenous infection, which could be solved through regular flushing of the drainage tube with normal saline. Gentamicin and saline can be used to regularly irrigate the drainage tube, and the accumulated liquid can also be suctioned by negative pressure so that the capsule area can shrink rapidly. If the symptoms of abdominal infection are serious or an abdominal abscess is formed and cannot be solved by conservative treatment, surgical treatment is required.

According to a multicenter (79 centers) retrospective study of NOSES in China, only 0.8% of patients developed abdominal infection after surgery. The result also indicates that NOSES can meet the aseptic principle as long as sufficient preparation is made and operating skills are mastered.

## 2. Anastomotic bleeding

Anastomotic bleeding is one of the early complications after surgery. Generally, stapled anastomosis is performed in laparoscopic surgery, and the main cause of anastomotic bleeding is incomplete mesenteric denudation at the site of the anastomosis, leaving blood vessels exposed. The failure of the stapler to effectively close these vessels results in bleeding. Anastomotic bleeding usually occurs within 48 hours after the operation, while bleeding due to pelvic hematoma breaking into the anastomosis wall usually occurs 7 days after the operation. According to the multicenter (79 centers) retrospective study of NOSES in China, only 0.9% of patients developed anastomotic bleeding after surgery.

Prevention is the key to the management of anastomotic bleeding. During the intraoperative anastomosis of the digestive tract, air and water injection test should be conducted to check the integrity of the anastomosis. If possible, laparoscopy could be used to detect the anastomotic status in operation. Anastomosis, especially the "danger triangle", could be sutured to reinforce if necessary.

Early symptoms of the majority of patients are persistent hematochezia, and the color varies from bright red to dark red depending on the location of anastomosis and the amount of bleeding. Physical examination may reveal that the drainage fluid is light pink or red. Some patients may be complicated with local tenderness. If anastomotic bleeding is severe or secondary infection occurs and anastomotic leakage is induced, clinical manifestations of anastomotic leakage, including rigor, hyperpyrexia, abdominal pain, peritoneal irritation, etc., may occur.

The vast majority of anastomotic bleeding can resolve spontaneously, and only a small number of patients require interventions. Intervention measures mainly include drug therapy, endoscopy treatment, and surgical treatment. Drug therapy includes oral or intramuscular administration of hemostatic drugs. When there is major bleeding, the bleeding point can be endoscopically visualized and clipped with hemostatic clips. If the endoscopy treatment fails, surgical treatment, ligation of bleeding point, and suture of anastomosis could be performed. In addition, for lower and ultra-low anus-preserving anastomotic bleeding, transanal reinforcement and suture of the anastomosis can be performed to stop the bleeding.

## 3. Intra-abdominal bleeding

Postoperative intra-abdominal bleeding of NOSES is usually caused by the insecurity of surgical hemostasis or vascular ligation, untreated coagulation dysfunction caused by blood system or other systemic diseases, or spontaneous hemorrhage caused by tissue necrosis or falling off of vascular clips.

The key to the prevention of intra-abdominal hemorrhage is to operate carefully and make sure that the ligation of vessels is properly performed. The operation should not be rushed at the cost of quality. For the elderly or patients with arteriosclerosis, avoid excessive isolation of blood vessels, and avoid intraoperative and postoperative blood pressure fluctuation in patients with hypertension. When bleeding occurs intraoperatively, exact hemostasis, particularly to large vessels, must be performed. For example, in the radical resection of rectal cancer, the management of inferior mesenteric artery bleeding requires relevant experience and skills. Different treatment methods should be taken according to different situations.

The clinical manifestation of intra-abdominal bleeding is determined by the site, amount, and duration of bleeding. Patients may be complicated with abdominal discomfort and mild abdominal distension. Bleeding sites have localized swelling, which may be accompanied by mild tenderness and increased local dullness. If the amount of bleeding is large, the patient may be positive for shifting dullness on percussion, and complicated with unstable vital signs, including increased pulse and respiratory rate, decreased blood pressure, with continued (or increased) bright red drainage. In general, bloody drainage often indicates active bleeding. It is not difficult to make the diagnosis according to the clinical manifestations.

In the event of mild bleeding after an operation, hemostatic drugs can be orally or intramuscularly administered, and the patient's condition should be closely observed. In the event of massive bleeding, blood pressure, pulse, and other vital signs should be closely observed and preparation should be ready for surgical exploration. Once active intra-abdominal bleeding is detected and the amount of bleeding is large, a second surgery should be timely conducted and surgical hemostasis should be performed. If surgical exploration is necessary, blood and blood clots should be suctioned as soon as possible. Check the original surgical site for bleeding points, clip or suture them, and then check the surgical site again. In patients requiring a second surgery due to postoperative bleeding, 60% to 70% do not have a clear source of bleeding. Thorough removal of the accumulated blood should be performed, followed by lavage and observation before closing the abdomen.

## 4. Anastomotic leakage

The occurrence of anastomotic leakage is associated with local factors, systemic factors, and technical factors. Systemic factors include poor nutritional status, long-term use of corticosteroids, preoperative radio-chemotherapy, concomitant diabetes, and other chronic diseases. Local factors include insufficient blood supply, excessive anastomotic tension, anastomosis infection, and anastomosis bowel edema. Technical factors include suture that is not tight, excessive tissue compression, and anastomotic device itself (such as stapler pin height). Therefore, attention should be paid to the

abovementioned points for the prevention of anastomotic leakage. Besides, air and water injection test is needed to check for patency of the anastomosis and to detect any bleeding or leakage. In hospitals where conditions permit, performing intraoperative colonoscopy can make the surgical procedure safer and more reliable.

The initial symptom of most of the patients with anastomotic leakage is fever or abdominal pain, which may be complicated with peritoneal irritation. Patients with severe abdominal infection may develop toxic shock and multiple organ failure. Fever can occur at any time, sometimes presenting as persistently high postoperative body temperature or a gradually increasing trend. Abdominal pain can be manifested as flatulence in the lower abdomen in the early stage or sudden onset of serious abdominal pain, which is complicated with tenderness, rebound tenderness, and other symptoms and signs of acute peritonitis. If the abdominal inflammation is limited, localized peritonitis or palpable swelling mass may occur. If there is a drainage tube, intestinal contents can be released from the drainage tube. A sudden increase in drainage liquid, turbidity, fecal matters, putrefactive odor, redness, and swelling around the drainage port, and sometimes air bubbles may appear.

Once diagnosed, the treatment of anastomotic leakage should be given as soon as possible. Local unobstructed drainage and infection control are the keys to early treatment. Most anastomotic leakage can be cured by drainage and irrigation. If the anastomotic leakage cannot heal for a long time, surgical treatment such as fecal diversion or bowel resection and anastomosis remake should be considered. Reasonable treatment can convert leakage into a controllable or localized leakage until it is healed.

According to the multicenter (79 centers) study of NOSES in China, 3.5% of patients developed anastomotic leakage after surgery. Although NOSES does not increase the incidence of anastomotic leakage, the surgeons must take good precautions. The key to its prevention is to ensure a tension-free and infection-free anastomosis with good blood supply. Moreover, surgeons should pay attention to the intestinal peristalsis tension. We do not encourage the common application of diverting colostomy for all patients with rectal cancer, as the stoma does not reduce the incidence of postoperative

anastomotic leakage. Instead, it may cause a series of problems. However, diverting colostomy is recommended for the following situations: poor preoperative bowel preparation, with incomplete intestinal obstruction; elderly patients with underlying diseases such as diabetes; patients with severe anemia and malnutrition; preoperative neoadjuvant radiochemotherapy; patients with narrow pelvis which is difficult to operate or high-risk constitution such as obesity; the location of the tumor is low, for which ultra-low anastomosis in anus-preserving surgery is required.

## 5. Rectovaginal fistula

Transvaginal specimen extraction has long been performed in laparoscopic surgery. In early studies, auxiliary incisions in the abdominal wall were needed. After many years of practice and follow-up, our team has validated the feasibility and safety of transvaginal specimen extraction.

During intestinal resection, some intestinal contents are highly likely to spill out, and during specimen extraction, compression of the bowel can cause fluid from the intestinal lumen to enter the abdominal cavity. Both of these situations increase the risk of intra-abdominal infection. If anastomotic leakage occurs on this basis with the presence of vaginal incision, the risk of the rectovaginal fistula is increased.

The causes of rectovaginal fistula can be divided into patient and iatrogenic factors. Underlying conditions such as comorbid diseases, malnutrition, immune deficiency, and age may increase the risk of fistula formation. Iatrogenic factors, especially surgical operation, are more closely related to the onset of rectovaginal fistula. Generally, lower location of rectal cancer, surgical traction, and vague visual field may increase the probability of the vagina's posterior wall being injured or being stapled in the anastomosis. Therefore, clear surgical field and confirmation of the location of the posterior vaginal wall before firing the stapler are important for the prevention of rectovaginal fistula. In addition, it should be noted that during the reinforcement and suture, the posterior vaginal wall and the anastomosis should not be sutured together.

Rectovaginal fistula is a complex complication, although its incidence is not high, this complex complication should not be ignored. Surgery timing for the repair of postoperative rectovaginal fistula, especially iatrogenic rectovaginal fistula, should be carefully chosen. Do not perform immediate surgery under the urgent demand of the patient. In the acute stage, one can expect natural healing with conservative treatment, vaginal douching, sitz baths, and keeping the area clean, and if the fistula is not too big, the chance of healing is higher. After the formation of an old fistula, it is recommended to wait for the local and systemic inflammation to subside and the scar to soften, and then repair the fistula after 3 months, and if the fistula is located lower, it can be repaired vaginally.

## 6. Intestinal obstruction

Intestinal obstruction is a common complication after abdominal surgery. Postoperative adhesion, internal hernia, distortion, infection, and other factors can lead to intestinal obstruction. Early postoperative symptoms concerning intestinal obstruction are mostly paralytic ileus. It is also associated with a poor physical condition, abdominal infection, liquid and electrolyte, and acid-base imbalances, etc. Late postoperative intestinal obstruction is often caused by intestinal adhesion, which is manifested as mechanical intestinal obstruction. Mechanical intestinal obstruction in the minority of patients may also be caused by intestinal volvulus or intussusception. According to the multicenter (79 centers) study of NOSES in China, 0.6% of patients developed intestinal obstruction after surgery. The main manifestations include abdominal pain, abdominal distension, vomiting, the arrest of exhaust and defecation, and other symptoms. Since the cause, type, location, and degree of intestinal obstruction vary, the clinical manifestations are different as well. In the event of strangulated intestinal obstruction, the disease progresses rapidly, and shock may occur. Therefore, early monitoring of the symptoms and signs of patients can provide an important basis for the treatment of obstruction.

As for the prevention of postoperative intestinal obstruction, intestinal contents flowing out should be avoided as far as possible on the technical level. Once contamination occurs in an operation, the abdominal cavity should be flushed thoroughly. Before the closure of the abdomen, careful examination should be performed to make sure that no foreign bodies are left in

the abdominal cavity, and the small intestine is replaced in normal physiological order and position, then covered by the greater omentum. Early ambulation should be encouraged to reduce the incidence of postoperative intestinal adhesions. In addition, some studies have reported cases of intestinal obstruction caused by trocar site hernia. Therefore, the closure of the trocar is also important.

Intestinal obstruction is a common complication of colorectal surgery, and its diagnosis and treatment are not difficult. The principle of treatment is to relieve the obstruction and correct the internal environment disorder. The selection of a therapeutic method should be made based on the cause, nature, location, the systemic condition, and the severity of the disease.

## 7. Intestinal volvulus

Intestinal volvulus can occur both in the early and late post- operative period. Usually, a bowel segment or even the total small bowel and its mesentery twist 360°-720° along the mesenteric axis. Therefore, both intestinal obstruction and mesenteric ischemia may occur. This is one of the most dangerous, most rapidly progressing, and most serious postoperative complications.

Postoperative bowel adhesions and too much intestinal contents are potential factors for the formation of volvulus. Strong intestinal peristalsis or sudden position change will lead to unsynchronized bowel loop movement, thereby causing volvulus of bowel loops. The prevention of postoperative intestinal volvulus should focus on the postoperative education to avoid the occurrence of intestinal volvulus caused by a sudden increase of abdominal pressure.

Intestinal volvulus can induce intestinal strangulation and necrosis in a short term. Timely surgical treatment can return the intestinal loop to normal position and reduce the mortality rate. It can also avoid short bowel syndrome due to the massive resection of the small bowel. For patients without obvious signs of peritonitis, colon necrosis, or intestinal wall necrosis (detected by colonoscopy), the soft catheters can be placed through the obstruction site with the guide of colonoscopy to reverse intestinal loops, exhaust large amounts of gas and feces, and replace the twisted bowel into a normal position.

However, surgery is needed if partial of the bowel wall is proved to be necrotic. If signs of peritonitis are obvious and the colon is considered necrotic, surgical treatment should be performed decisively. Surgical treatments contain separation of adhesion, resection of the necrotic colon and lengthy colon, and replacement of the colon into a normal position.

## 8. Internal abdominal hernia

An internal hernia refers to the condition in which an abdominal organ passes through a congenital or secondary opening in the abdominal cavity (such as the mesenteric defect or omental foramen) into another abdominal space, without protruding to the body's surface. Internal abdominal hernia lacks obvious clinical manifestation and it is therefore prone to being misdiagnosed. Abdominal distension, pain, and discomfort are the main manifestations of internal hernia, and some are complicated with chronic intestinal obstruction. Therefore, appropriate preoperative imaging examinations are the keys to improve the diagnosis rate and contribute to make proper surgical decisions. In order to prevent the occurrence of internal abdominal hernia, the mesenteric hiatus may be closed in the operation.

X-ray examination shows only intestinal obstruction signs like air-fluid levels and bowel dilatation. Thus, CT scan is generally recommended to help determine the location, extent and size of internal hernia. Even if the hernia location is concealed, CT scan can still provide an accurate reference for the diagnosis. Once the diagnosis is clear, timely surgical treatment is required to avoid intestinal ischemia and necrosis. The prevention of internal abdominal hernia lies in fine operation and closure of the mesenteric hiatus as far as possible. Surgeons cannot be overconfident. After the operation is completed, careful inspection should be made to identify any potential risk factors, and any issues should be addressed promptly.

## 9. Tumor implantation of trocar sites and vaginal incision

Due to the absence of auxiliary incision in the abdominal wall, the trocar sites and vagina incision become the potential location of tumor implantation. It is generally believed that the pneumoperitoneum could cause the tumor cells to spray and promote the tumor

metastasis. During the operation, preventive measures include tumor-free manipulation, the use of a protective sleeve to isolate the tumor during specimen extraction, and intra-abdominal gas should be released slowly through the suction connected with the valve of the trocar. At the end of the operation, trocars are pulled out only when the gas is completely released to avoid the chimney effect caused by direct gas evacuation through the trocar hole. Threaded but not smooth trocars should be used to prevent the trocar from sliding. If there is air leak around the trocar, the trocars should be replaced or fixed to the abdominal wall to maintain the air-tightness of the pneumoperitoneum. In addition, in order to reduce the incidence of abdominal implantation, NOSES is not recommended for $T_4$ stage patients. The author usually irrigates the abdominal cavity and vagina with dilute iodine solution and distilled water. Distilled water is hypoosmotic and irrigation of the abdominal cavity can lead to tumor cell swelling, rupture, and thus inactivation. At the same time, the tumor tissue, when heated, causes cancer cells to form emboli in the microvasculature, leading to hypoxia, acidosis, and metabolic disorders, ultimately resulting in cell lysis. In contrast, normal tissue cells can remain normal through vasodilation and heat dissipation, etc. The strict tumor-free operation is not only the basic requirement of NOSES, but also one of the key points to improve the prognosis of patients.

## 10.  Duodenal stump leakage

Duodenal stump leakage is a severe complication that may occur in patients with gastric cancer after undergoing NOSES with Billroth Ⅱ anastomosis or total gastrectomy. Duodenal stump leakage is one of the main factors affecting postoperative recovery or even the cause of death. In addition to anemia, malnutrition, and other systemic factors, duodenal stump leakage may be caused by the falling off of stapler cartridge from the stump, thermal injury of the duodenum by ultrasonic scalpel, incomplete obstruction of the afferent loop, and excessive tension in the NOSES for gastric cancer. Correct management of the duodenal stump is one of the keys to prevent duodenal stump leakage. For skilled surgeons, perform purse-string suture to embed the duodenal stump with barbed suture under laparoscopy is a simple and effective approach. Duodenal stump leakage

usually occurs 3-8 days after the operation, with sudden onset of epigastric pain or distension, accompanied by fever and tachycardia, abdominal tenderness and rigidity in the right upper abdomen, and leukocytosis. For patients with drainage tube in the abdominal cavity, bile-containing intestinal fluid can be drained out, ascites is detectable by ultrasonography, and yellow bile or pus can be obtained by paracentesis. For the treatment, most patients can be cured by conservative treatment such as adequate abdominal drainage and parenteral nutrition. If the duodenal stump leakage is caused by afferent loop obstruction, the second operation is required to perform Roux-en-Y anastomosis.

## 11.  Afferent loop obstruction

Afferent loop obstruction after gastric cancer resection is rare. It is a special high intestinal obstruction that occurs after gastric cancer resection. It is mainly caused by the stasis of bile, pancreatic, and intestinal secretions in the bowel lumen above the anastomosis. As a closed-loop mechanical intestinal obstruction, it is prone to cause strangulation of the bowel, which requires surgery to relieve the obstruction. Typical symptoms include sudden and severe epigastric pain, frequent nausea and vomiting, vomiting of small amount of bile-free gastric contents, tenderness in the right upper quadrant, with possible palpable mass. Digestive tract radiography shows that the contrast medium can enter the efferent loop jejunum smoothly through the anastomosis, but cannot enter the afferent loop jejunum, or only a small amount of contrast medium can slowly enter the afferent loop and shows obvious dilatation changes. Ultrasonography reveals dilatation of the duodenum with a liquid anechoic area. For patients without strangulation of the bowel, the principle of operation is to eliminate the etiology, relieve the obstruction, and establish a physiological channel. For patients with strangulation of bowel, the affected intestinal segments should be resected, the obstruction should be relieved, and the drainage should be strengthened during the operation. Pancreatoduodenectomy is inevitable if the second and third segments of the duodenum are necrotic.

## 12.  Efferent loop obstruction

Efferent loop obstruction after gastric cancer

resection is uncommon. Its causes include angulation of the efferent loop caused by intra-abdominal adhesions or compression of the bowel by the adhesive band, retrograde intussusception of the efferent loop, angulation of the bowel segment of the efferent loop and the anastomosis, and internal hernia of the efferent loop, etc. The main manifestations are the signs of high small intestinal obstruction, including epigastric fullness, accompanied by nausea and vomiting of food and bile. The diagnosis is made based on upper gastroenterography, and CT can show the dilated bowel. Conservative treatment can be performed first. If there is no improvement after conservative treatment or mechanical intestinal obstruction cannot be ruled out, surgical exploration can be considered. The principle of operation is to eliminate the cause of intestinal obstruction, perform resection of necrotic bowel segment, and restore bowel patency.

## 13. Postoperative pancreatitis and pancreatic fistula

With the extensive development and popularization of laparoscopic $D_2$ radical gastrectomy for gastric cancer in China, the incidence rates of postoperative pancreatic fistula and pancreatitis have been increasing with the application of high-frequency electric scalpel and ultrasonic scalpel in NOSES for gastric cancer. It has been reported that the incidence of pancreatic fistula after laparoscopic gastrectomy is 0.9%. Pancreatic fluid is corrosive and can lead to complications such as organ perforation, bleeding, and severe infection. Pancreatitis after gastric cancer surgery is difficult to diagnose. The lack of timely discovery and delay in treatment are prone to cause aggravation of the condition or even death. In the gastric cancer surgery, the anatomical characteristics of the operative area and the iatrogenic mechanical injury of the operation itself may lead to the onset of postoperative pancreatic fistula and pancreatitis. The clinical symptoms of post- operative pancreatitis and pancreatic fistula lack specificity. They usually occur on day 3-10 after the operation. They are mainly manifested as epigastric pain, but the location of the pain is vague and often accompanied by radiating pain in the lower back. Other manifestations include nausea, vomiting, and abdominal distension, which are difficult to explain by

other causes. The recovery of gastrointestinal function is slow, which is not consistent with the recovery of the disease course. Patients may also experience persistent fever or leukocytosis. In severe cases, the condition may progress to sepsis or lead to multiple organ dysfunction. The diagnosis of the pancreatic fistula is mainly based on peritoneal drainage fluid amylase, serum and urine amylase and clinical symptoms. Elevation of peritoneal drainage fluid amylase is defined as amylase concentration in the peritoneal drainage fluid being more than 3 times the upper limit of normal serum amylase concentration at or more than 3 days after the operation. Dynamic contrast-enhanced CT is the gold standard for clinical diagnosis of necrosis and the degree of necrosis in the pancreatitis of after gastric cancer resection. Once pancreatic fistula occurs, unobstructed abdominal drainage should be established, fasting, gastrointestinal decompression, and drugs that inhibit pancreatic secretion should be applied promptly. Surgical drainage and lavage should be performed if necessary.

## 14. Postoperative lymphatic leakage

The chylous effusion caused by the breakage of the main branches of lymphatic vessels after the gastric cancer resection is called lymphatic leakage, which is also referred to as chyle leakage. NOSES of gastric cancer apply ultrasonic scalpel for transection and dissection. In theory, the incidence of lymphatic leakage is lower than that of conventional surgery. The occurrence of lymphatic leakage is closely related to the intraoperative management of lymphatic vessels. Therefore, intraoperative prevention is key to avoiding postoperative lymphatic leakage. Diagnosis is confirmed by an increase in milk-like drainage with no concomitant symptoms (e.g., fever, pain), and presence of chylomicrons in drainage fluid when the patient starts feeding after operation. The treatment is mainly non-surgical, including total parenteral nutrition, internal environment maintenance, albumin supplementation, and tentative closure of catheter for observation. Most cases of lymphatic leakage heal within 2 weeks after conservative treatment and rarely require surgery.

## 15. Postoperative gastroparesis

Postoperative gastroparesis is a syndrome of gastric

emptying disorder after gastrointestinal surgery. It mainly occurs in gastric surgery, but also occurs in the intestinal, pancreatic, and other abdominal and gynecological operations. The incidence of delayed gastric emptying varies from 0.6%-7.4% in foreign literatures and 5.0%-10.0% in Chinese literatures due to different surgical methods, the extent of resection, and other factors. The pathogenesis of postoperative delayed gastric emptying is still unclear, which may be related to the changes of normal neurohormones and myogenic factors on gastric emptying. It usually occurs 2-3 days after operation, when the diet is changed from fasting to liquid or from liquid to semiliquid. Patients experience nausea and vomiting of remnant gastric contents. The diagnostic criteria of postoperative gastroparesis have not been unified, but the core criterion is to exclude the mechanical obstruction of the remnant gastric outflow tract. In terms of treatment, fasting, continuous gastrointestinal decompression, promotion of gastrointestinal peristalsis, strengthening of parenteral nutrition, and other measures are taken, and communications with patients are conducted to establish their confidence. The patients can be cured after conservative treatment. In recent years, traditional Chinese medicine has achieved some success in the treatment of postoperative delayed gastric emptying. Acupuncture, moxibustion, and application of traditional Chinese medicine can be combined to accelerate the recovery of postoperative gastroparesis.